The Menopause and Postmenopause

The Menopause and Postmenopause

The Proceedings of an International Symposium held in Rome, June 1979

Edited by

N. Pasetto
Patologia Ostetrica e Ginecologica, Università di Roma, Italy

R. Paoletti
Istituto di Farmacologia, Università di Milano, Italy
and
J. L. Ambrus
Department of Health, Buffalo, New York, USA

University Park Press
Baltimore

Published in USA and Canada by
University Park Press
233 East Redwood Street
Baltimore, Maryland 21202

Published in UK by
MTP Press Limited
Falcon House
Lancaster, England

First published 1980

ISBN-13: 978-94-011-7232-5   e-ISBN-13: 978-94-011-7230-1
DOI: 10.1007/978-94-011-7230-1
LCCN: 79-93427

Filmset by Mather Bros (Printers) Ltd, Preston, England

Contents

CONTENTS

List of Contributors

C. M. Ambrus
Department of Health, State of New York,
Roswell Park Memorial Institute,
Buffalo, New York 14263, USA

J. L. Ambrus
Department of Health, State of New York,
Roswell Park Memorial Institute,
Buffalo, New York 14263, USA

L. Baschieri
Cattedra di Patologia Ostetrica e
  Ginecologica,
Università di Roma, V. le Regina Elena,
324-00161 Roma, Italy

K. I. Bland
Department of Surgery,
University of Louisville School of Medicine,
Louisville, Kentucky, USA

P. Boemi
Istituto di Patologia Ostetrica e Ginecologica,
Università di Catania,
95124 Catania, Italy

H. M. Bolt
Department of Obstetrics and Gynecology
  and Institute of Toxicology,
University of Tübingen,
7400 Tübingen, West Germany

F. Boselli
Istituto di Clinica Ostetrica e Ginecologica,
Università di Modena,
41100 Modena, Italy

R. Bradley
Department of Pathology,
Harvard Medical School,
Massachusetts General Hospital,
Boston, MA. 02114, USA

M. Braun
Department of Health, State of New York,
Roswell Park Memorial Institute,
Buffalo, New York 14263, USA

J. B. Buchanan
Department of Radiology,
University of Louisville School of Medicine,
Louisville, Kentucky, USA

S. Campbell
Department of Obstetrics and Gynaecology,
Kings College Hospital Medical School,
Denmark Hill, London SE5 8RX, UK

G. B. Candiani
Istituto di Clinica Ostetrica e Ginecologica,
Università di Milano,
Via Commenda, 12-Milano, Italy

S. G. Carinelli
Istituto di Clinica Ostetrica e Ginecologica,
Università di Milano,
Via Commenda, 12-Milano, Italy

S. Cianci
Istituto di Clinica Ostetrica e Ginecologica,
Università di Catania,
95124 Catania, Italy

A. Coppen
MRC Neuropsychiatry Laboratory,
West Park Hospital,
Epsom KT19 8PB, Surrey, UK

R. Deghenghi
Ayerst Research Laboratories,
1025 Lauretien Boulevard,
Saint-Laurent, Montreal,
Quebec, Canada

LIST OF CONTRIBUTORS

A. R. Feinstein
Department of Internal Medicine,
Yale University, School of Medicine,
New Haven, Connecticut, USA

J. Fishman
Rockefeller University,
1230 York Avenue,
New York, NY 10021, USA

R. Don Gambrell, Jr
Medical College of Georgia,
Augusta, Georgia 30901, USA

M. Gilette
Department of Health, State of New York,
Roswell Park Memorial Institute,
Buffalo, New York 14263, USA

A. Goles
Istituto di Clinica Ostetrica e Ginecologica,
Università di Modena,
41100 Modena, Italy

G. S. Gordan
Department of Medicine,
University of California, Medical Center,
San Francisco, California, USA

R. Göser
Universitäts-Frauenklinik,
7400 Tübingen, West Germany

A. Grasso
Istituto di Clinica Ostetrica e Ginecologica,
Università di Modena,
41100 Modena, Italy

L. A. Gray, Sr
Department of Obstetrics and Gynecology,
University of Louisville,
School of Medicine,
Louisville, Kentucky, USA

P. Hale
Department of Health, State of New York,
Roswell Park Memorial Institute,
Buffalo, New York 14263, USA

R. I. Horwitz
Department of Internal Medicine,
Yale University, School of Medicine,
New Haven, Connecticut, USA

C. C. Huang
Department of Health, State of New York,
Roswell Park Memorial Institute,
Buffalo, New York 14263, USA

O. Jung
Department of Health, State of New York,
Roswell Park Memorial Institute,
Buffalo, New York 14263, USA

R. J. B. King
Hormone Biochemistry Department,
Imperial Cancer Research Fund,
Lincoln's Inn Fields,
London WC2A 3PX, UK

H. P. Klotz
9 Boulevard Delessert,
Paris 75106, France

R. Lindsay
Beecham Pharmaceuticals,
Nutritional Research Centre,
Walton Oaks, Tadworth,
Surrey KT20 7NT, UK

G. Maccarrone
Istituto di Clinica Ostetrica e Ginecologica,
Università di Modena,
41100 Modena, Italy

J. McQueen
Chelsea Hospital for Women,
Dovehouse Street, Chelsea,
London SW3, UK

M. Maneschi
Istituto di Clinica Ostetrica e Ginecologica,
Università di Palermo,
90127 Palermo, Italy

C. P. Martucci
Rockefeller University,
1230 York Avenue,
New York, NY 10021, USA

R. Maturi
Cattedra di Patologia Ostetrica e
Ginecologica,
Università di Roma, V. le Regina Elena,
324-00161 Roma, Italy

V. Mazza
Istituto di Clinica Ostetrica e Ginecologica,
Università di Modena,
41100 Modena, Italy

V. Messana
Istituto di Clinica Ostetrica e Ginecologica,
Università di Palermo,
90127 Palermo, Italy

LIST OF CONTRIBUTORS

J. Minardi
Chelsea Hospital for Women,
Dovehouse Street, Chelsea,
London SW3, UK

D. G. Montanari
Istituto di Clinica Ostetrica e Ginecologica,
Università di Modena,
41100 Modena, Italy

C. Nolan
Department of Health, State of New York,
Roswell Park Memorial Institute,
Buffalo, New York 14263, USA

A. Novick
Department of Health, State of New York,
Roswell Park Memorial Institute,
Buffalo, New York 14263, USA

B. Paigen
Department of Health, State of New York,
Roswell Park Memorial Institute,
Buffalo, New York 14263, USA

R. Paoletti
Istituto di Farmacologia,
Università di Milano,
Via Vanvitelli, 32-Milano, Italy

F. Pasetto
Cattedra di Patolgia Ostetrica e Ginecologica,
Università di Roma, V. le Regina Elena,
324-00161 Roma, Italy

N. Pasetto
Cattedra di Patologia Ostetrica e Ginecologica,
Università di Roma, V. le Regina Elena,
324-00161 Roma, Italy

M. E. L. Paterson
Birmingham and Midland Hospital
for Women,
Sparkhill, Birmingham B11 4HL, UK

P. P. Pellegri
Istituto di Clinica Ostetrica e Ginecologica,
Università di Modena,
41100 Modena, Italy

E. Piccione
Cattedra di Patolgia Ostetrica e Ginecologica,
Università di Roma, V. le Regina Elena,
324-00161 Roma, Italy

A. Poli
Istituto de Farmacologia,
Università di Milano, Via Vanvitelli 32,
Milano, Italy

S. Regalla-Spavento
Department of Health, State of New York,
Roswell Park Memorial Institute,
Buffalo, New York 14263, USA

S. J. Robboy
Department of Pathology,
Harvard Medical School,
Massachusetts General Hospital,
Boston, MA. 02114, USA

S. M. Rubino
Istituto di Clinica Ostetrica e Ginecologica,
Università di Palermo,
90127 Palermo, Italy

A. E. Schindler
Universitäts-Frauenklinik,
7400 Tübingen, West Germany

S. R. Sirianni
Department of Health, State of New York,
Roswell Park Memorial Institute,
Buffalo, New York 14263, USA

P. Smith
Department of Urology,
Bristol Royal Infirmary,
Bristol, UK

P. Spavento
Department of Health, State of New York,
Roswell Park Memorial Institute,
Buffalo, New York 14263, USA

J. W. W. Studd
King's College Hospital,
Denmark Hill, London SE5 9RS, UK

C. Suchetzky
Department of Health, State of New York,
Roswell Park Memorial Institute,
Buffalo, New York 14263, USA

M. H. Thom
Dulwich Hospital,
London SE22, UK

J. P. Thomas
Hôpital Universitaire Brugman,
Service de Gynecologie et Obstetrique,
Place A. Von Gehuchten 4,
1020 Bruxelles, Belgium

LIST OF CONTRIBUTORS

P. T. Townsend
Department of Obstetrics and Gynaecology,
King's College Hospital Medical School,
Denmark Hill, London SE5 8RX, UK

C. Vaughan
University Hospital,
New York University Medical Centre,
New York, USA

R. Vokaer
Hôpital Universitaire Brugman,
Service de Gynecologie et Obstetrique,
Place A. Von Gehuchten 4,
1020 Bruxelles, Belgium

W. Völker
Frauenklinik der Med.,
Hochschule Hannover,
Podbielskistrasse 380,
D3000 Hannover 51, West Germany

A. Volpe
Istituto di Clinica Ostetrica e Ginecologica,
Università di Modena,
41100 Modena, Italy

T. Wade-Evans
Birmingham and Midland Hospital
for Women,
Sparkhill, Birmingham B11 4HL, UK

B. F. Weisberg
University of Louisville,
School of Medicine,
Louisville, Kentucky, USA

J. M. Wenderlein
Universitäts-Frauenklinik,
Krankenhaus Strasse 21–23,
D8520 Erlangen, West Germany

M. I. Whitehead
Department of Obstetrics and Gynaecology,
King's College Hospital Medical School,
Denmark Hill, London SE5 8RX, UK

K. Wood
MRC Neuropsychiatry Laboratory,
West Park Hospital,
Epsom KT19 8PD, Surrey, UK

M. Zwirner
Universitäts-Frauenklinik,
7400 Tübingen, West Germany

Preface

The treatment of menopausal and postmenopausal symptoms is a focus of considerable debate, on account of both the medical and social factors involved. And perhaps the cause of the greatest current interest and concern is not so much the effectiveness of present-day treatment but its safety. Opinions on the subject vary; and to resolve the arguments we must turn to the results of scientific experiment, both the clinical and biological. It is only by comparing experimental results that it is possible to move forward, albeit slowly, towards a generally agreed consensus based upon objective scientific data.

It is for this reason that we are particularly grateful to Ayerst Laboratories whose support and help have enabled us to turn our original proposal for an International Symposium into a reality. We are also grateful to the publishers for the efficiency with which they have organized the publication of the Proceedings.

It is our hope and that of all the distinguished participants that all readers of this volume will be able to find something in it which will stimulate further thought and discussion – even though they may not necessarily agree with all the conclusions expressed – for the success of a Symposium turns not only on the subject under examination but also on the quality of debate and discussion it encourages.

N. PASETTO, R. PAOLETTI and J. L. AMBRUS

Section I
Pharmacological
Update

1
Chemistry and Biochemistry of Natural Estrogens

R. DEGHENGHI

A very large number of substances are known to possess estrogenic activity[1] as defined by certain biological effects, usually growth and development, on target tissues and organs related to reproductive function in the female.

Natural estrogens are defined, for the purpose of this presentation, as

Table 1.1 Commercially available natural estrogens

Chemical name	Available preparations
17β-Estradiol	Pellets for implantation; Suspension for injection; Suppositories (vaginal); Tablets for oral administration; Percutaneous gel
17β-Estradiol benzoate	Solution for injection
17β-Estradiol cyclopentylpropionate	Solution for injection
17β-Estradiol dipropionate	Solution for injection
17β-Estradiol valerate	Solution for intramuscular injection; Oral tablets
Estriol	Cream; Lotion; Solution for injection; Tablets for oral use
Conjugated estrogens (equine)	Cream for vaginal application; Solution; Tablets for oral use
Estrone	Suspension for injection; Pellets; Suppositories (vaginal); Tablets for oral use
Piperazine estrone sulfate	Elixir for oral use; Tablets for oral use
Zeranol	Oral tablets; Ear implants (veterinary)

substances present in nature, but not necessarily obtained from natural sources, and of therapeutic interest. First-order derivatives of some natural estrogens such as man-made esters and salts will also be included if it is known that, by virtue of metabolism, the parent natural estrogen is generated *in vivo*.

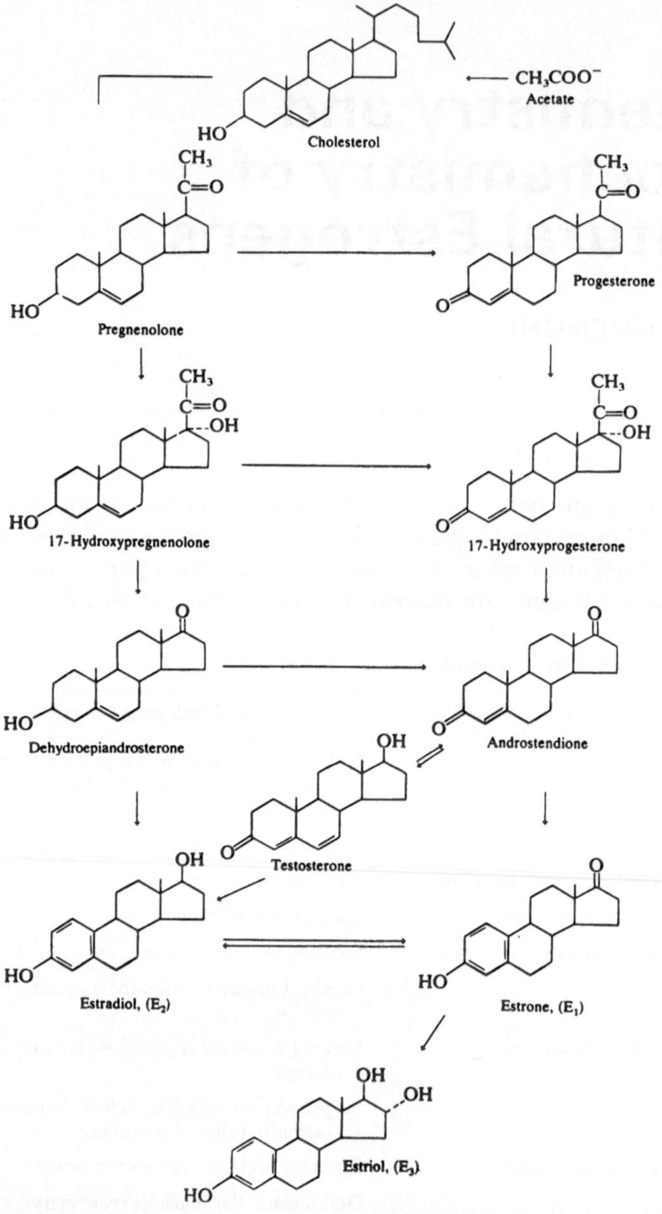

Figure 1.1   Derivation of estrone (E$_1$), estradiol (E$_2$) and estriol (E$_3$) from cholesterol

Table 1.1 lists commercially available natural estrogens and certain derivatives. All but the last one are steroids, like the ovarian steroidal hormones estrone, estradiol and estriol.

Table 1.2 lists some commercially available estrogens which we define as 'non-natural' by virtue of being synthetic chemical compounds whose metabolites, at least the major ones, are not the primary ovarian hormones. They will be referred to by comparison only.

Table 1.2   Commercially available synthetic estrogens

Chemical name	Available preparations
Ethynyl estradiol (EE)	Oral tablets or capsules
Mestranol	Oral tablets or capsules
Quinestrol	Oral tablets or capsules
Diethylstilbestrol (DES)	Oral tablets or capsules
Chlorotrianisene (TACE)	Oral tablets or capsules
Clomiphene	Oral tablets or capsules

It is of course well known that estrone (E_1), estradiol (E_2) and estriol (E_3) originate biogenetically from cholesterol, as shown in Figure 1.1. An important constituent of conjugated estrogens from equine sources, equilin (see Figure 1.2), does not, however, derive from cholesterol, but from earlier precursors by a pathway which is still being elucidated today.

The same conjugated estrogens (equine) contain additional compounds such as the 17α-dihydro derivatives of estrone, equilin and equilenin which differ from estradiol by having a 17α-hydroxyl function. We will discuss later some peculiar properties of these compounds.

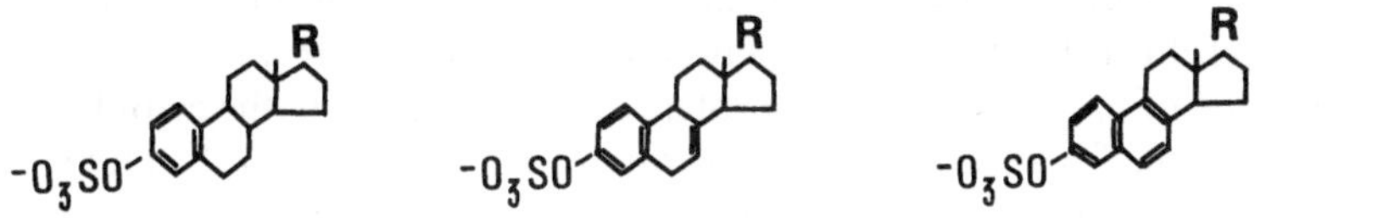

R	Name	R	Name	R	Name
O ‖	estrone SO₄⁻	O ‖	equilin SO₄⁻	O ‖	equilenin SO₄⁻
OH │	17β-estradiol SO₄⁻	OH │	17β-dihydroequilin SO₄⁻	OH │	17β-dihydroequilenin SO₄⁻
OH ⋮	17α-estradiol SO₄⁻	OH ⋮	17α-dihydroequilin SO₄⁻	OH ⋮	17α-dihydroequilenin SO₄⁻

Figure 1.2   Structure of conjugated equine estrogens

The only non-steroidal estrogen in Table 1.1 is Zeranolol or Zeranol, produced by the mold *Gibberella zeae* and commercially available as a growth promotion agent in feed animals, but also available in certain countries for human therapy (see Figure 1.3). It is a rather weak estrogen which has shown antitumor activity in animals[2].

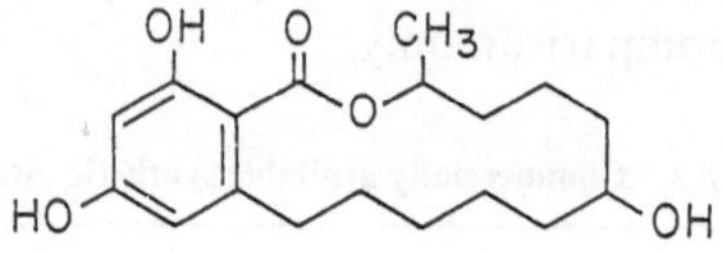

Figure 1.3   Structure of Zeranolol or Zeranol

Some of the biological effects of estrogens on various target organs are listed in Table 1.3.

Table 1.3   Biological effects of estrogens on various target organs or tissues

Ovary	Stimulate follicular growth; small doses cause weight increase of the ovary whereas large doses cause atrophy
Uterus	Endometrial growth
Vagina	Cornification of epithelial cells, accompanied by thickening and stratification of epithelium
Cervix	Increased amount of cervical mucus with a lowered viscosity
Pituitary	Small doses promote secretion of pituitary gonadotropins (supportive effect): larger doses cause inhibition
Bone	Anti-osteolytic effect

The subcellular mechanism of action responsible for most, if not all, biological effects has been extensively studied in recent years and involves the interaction of the estrogen with a protein receptor present in the cytoplasm of the target cell. The cytoplasmic estrogen-receptor complex translocates in the nucleus where it stimulates the transcription of particular genes and the synthesis of RNA which is then translated into proteins. Very schematically, this is represented in Figure 1.4.

The magnitude of a cell's response appears to be related to the intracellular concentration of receptor proteins. The potency of estrogens, on the other hand, has been correlated to the molecular structure responsible for receptor recognition and binding affinity, but also to the retention time in the nucleus of the estrogen-receptor complex. Since this appears to be true for both estrogens and anti-estrogens, additional nuclear events, such as specificity of binding sites to the chromatin, are of importance. It has also been proposed that a potent estrogen is responsible for the cytoplasmic resynthesis or replenishment of receptors following the initial depletion due to translocation in the nucleus.

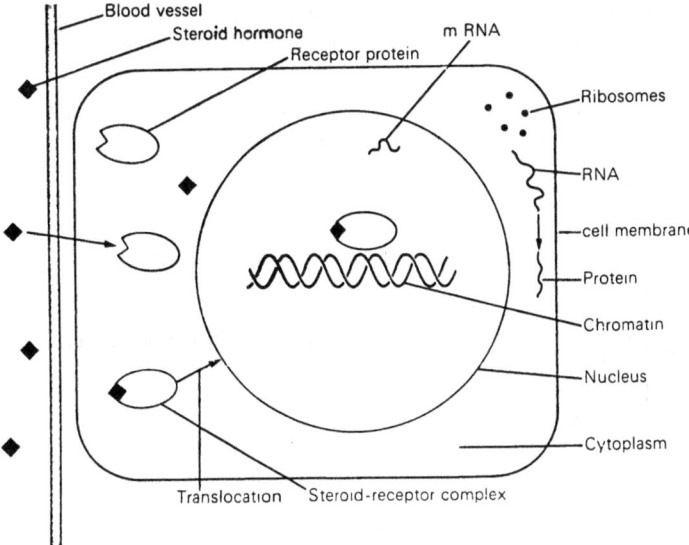

Figure 1.4 A model of steroid hormone interactions on a target cell

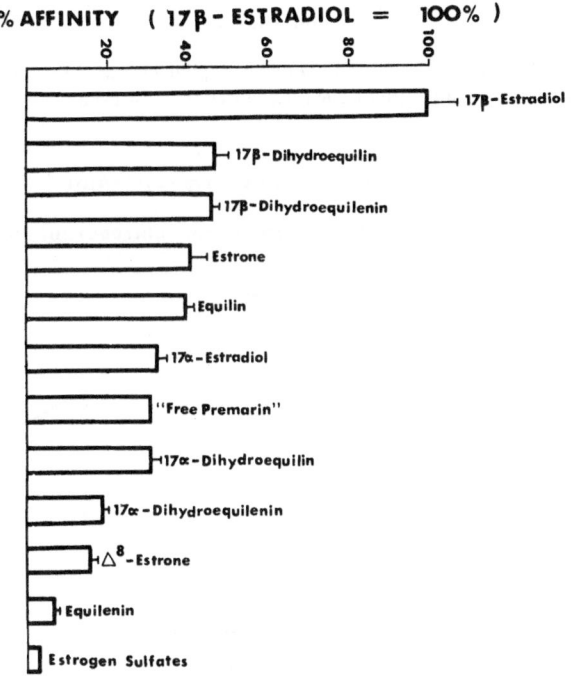

Figure 1.5 Relative binding affinities of some estrogens

In our laboratories, we have recently studied[3] the relative *in vitro* binding affinities of various estrogens using rabbit uterine cytosol as the source of receptor (Figure 1.5).

The binding characteristics of various estrogens can also be assessed *in vivo*. Immature rats receive a single injection of estrogen and are sacrificed at

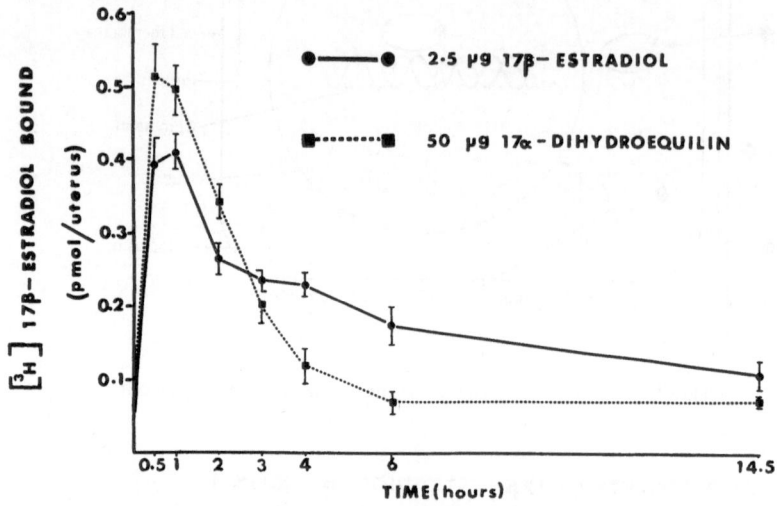

Figure 1.6 *In vivo* uptake of 17β-estradiol and 17α-dihydroequilin in immature rat uterus: levels of nuclear estrogen-receptor complex after a single s.c. injection of estrogen

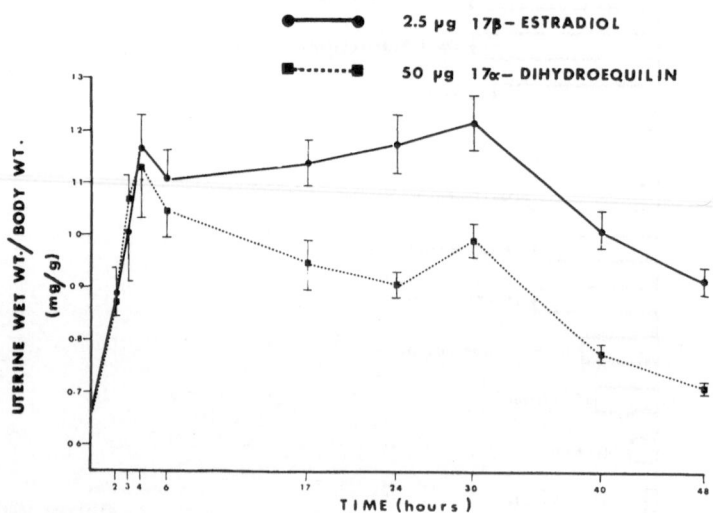

Figure 1.7 Change in uterine wet weight after a single dose of estrogen

various times thereafter. The uterine weight is recorded and uteri processed to measure the nuclear receptor content. The data and the correlation are shown in Figures 1.6 to 1.11.

In vitro or *in vivo* receptor studies can easily be accomplished in the laboratories and they have proven their usefulness not only to elucidate a possible

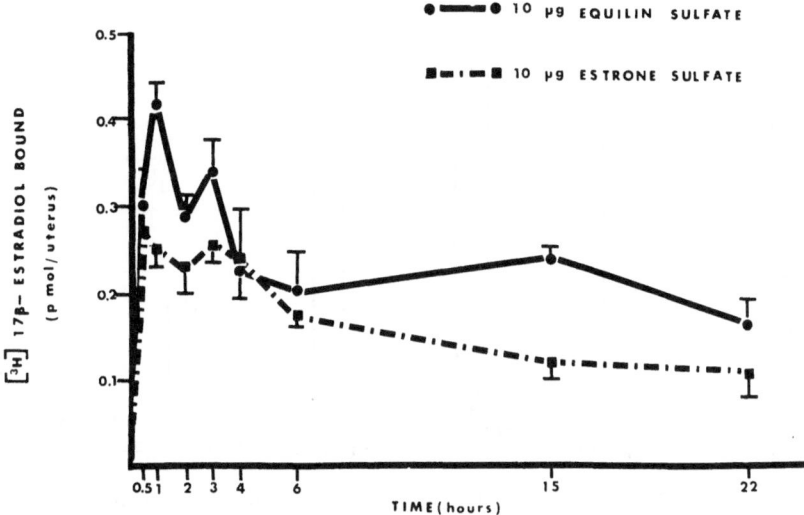

Figure 1.8 *In vivo* uptake of estrone sulfate and equilin sulfate: levels of nuclear estrogen-receptor complex after a single s.c. injection of estrogen

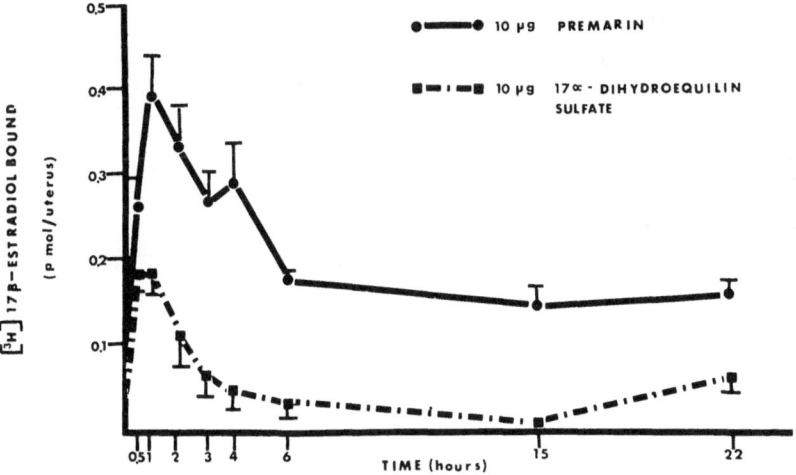

Figure 1.9 *In vivo* uptake of 17α-dihydroequilin sulfate and Premarin: levels of nuclear estrogen-receptor complex after a single s.c. injection of estrogen

mechanism of action but also to correlate estrogen effects in a clinical situation. Other measurements, however, are more commonly evaluated in a clinical set-up and these include serum estrogen levels. From those, it is

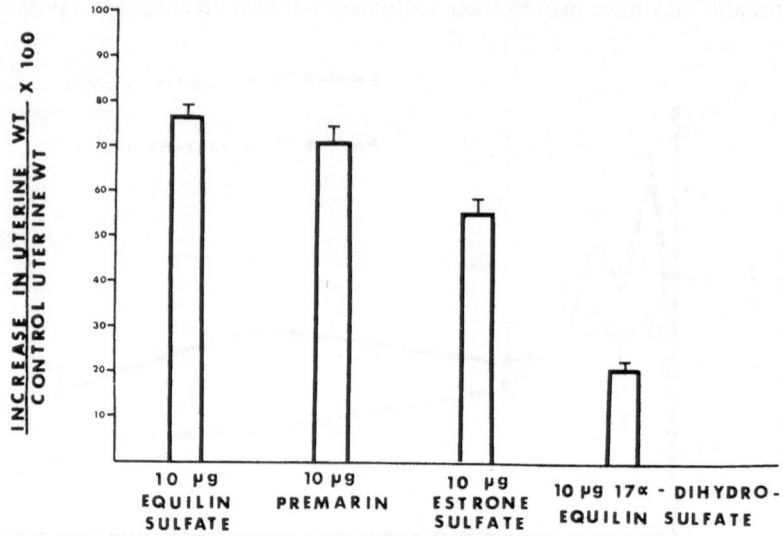

Figure 1.10   Percentage increase in uterine wet weight 22 hours after a single injection of estrogen

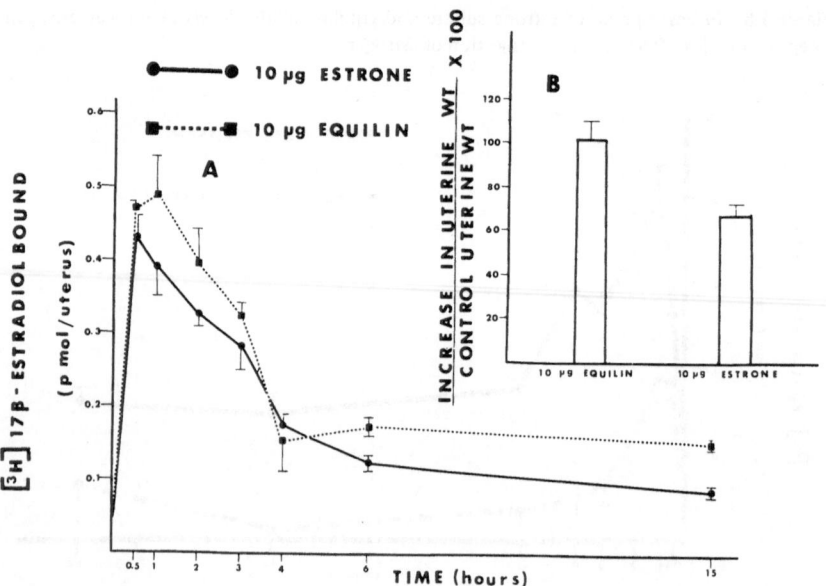

Figure 1.11   Uptake and uterotrophic effects of unconjugated estrone and equilin on A: nuclear estrogen-receptor levels; and B: uterine wet weight 22 hours post-injection

possible to determine a pharmacokinetic profile and the extent of absorption and metabolism of various estrogen preparations.

It has been generally accepted that serum levels obtained with effective therapeutic doses of natural estrogens should be at least comparable to the mean concentration of endogenous ovarian estrogens under normal or ideal physiological conditions (Table 1.4). It carí be argued, however, that bioavailability profiles, important as they are, may not be sufficient to account for pharmacological and therapeutic differences between natural and synthetic estrogens. This is well recorded in the literature and common in everyday clinical practice.

Table 1.4   **Mean concentration of ovarian steroids in physiological conditions (serum levels in pg/ml)**

	E_1	E_2	E_3	Progesterone
Normal women				
Follicular phase	50	60	—	50
Mid-cycle	200	400	150	—
Luteal phase	140	250	120	12000
Post-menopausal	30	10	7	5
Pregnancy (3rd month)	1100	2600	970	35000
Normal men	60	20	10	120

Below we examine some of these differences.

Effects on liver function

The mammalian liver is known to possess estrogen receptors[4], and binding by estradiol or 17-ethynyl estradiol has been correlated to increased renin substrate and triglycerides. Ethynyl estradiol is ten times more potent than estradiol in increasing plasma renin substrate in rats[5]. Significantly, ethynyl estradiol and its metabolites were found to bind more irreversibly than estradiol to human liver microsomal proteins.

Effects on lipids

The differences between the serum lipid patterns of pre- and postmenopausal women[6] are often ascribed to ovarian function, i.e. to a decrease in estrogen production. However, the administration of estrogens to estrogen-deficient women does not always bring about changes resembling that of younger women. Indeed, it has been shown that triglyceride and cholesterol concentrations were higher in women taking oral contraceptives or estrogens compared to non-users[7]. It has also been shown that natural conjugated estrogens (oral) stimulate VLD-triglyceride (TG) production rate and, to some extent, VLD-TG removal rate[8]. Several groups, however, have argued that effects on lipids are a function of the route of administration. Thus, serum triglycerides are not elevated in women taking an injectable contraceptive (estradiol-17-enanthate and dihydroxy-progesterone acetophenide) contrary to women receiving oral ethynyl estradiol–norgestrel combinations[9]. Percutaneous administration of estradiol did not give rise to triglycerides and in some cases a fall of high TG basal levels was observed[10].

In another study, serum triglyceride and protein concentrations were elevated in women taking oral ethynyl estradiol, but not in women given a single intramuscular dose of estradiol cypionate[11] or conjugated estrogens[12]. In the rat, injected estradiol or ethynyl estradiol both produce hyper-triglyceridemia, but estradiol had no effect on liver triglycerides while ethynyl estradiol lowered them and tended to elevate cholesterol[13]. Thus it appears that both route of administration and the molecular structure of estrogens determine their effect on lipids.

Effects on prolactin

Estrogens, such as estradiol[14] and ethynyl estradiol[15], are known to increase prolactin secretion in humans. However, both estrone and estrone sulfate[16] failed to alter prolactin secretion or levels and, later, actually suppressed it. Conjugated estrogens given i.v. also had no effect on prolactin levels[17]. In all probability, a different pharmacokinetic profile between various estrogens is responsible for the effect, or lack thereof, on prolactin.

Thromboembolic and coagulation effects

Thromboembolic and coagulation effects are not the same for all estrogens. Numerous studies have reported an association between the use of estrogens and risk of various thromboembolic diseases. Most of these changes, however, have been reported for the synthetic estrogens such as ethynyl estradiol or mestranol[18] and infrequently or none at all for conjugated estrogens[19].

Effects on carbohydrate metabolism

A decrease in tolerance to oral glucose after prolonged use of synthetic estrogen containing oral contraceptives has been reported, but these effects were much less or absent in women taking natural conjugated estrogens[20].

CNS effects of estrogens

Since the earliest therapeutic applications of estrogens, a definite, if ill-defined, CNS effect was noted. Only recently this 'feeling of well-being' and, in certain cases, an antidepressant effect have been studied and quantified[21]. Improvements of estrogen-treated patients were noted in cases of anxiety, sleep disturbances, fatigue, restlessness, irritability, depression, concentration and memory disturbances when compared to placebo treatment. A similar double-blind controlled study[22] of the effect of estrone (piperazine) sulfate revealed only placebo effects on depression, anxiety and hot flushes, but an objective decrease in the brokenness of sleep in perimenopausal women complaining of insomnia.

The existence of brain receptors sensitive to certain steroids and estrogens (similar to the opioid brain receptors) has been described[23, 24]. It is noteworthy that of many estrogens tested, only 17α-derivatives, such as 17α-dihydro-equilin, 17α-dihydroequilenin and 17α-estradiol, all present as sulfates in conjugated estrogens (equine), have shown opiate receptor binding activity. Additional studies are needed to ascertain a clinical relevance of these findings.

ABSORPTION OF ESTROGENS

Therapeutically effective estrogens are administered in a number of ways, as previously shown in Table 1.1. Not only does their absorption vary according to the route of administration, but extensive metabolism is known to occur even before estrogens are systemically available. When estrogens are taken orally, they may be subjected to intensive metabolism by the intestinal micro-flora[25]. Thus, oral estradiol (micronized) is converted extensively into estrone which predominates in serum[26]. Similarly, estradiol valerate, when given orally, gives serum estrone levels higher than estradiol[27].

Conjugated estrogens are readily absorbed, although extensive hydrolysis of the sulfate esters is presumed. In addition to intestinal metabolism, oral absorption results in higher steroid levels in the portal system and relative higher 'first pass' hepatic metabolism.

Vaginal absorption of estrogens is rapid and efficient[28]. Contrary to oral ingestion, serum levels of estradiol are higher than estrone when estradiol is applied intravaginally. Epidemiologically, no causal association was found between intravaginal estrogen creams and endometrial cancer[29], a finding that could, however, be related to duration of therapy.

The percutaneous absorption of steroid hormones through the animal skin has been reported by Zondek 50 years ago[30]. Numerous studies in animals[31] and humans[32] have since been reported. More recently[10], the systemic blood levels and effects on lipids of a dermal gel containing estradiol have been published. The absorbed estradiol, as measured in plasma, is about one hundredth of the topically applied dose[10]. Additional data on pharmaco-kinetics and metabolism of estradiol in human skin are anticipated with interest.

Differences in absorption, when the same route of administration is used, are due to differences in formulation or in the physical properties of the product, *cf.* the increased oral absorption of micronized *vs.* non-micronized estradiol. Even when one has chemical and compendial equivalence of the drug substance, clinical differences between estrogen formulations may be due to different content uniformity standards between formulation lots and also to different stability of the commercial preparations. Such 'bio-inequivalence' between four conjugated estrogens tablets USP products was recently documented[33].

CONCLUSIONS

Although the clinical use of estrogens in modern therapy is not yet 50 years old, there is clear evidence[34] that as early as the eleventh century AD the Chinese were using estrogens in therapeutically effective doses obtained from placental preparations or from urine fractionation and sublimation.

So we can say that the usefulness of estrogens in therapy has been known a long time. In the past few decades, our knowledge of this class of substances has increased enormously. Not only do we know them well enough chemically to produce them reliably, but we have learned how to measure them in the smallest amounts in biological fluids. We have a satisfactory, if not complete, mechanism of action to explain how they work at the subcellular level. More important, I believe, is the knowledge of their dissimilarity. Estrogens do act differently according, not only to differences in their chemistry and biochemistry, but to the way they are administered. Armed with this knowledge, we should be able to improve further the therapeutic use of these valuable substances.

Acknowledgments

To the following colleagues at Ayerst Laboratories: Drs M. Gahwyler and J. Morrison (New York, NY), G. Milosovich (Rouses Point, NY), D. Dvornik, D. Lee, M. L. Givner and M. D. Stern (Montreal, Canada), I am indebted for suggestions and information.

References

1. cf. Deghenghi, R. and Givner, M. L. (1979). The female sex hormones and analogs. *Burger's Medicinal Chemistry*, 4th Ed., pp. 917–939
2. Teller, M. N., Stock, C. C., Borie, M. and McMahon, S. (1979). Resorcylic acid lactones: new compounds active against DMBA-induced rat mammary carcinomas. *Am. Assoc. Cancer Res. Annual Meeting*, May 16–19, New Orleans
3. Stern, M. D. and Givner, M. L. (1978). Studies on the mechanism of action of conjugated equine estrogens. *Endometrial Cancer*, pp. 309–322 (London: Baillière Tindall)
4. Eisenfeld, A. J., Aten, R., Weinberger, M., Haselbacher, G., Halpern, K. and Krakoff, L. (1976). Estrogen receptor in the mammalian liver. *Science*, **191**, 862

5. Ménard, J., Corvol, P., Foliot, A. and Raynaud, J. P. (1973). Effects of estrogens on renin substrate and uterine weights in rats. *Endocrinology*, **93**, 747

6. Furman, R. H., Alanpovic, P. and Howard, R. P. (1967). Effects of androgens and estrogens on serum lipid and the composition and concentration of serum lipoprotein in normal normolitemic and hyperlipidemic states. *Prog. Biochem. Pharmacol.*, **2**, 215–249 (Basel and New York: Karger)

7. (a) Wallace, R. B., Hoover, J., Sandler, D., Rifkind, B. M. and Tyroler, H. A. (1977). Altered plasma-lipids associated with oral contraceptive or estrogen consumption. *Lancet*, **ii**, 11

   (b) Barrett-Connor, E., Brown, V., Turner, J., Austin, M. and Criqui, M. H. (1979). Heart disease risk factors and hormone use in postmenopausal women. *J. Am. Med. Assoc.*, **241**, 2167

8. Glueck, C. J., Fallat, R. W. and Scheel, D. (1975). Effects of estrogenic compounds on triglyceride kinetics. *Metabolism*, **24**, 537

9. Donde, U. M. and Virkar, K. (1975). Effect of contraceptive steroids on serum lipids. *Am. J. Obstet. Gynecol.*, **123**, 736

10. Loeper, J., Loeper, J., Ohlghiesser, C., de Lignières, B. and Mauvais-Jarvis, P. (1977). Influence de l'estrogènothérapie sur les triglycérides. *Nouv. Presse Méd.*, **6**, 2747

11. Buckman, M. T., Johnson, J., Ellis, H., Srivastava, L. and Peake, G. T. (1979). Lipemic and proteinemic effect of estrogen is dependent on route of estrogen administration. *Endocrine Society 61st Annual Meeting*, Abstr. 956

12. Bolton, C. H., Ellwood, M., Hartog, M., Martin, R., Rowe, A. S., Wensley, R. T. (1975). Comparison of the effects of ethinyl estradiol and conjugated equine estrogens in oophorectomized women. *Clin. Endocrinol.*, **4**, 131

13. Hill, P. and Dvornik, D. (1969). Estrogen-induced hypertriglyceridemia in female rats. *Circulation*, Suppl. III to **39** and **40**, 106

14. Yen, S. S. C., Vandenberg, G. and Siler, T. M. (1974). Modulation of pituitary responsiveness to LRF by estrogen. *J. Clin. Endocrinol. Metab.*, **39**, 170

15. Wiedemann, E., Schwartz, E. and Frantz, A. G. (1976). Acute and chronic estrogen effects upon serum somatomedin activity, growth hormone, and prolactin in man. *J. Clin. Endocrinol. Metab.*, **42**, 942

16. Kandeel, F., Butt, W. R. and London, D. R. (1977). Regulation of serum prolactin by estrone and estrone sulfate in normally menstruating women. *Acta Endocrinol.*, **212** (Suppl.), 42

17. L'Hermite, M., Delogne-Desnoeck, J., Michaux-Duchene, A. and Robyn, C. (1978). Alteration of feedback mechanism of estrogen on gonadotropin by sulpiride-induced hyperprolactinemia. *J. Clin. Endocrinol. Metab.*, **47**, 1132

18. Von Kaulla, E., Droegemueller, W. and Von Kaulla, K. N. (1975). Conjugated estrogens and hypercoagulability. *Am. J. Obstet. Gynecol.*, **122**, 688

19. Notelovitz, M. and Greig, H. B. W. (1976). Natural estrogen and anti-thrombin III activity in postmenopausal women. *J. Reprod. Med.*, **16**, 87

20. Notelovitz, M. and Greig, H. B. W. (1975). The effect of natural estrogens on coagulation. *S. Afr. Med. J.*, **49**, 101

21. Fedor-Freybergh, P. (1977). The influence of estrogens on the well-being and mental performance in climacteric and postmenopausal women. *Acta Obstet. Gynecol. Scand.*, **64** (Suppl.), 1

22. Thomson, J. and Oswald, I. (1977). Effect of estrogen on the sleep, mood and anxiety of menopausal women. *Br. Med. J.*, **2**, 1317

23. La Bella, F. S., Kim, R. S. and Templeton, J. (1978). Opiate receptor binding activity of 17α-estrogenic steroids. *Life Sci.*, **23**, 1797

24. Pugsley, T. and Lippmann, W. (1978). Effect of somatostatin analogues and 17α-dihydroequilin on rat brain opiate receptors. *Res. Commun. Chem. Pathol. Pharmacol.*, **21**, 153

25. Adlercreutz, H., Martin, F., Pulkkinen, M., Dencker, H., Rimer, U., Sjöberg, N.-O. and

Tikkanen, M. J. (1976). Intestinal metabolism of estrogens. *J. Clin. Endocrinol. Metab.*, **43**, 497

26. Yen, S. S. C., Martin, P. L., Burnier, A. M., Czekala, N. M., Greaney, M. O. Jr. and Callantine, M. R. (1975). Circulating estradiol, estrone and gonadotropin levels following the administration of orally active 17β-estradiol in postmenopausal women. *J. Clin. Endocrinol. Metab.*, **40**, 518

27. Englund, D. E. and Johansson, E. D. B. (1977). Pharmacokinetic and pharmacodynamic studies on estradiol valerianate administered orally to postmenopausal women. *Acta Obstet. Gynecol. Scand.*, **65** (Suppl.), 27

28. (a) Englund, D. E. and Johansson, E. D. B. (1978). Plasma levels of estrone, estradiol and gonadotrophins in postmenopausal women after oral and vaginal administration of conjugated equine estrogens (Premarin). *Br. J. Obstet. Gynaecol.*, **85**, 957
(b) Schiff, I., Tulchinsky, D. and Ryan, K. J. (1977). Vaginal absorption of estrone and 17β-estradiol. *Fertil. Steril.*, **28**, 1063
(c) Rigg, L. A., Hermann, H. and Yen, S. S. C. (1978). Absorption of estrogens from vaginal creams. *N. Engl. J. Med.*, **298**, 195; see also ref. 31

29. Horwitz, R. I. and Feinstein, A. R. (1979). Intravaginal estrogen creams and endometrial cancer. *J. Am. Med. Assoc.*, **241**, 1266

30. Zondek, B. (1929). Folliculin. *Klin. Wochensch.*, **142**, 895

31. Tresca, J.-P., Ponsard, G. and Jayle, M.-F. (1977). Cinétiques de pénétration transcutanée et de fixation du 3-propyl éther, 17-méthyl éther estradiol et de l'estradiol au niveau de différents tissus chez la ratte. *Canad. J. Biochem.*, **55**, 1096

32. (a) Goldzieher, J. W. and Baker, R. E. (1960). The percutaneous absorption of estradiol and progesterone. *J. Invest. Dermatol.*, **35**, 215
(b) Wepierre, J. and Marty, J. P. (1979). Percutaneous absorption of drugs. *TIPS – Trends in Pharm. Sci.* (inaugural issue), p. 23

33. Adams, W. P., Johnson, R. N., Hasegawa, J. and Haring, R. C. (August 1979). Conjugated estrogens bioinequivalence – a comparison of four products in postmenopausal women. *J. Pharm. Sci.* (in press)

34. Needham, J. and Gwei-Djen, L. (1968). Sex hormones in the Middle Ages. *Endeavour*, **27**, 130

2
Estrogens and Prostaglandins

R. PAOLETTI and A. POLI

The menopausal period is characterized by several symptoms, such as labile temperature control, vasodilatation with flushing, lowered pain threshold and osteoporosis[1], which may be correlated with either an excessive production of endogenous prostaglandins or with an alteration of the ratio among the different prostaglandins in the brain or in the sexual organs.

These clinical observations should be correlated with the experimental investigations on the possible relations existing among estrogens, progesterone and prostaglandins.

In this review the metabolism of gonadal prostaglandins and their possible functions in reproduction, pregnancy and menopause will be discussed.

PROSTAGLANDIN METABOLISM

Prostaglandins are cyclic derivatives of a polyunsaturated fatty acid, arachidonic acid. This fatty acid is a constituent of plasma phospholipids and it is released from such membrane constituents by the action[2] of the selective phospholipase A_2.

Free arachidonic acid may be attached by a specific enzyme, cyclooxygenase, which by introducing an oxygen molecule in its structure gives origin to the basic compounds of the prostaglandin series, that is cyclic endoperoxides[2]. These compounds have a short halflife and are transformed in a time of minutes into the stable prostaglandins (PGE, PGF, PGA). The various classes of prostaglandins, which differ from one another in the number of double bonds and in oxygenated substituents (enolic or chetonic form) are characterized by an extremely wide and differentiated spectrum of action, affecting mobility, reactivity and blood supply of a number of organs in various manners.

Recently the picture of metabolites of arachidonic acid has been enriched by the discovery of two new groups of substances: unstable intermediates and compounds generated by lipo-oxygenase. Two new unstable compounds have been described recently: thromboxane A_2 and prostacyclin (PGI_2)[3,4]. These substances, short-lived and spontaneously transformed into characteristic metabolites, affect in opposite ways most of the prostaglandin-sensitive systems: while the former has a vasoconstrictive action, the latter is a vasodilatator; platelets are aggregated by thromboxane whereas prostaglandin I_2 prevents aggregation; smooth muscle is usually contracted by TXA_2 and released by prostacyclin[5-7]. An imbalance between these two antagonistic compounds may represent the biochemical base of many physiological and pathological situations.

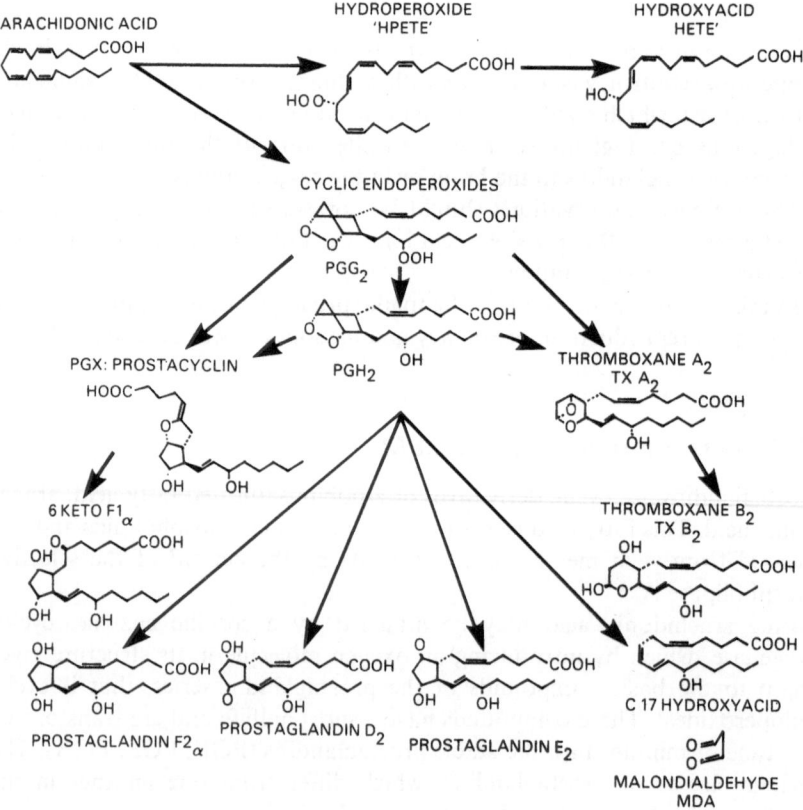

Figure 2.1a Metabolic pathway of arachidonic acid

The second group of new derivatives is originated by the introduction of two atoms of oxygen in the molecule of arachidonic acid, catalysed by the lipo-oxygenase[8], which is not a cyclizing enzyme but an enzyme which also utilizes arachidonic acid as a substrate. The main member of this group is HETE, a stable compound with algogenic and chemotactic properties[9]. It has recently been shown that SRS-A, a physiological mediator of inflammation, is constituted by a molecule of a polyunsaturated hydroxy fatty acid and one of cysteine linked with a tiglic bond[10].

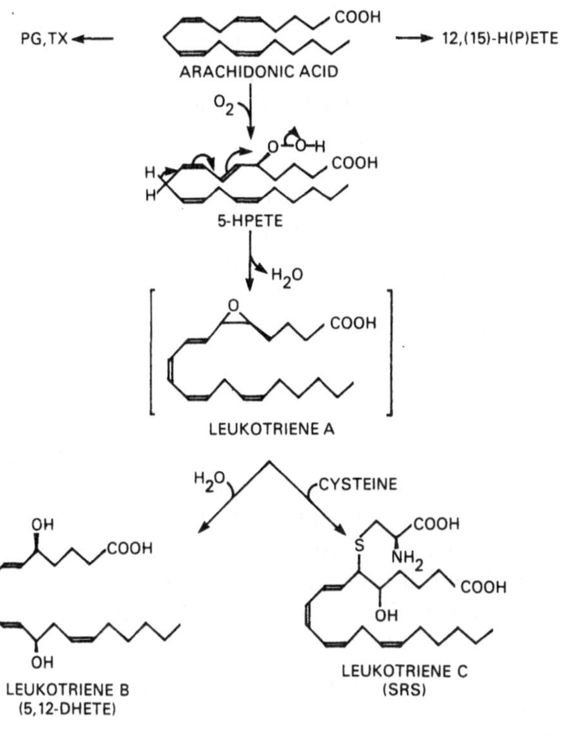

Figure 2.1b Scheme of oxygenative transformations of arachidonic acid. 5(6)-Oxido-7,9,11,14-eicosatetraenoic acid (5) (leukotriene A), 5(S),12(R)-(E,Z,E,Z)-6,8,10,14-eicosatetraenoic acid (2) (leukotriene B) and 5-hydroxy-6-sulfidocysteinyl-7,9,11,14-eicosatetraenoic acid (1) (leukotriene C)

The biosynthesis of arachidonic acid derivatives by lipo-oxygenase is greatly enhanced by the administration of compounds of the acetylsalicylic group, which inhibit in a irreversible form the cyclo-oxygenases[11, 12].

Arachidonic acid cleaved from phospholipids primarily follows – under these conditions – the lipo-oxygenase pathway, and HETE-related compounds are accumulated. Also the glucocorticoid steroids prevent prostaglandin formation, but they act at a higher level by reducing the availability of arachidonate to its metabolic system[13, 14]. Both cyclo-oxygenase and lipo-oxygenase compounds synthesis are therefore depressed and this explains the most effective and complete anti-inflammatory effects of these compounds in many systems. The metabolic pathways of arachidonic acid are shown in Figures 2.1a and 2.1b.

PROSTAGLANDINS IN PREGNANCY AND REPRODUCTION

Stable prostaglandins have been measured in the gonads and sexual organs under several physiological and pathological conditions, and they play an important role in human and animal reproduction.

Prostaglandins are also involved in the release of LH, as originally shown by Orczyk and Behrman[15] and by Armstrong and Grinwich[16]. PGE_1 and PGE_2 act directly on the hypothalamus on the release of LH[17, 18]. Indomethacin, an inhibitor of cyclo-oxygenase, decreases plasma LH levels in ovariectomized rats, and this inhibition is counteracted by administration of LH-RH[19, 20]; finally, PGE_2 releases LH-RH in rats[19, 20]. The experimental evidence indicates that PGE_2 in the rat, and possibly $PGF_{2\alpha}$ in other species, induce LH-RH release by acting at the hypothalamic level.

Prostaglandins are also effective in physiological ovulation, which is inhibited by indomethacin, an effect fully antagonized by exogenous PGE_2[21, 22]. A follicular increase of PGF and PGE has been shown after LH administration or after mating, and this effect is prevented by indomethacin[23]. The same prostaglandin inhibitor or the intrafollicular administration of $PGF_{2\alpha}$ antiserum blocks ovulation in rabbits[24]. The precise mode of action of prostaglandins in ovulation is, however, not yet fully elucidated. In human endometrium the levels of prostaglandin and the ratio PGF:PGE is higher (from 1 to 3) in the luteal phase than in the proliferative phase[25, 26]. However, the wide range of values observed in human tissues makes it impossible to draw conclusions concerning the possible role of these compounds in menstruation. The indomethacin treatment alleviates the symptoms of dysmenorrhea and reduces the abnormally high levels of PGFs, indicating that disorders of menstruation may be associated with an overproduction of one or more prostaglandins[27].

$PGF_{2\alpha}$ is also secreted by the uterus, and exerts a luteolytic effect in many mammalian species but not in the human[28]. In human subjects $PGF_{2\alpha}$ infusion reduces the progesterone output with modest effects on estrogens during the late, but not in the early, phase of the luteal cycle[29]. The physiological stimulus for $PGF_{2\alpha}$ formation and release in uterus is probably a combination of estrogens and progesterone released from the ovaries, estradiol also increasing the uterine capacity of producing $PGF_{2\alpha}$ by increasing the concentration of the prostaglandin-synthesizing enzymes[30].

In early pregnancy in mice indomethacin prevents implantation, an effect frequently reversed with the administration of PGE_2 or $PGF_{2\alpha}$[31]. Indomethacin also prevents implantation when given in days two or three of pregnancy in mice[32].

During early pregnancy much less $PGF_{2\alpha}$ is released by the guinea-pig uterus than by the non-pregnant uterus[28], explaining the lack of luteolysis during pregnancy. A metabolite of $PGF_{2\alpha}$, 15-keto-13,14-dihydro-$PGF_{2\alpha}$, appears in pulses in the peripheral plasma during the last days of the normal cycle, in coincidence with a decrease of progesterone levels. In pregnant cows progesterone levels remain high and the increase of $PGF_{2\alpha}$ metabolites in plasma is not observed, indicating that during early pregnancy the $PGF_{2\alpha}$ released from the uterus is reduced, and explaining luteal maintenance[33].

An important role of $PGF_{2\alpha}$ is shown in parturition. Indomethacin or aspirin treatment prolongs gestation in several mammalian species[34-36]. In humans a retrospective study indicated a significant inhibiting effect on labour by aspirin[37].

On the other hand, peripheral plasma levels of 15-keto-13,14-dihydro-$PGF_{2\alpha}$ increase in women 10–30-fold during labour[38].

PROSTACYCLIN IN PREGNANT HUMAN UTERUS

In recent years evidence has been obtained in several laboratories that not only stable prostaglandins, but also prostacyclin (PGI_2), are formed in rat uterus at the end of the gestation period[39]. This compound, as shown in our laboratory, inhibits the spontaneous motility of isolated normal human myometrium and specifically antagonizes the contractions induced by $PGF_{2\alpha}$[40]. Human myometrium, both pregnant and non-pregnant, generates PGI_2, as

Table 2.1 Cyclic AMP formation in human myometrial system: effects of pregnancy and prostacyclin

PGI_2	Cyclic AMP (pmol/mg protein)	
	Non-pregnant uterus	Pregnant uterus
Control	0.63 ± 0.15	1.72 ± 0.21
10^{-5} mol/l	1.66 ± 0.09	4.03 ± 0.38
10^{-4} mol/l	3.25 ± 0.19	4.97 ± 0.34

shown by Omini et al.[41]. This compound may have a physiological role by determining the motility of myometrium and modulating the uterine responses to the stimulatory activity of prostaglandins and other hormones during pregnancy. The lowering of uterine tone and contractility induced by PGI_2 may be explained by the increase of cAMP in the myometrial fibres induced by PGI_2 which is known to stimulate adenylyl cyclase activity also in other tissues[42] (Table 2.1).

CONCLUDING REMARKS

The amount of experimental data available in human tissues and in animal models is rapidly growing for the periods of the physiological cycle and pregnancy. In contrast, few data are available for the menopausal period in the human or in animals after castration. Treatment of ovariectomized hamster with estrogens decreased, and with progesterone increased, the binding of prostaglandin E_1 and $F_{2\alpha}$ to their receptors[43], suggesting that in the reproductive tract there is a protein specifically binding prostaglandins and indicating that female gonadal hormones affect the affinity of prostaglandins for such protein. For future research it is of great importance to investigate the uterine response and that of other smooth muscle preparations of the reproductive tract to exogenous prostaglandins after castration or during the menopausal period. These data should be also correlated with biosynthesis, release and binding of endogenous prostaglandins in the same systems. The study of the effects of natural and synthetic estrogens and progesterone on the same parameters will be also essential for the understanding of the possible role of prostaglandins and other arachidonic acid metabolites on the onset of the principal symptoms of menopause.

References

1. International Symposium on the Menopause and the Postmenopause, Rome, 1979
2. Vane, J. R. (1978). In F. Coceani and P. M. Olley (eds), *Advances in Prostaglandins and Thromboxane Research*, vol. 4, p. 27. (New York: Raven Press)
3. Hamberg, M., Svensson, J. and Samuelsson, B. (1976). In B. Samuelsson and R. Paoletti (eds), *Advances in Prostaglandin and Thromboxane Research*, vol. 1, p. 19. (New York: Raven Press)
4. Moncada, S., Herman, A. G., Higgs, E. A. and Vane, J. R. (1977). *Thromb. Res.*, **11**, 323
5. Piper, P. J. and Vane, J. R. (1969). *Nature*, **223**, 29
6. Needleman, P., Moncada, S., Bunting, S., Vane, J. R., Hamberg, M. and Samuelsson, B. (1976). *Nature*, **261**, 559
7. Moncada, S., Gryglewski, R., Bunting, S. and Vane, J. R. (1976). *Prostaglandins*, **12**, 715
8. Hamberg, M. and Samuelsson, B. (1974). *Proc. Natl. Acad. Sci. USA*, **71**, 3400
9. Turner, S. R., Tainer, J. A. and Lynn, W. S. (1975). *Nature*, **257**, 580
10. Borgeat, P. and Samuelsson, B. (1979). Fourth International Conference on Prostaglandins, Washington, DC, USA
11. Smith, J. B. and Willis, A. L. (1971). *Nature (New Biol.)*, **231**, 239
12. Ferreira, S. H., Moncada, S. and Vane, J. R. (1971). *Nature (New Biol.)*, **231**, 237
13. Lewis, G. P. and Piper, P. J. (1975). *Nature*, **254**, 308
14. Gryglewski, R., Panczeko, B., Korbut, R., Grodzinska, L. and Ocetkiewicz, A. (1975). *Prostaglandins*, **10**, 343
15. Orczyk, G. P. and Behrman, H. R. (1972). *Prostaglandins*, **1**, 3
16. Armstrong, D. T. and Grinwich, D. L. (1972). *Prostaglandins*, **1**, 21
17. Harms, P. G., Ojeda, S. R. and McCann, S. M. (1973). *Science*, **181**, 760
18. Spies, H. G. and Norman, R. L. (1973). *Prostaglandins*, **4**, 131
19. Ojeda, S. R. (1976). *Prostagl. Ther.*, **2**, 3
20. Eskay, R. L., Warberg, J., Mical, R. S. and Porter, J. C. (1975). *Endocrinology*, **97**, 816

21. O'Grady, J. P., Caldwell, B. V., Auletta, F. J. and Speroff, L. (1972). *Prostaglandins*, 1, 97
22. Tsafriri, A., Lindner, H. R., Zor, A. and Lamprecht, S. A. (1972). *Prostaglandins*, 2, 1
23. Yang, N. S. T., Marsh, J. M. and Lemaire, W. J. (1973). *Prostaglandins*, 4, 395
24. Armstrong, D. T., Grinwich, D. L., Moon, Y. S. and Zamechik, J. (1974). *Life Sci.*, 14, 129
25. Pickles, V. R., Hall, W. J., Best, F. A. and Smith, G. N. (1965). *J. Obstet. Gynaecol. Br. Commonw.*, 72, 185
26. Downie, J., Poyser, N. L. and Wunderlich, M. (1974). *J. Physiol. (Lond.)*, 236, 465
27. Halbert, D. R., Demers, L. M., Fontana, J. and Jones, D. E. D. (1975). *Prostaglandins*, 10, 1047
28. Horton, E. W. and Poyser, N. L. (1976). *Physiol. Rev.*, 56, 595
29. Hillier, K., Dutton, A., Corker, C. S., Singer, A. and Embrey, M. P. (1972). *Br. Med. J.*, 4, 333
30. Poyser, N. L. (1976). In B. Samuelsson and R. Paoletti (eds), *Advances in Prostaglandins and Thromboxane*, vol. 2, p. 633. (New York: Raven Press)
31. Lau, I. F., Saksena, S. K. and Chang, M. C. (1973). *Prostaglandins*, 4, 795
32. Chatterjee, A. (1973). *Proc. Ind. Nat. Sci. Acad.*, 39, 408
33. Kindahl, H., Edqvist, L. E., Ban, A. and Granström, E. (1970). *Acta Endocr. (Copenh.)*, 82, 134
34. Aiken, J. W. (1972). *Nature (Lond.)*, 240, 21
35. Chester, R., Dukes, M., Slater, S. R. and Walpole, A. L. (1972). *Nature (Lond.)*, 240, 37
36. Novy, M. J., Cook, M. J. and Manaugh, L. (1974). *Am. J. Obstet. Gynecol.*, 118, 412
37. Flowers, R. J. (1974). *Pharmacol. Rev.*, 26, 33
38. Green, K., Bygdeman, M., Toppozoda, M. and Wiqvist, N. (1975). *Am. J. Obstet. Gynecol.*, 120, 25
39. Williams, K. I., Dembinska-Kiec, A., Zmuda, A. and Gryglewski, R. J. (1978). *Prostaglandins*, 15, 343
40. Berti, F., Fano, M., Folco, G. C., Longiave, D. and Omini, C. (1978). *Prostaglandins*, 15, 867
41. Omini, C., Folco, G. C., Pasargiklian, R., Fano, M. and Berti, F. (1979). *Prostaglandins*, 17, 1
42. Gorman, R. R., Bunting, S. and Miller, O. V. (1977). *Prostaglandins*, 13, 377
43. Wakeling, A. E. and Wyngarden, L. J. (1974). *Endocrinology*, 95, 55

3
Plasma Concentration of Estrogens after Application of various Estrogen Preparations

A. E. SCHINDLER, M. ZWIRNER, R. GÖSER
and H. M. BOLT

In spite of the extensive use of natural and synthetic estrogens in pre- and postmenopausal women, limited data are available about the circulating plasma levels of the parent compounds and their metabolites regarding extent and time course of absorption as well as clearance, recirculation and metabolism. There are different types of applications (oral, parental, mucosal), differences in steroid moiety (free, sulfoconjugated, esterified) and different types of estrogens (estrone, estradiol, estriol) creating a variety of results.

The purpose of this study was to investigate the oral route of application of sulfoconjugated and free estrone using identical experimental conditions in order to study absorption, disappearance and metabolism of these steroid moieties.

MATERIALS AND METHODS

Fourteen women volunteers aged 19–42 (mean 27.6 years) with normal menstrual cycles without medication participated in the study. Three preparations were used: (1) 3.75 mg Presomen ᴿ (conjugated equine estrogens); (2) 2.63 mg free estrone dissolved in alcohol; and (3) 3.87 mg estrone sulfate (K⁺) corresponding to 2.63 mg free estrone dissolved in alcohol. These hormone preparations were taken orally on the 25th day of the cycle and antecubital vein blood was drawn in heparinized tubes at zero time and 1, 2, 4, 6, 8, 10, 12, 16, 24, 48 h after intake of the medication. Free estrone (E_1 free) and estradiol (E_2 free) were measured by specific radioimmunoassays after ether extraction using antisera obtained against estrone-6-oxo:BSA and estradiol-6-oxo:BSA respectively[1]. Total estrone (E_1 total) was radioimmuno-assayed after enzyme hydrolysis and ether extraction using the same anti-serum as for E_1 free.

RESULTS

The concentration changes during the time of study of E_1 free for the three experimental preparations are shown in Figure 3.1. The fastest increase was seen with ingestion of E_1 free dissolved in alcohol reaching the measured maximum within 2 h and demonstrating between 6 and 8 h a shoulder which

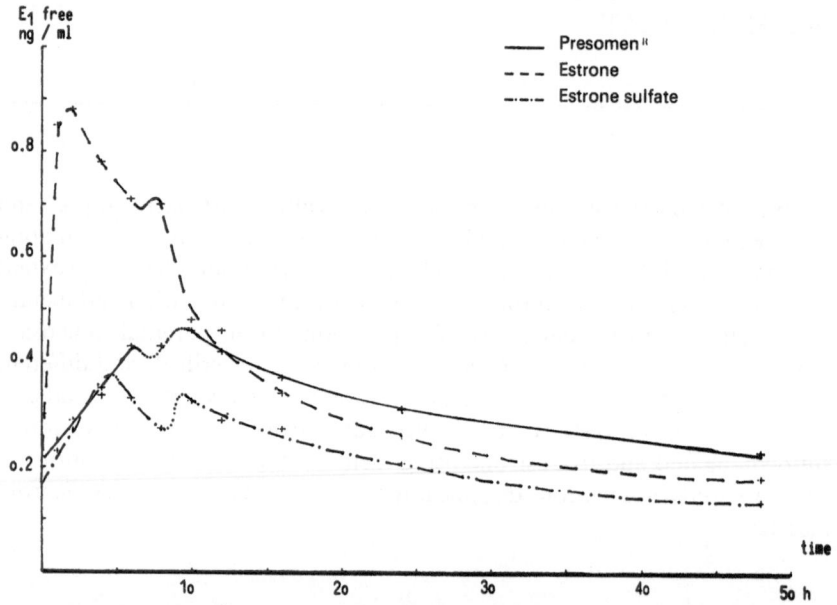

Figure 3.1   The concentration of plasma unconjugated estrone (E_1 free)

could be comparable with enterohepatic recirculation. Such recirculation is obvious from the data obtained with preparations 1 and 3. With all three preparations the pretreatment values of E_1 free were reached within 48 h.

Figure 3.2 demonstrates the data of E_1 total. The most striking finding is the rapid rise of E_1 total after application of E_1 free indicating rapid absorption and conjugation of E_1 using preparation 2. Similar to the data of E_1 free,

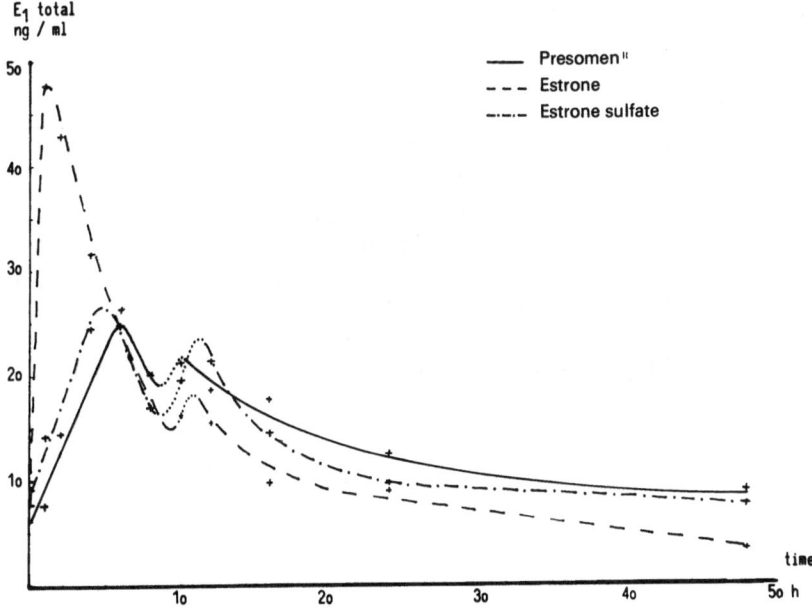

Figure 3.2 The concentration of plasma total estrone (E_1 total)

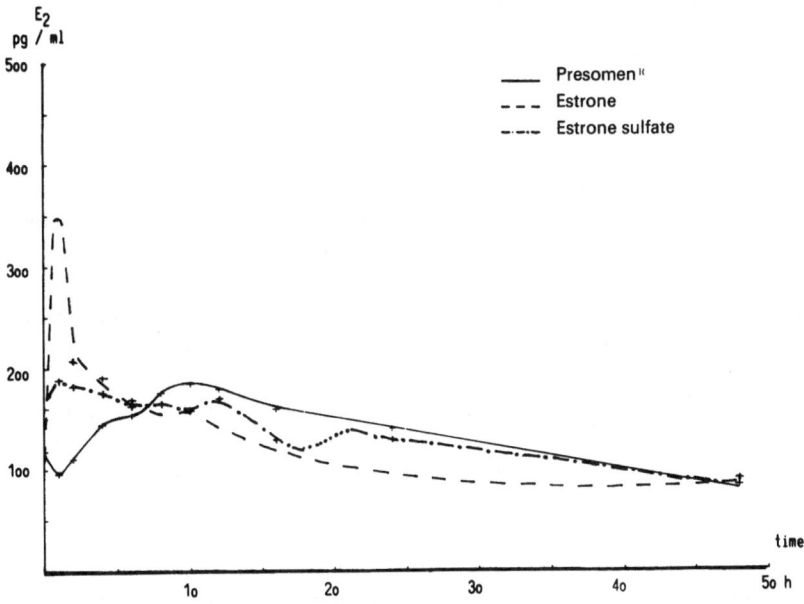

Figure 3.3 The concentration of plasma unconjugated estradiol (E_2 free)

enterohepatic recirculation of conjugated E_1 appears to occur between 8 and 12 h. E_1 total also reached treatment levels again within 48 h.

In Figure 3.3 the data of plasma E_2 free are summarized. The preparations 2 and 3 dissolved in alcohol demonstrate a maximum of E_2 free concentration within 1 h with the possibility of enterohepatic recirculation between 8 and 12 h, while with the commercially available conjugated estrogen preparation the maximal E_2 free level is reached at about 10 h and elevated levels are maintained over a 24 h period, while for preparations 2 and 3 the concentration of E_2 free was below the pretreatment values at that time (Figure 3.3).

Taking the $E_1 : E_2$ ratio into account, the least increment of E_1 free over E_2 free is found with preparation 1 (Table 3.1).

Table 3.1 $E_1 : E_2$ ratios after oral intake of three estrogen preparations

Time (h)	$E_1 : E_2$ ratio		
	Preparation 1	Preparation 2	Preparation 3
0	1.9	1.5	1.0
1	2.3	2.4	1.3
2	2.4	4.2	1.5
4	2.4	4.1	1.9
6	2.7	4.2	2.0
8	2.4	4.6	1.6
10	2.5	3.1	2.0
12	2.3	3.3	1.7
16	2.3	2.9	2.1
24	2.2	2.5	1.6
48	2.8	2.0	1.4

DISCUSSION

Normal menstruating volunteers on the 25th day of the menstrual cycle were chosen in order to avoid bleeding abnormalities when using the estrogen preparations and to be able to compare the data with results obtained using ethinyl estradiol under identical conditions[2].

Similar to data obtained in postmenopausal women with oral conjugated equine estrogens[3], an E_1 free : E_2 free ratio around 2.5 was found in this study (Table 3.1). Indeed, oral application results in particular patterns of circulating E_1 free and E_2 free. There is a greater increment of plasma E_1 than E_2 when micronized estradiol or estradiol valerianate is used[4, 5, 6, 7, 11]. Using estrone sulfate the rise of plasma E_1 and E_2 is not so divergent as shown in this study and by others[8]. This indicates a rapid conversion of estradiol to estrone by the gastrointestinal tract and/or liver leading to high $E_1 : E_2$ ratios[5] between 5 to 8, while oral use of estrone sulfate results in an $E_1 : E_2$ ratio between 2.0 and 2.7, as shown in this study (Table 3.1), reflecting relatively high conversion of estrone sulfate to E_2. In addition, the results of this investigation indicate a more favourable plasma $E_1:E_2$ ratio being obtained with estrone sulfate than with free E_1.

From a clinical point of view, it can be concluded that with oral use of conjugated equine estrogens or estrone sulfate the $E_1:E_2$ ratio remains closer to the physiological condition than when using estradiol orally. This applies for short term treatment, as shown in this study, and long term application[6] as well. Considering plasma estrone sulfate, similar concentrations were found when either 1.5 mg piperazine estrone sulfate or 2 mg estradiol valerianate were ingested[7].

Evidence has been obtained in this study that enterohepatic recirculation occurs between 8 and 12 h in normal menstruating women, independent of the steroid moiety used (Figures 3.1–3.3). This is in accordance with findings obtained using ethinyl estradiol in a similar study group[2].

Aside from the oral intake, intramuscular or vaginal application of E_2 results in a predominance of the plasma E_2 concentration[8,9]. Vaginal application of conjugated equine estrogen did increase the plasma E_1 and E_2 concentration, but did not change the pretreatment $E_1:E_2$ ratio[9].

Intranasal administration of micronized E_2 induced a short-lasting rise of circulating E_2 followed by a progressive increase of the $E_1:E_2$ ratio which rose above unity after 1 h and reached about 2.0 to 2.5 after 6–8 h[10].

Therefore, it is obvious that the circulating estrogen levels are dependent from local metabolism at the absorption site. Estrogens taken orally in addition are subjected to primary passage through the liver. In contrast to a previous report in amenorrheic women[11], we have found free E_2 elevations after all the estrogen preparations tested. The differences in results could perhaps reflect changes in metabolism of conjugated estrone in amenorrheic patients in comparison to normal menstruating women.

Overall, the biologically most favourable plasma concentration curve of free E_2 was obtained with conjugated equine estrogens (Figure 3.3).

Acknowledgments

The expert technical assistance of Mrs G. Hochlehnert and Miss E. Mark is greatly appreciated. The study was supported in part by Kali Chemie Pharma GmbH, Hanover.

References

1. Friedrich, E., Jaeger-Whitegiver, E. R., Bieder, M., Halverscheidt, H., Penke, B., Pallai, P., Keller, E. and Schindler, A. E. (1974). Standardization of specific radioimmunoassays for plasma estrone, estradiol, progesterone and androstenedione. *J. Steroid Biochem.*, **5**, 305
2. Bolt, H. M., Löffler, S., Rowe, P. H. and Schindler, A. E. (1979). Influence of enterohepatic circulation on pharmacokinetics of estrogenic hormones. *Naunyn-Schmiedeberg's Arch. Pharmacol.*, **307** (Suppl.), 307

3. Strecker, J. R., Lauritzen, Ch. and Goessens, L. (1979). Plasma concentrations of unconjugated and conjugated estrogens and gonadotropins following application of various estrogen preparations after oophorectomy and in the menopause. *Maturitas*, 1, 183

4. Yen, S. S. C., Martin, P. L., Burnier, A. M., Czekala, N. M., Greaney, M. O. and Callantine, M. R. (1975). Circulating estradiol, estrone and gonadotropin levels following the administration of orally active 17β-estradiol in postmenopausal women. *J. Clin. Endocrinol. Metab.*, 40, 518

5. Englund, D. E. and Johansson, E. D. B. (1977). Pharmacokinetic and pharmacodynamic studies on estradiol valerianate administered orally to postmenopausal women. *Acta Obstet. Gynecol. Scand.*, **Suppl.** 65, 27

6. Larsson-Cohn, U., Johansson, E. D. B., Kágedal, B. and Wallentin, L. (1977). Serum FSH, LH and estrone levels in postmenopausal patients on estrogen therapy. *Br. J. Obstet. Gynaecol.*, 85, 367

7. Anderson, A. B. M., Sklovsky, E., Sayers, L., Steele, P. A. and Turnbull, A. G. (1978). Comparison of serum estrogen concentrations in postmenopausal women taking estrone sulphate and estradiol. *Br. Med. J.*, 1, 140

8. Englund, D. E. and Johansson, E. D. B. (1976). Plasma levels of estrone and estradiol after oral, intramuscular and vaginal administration of natural estrogens. *Proceedings from a Gynaecological Symposium held in Malmö, September 6–7.* Part I, 17

9. Whitehead, M. I., Minardi, J., Kitchin, Y. and Sharples, M. J. (1978). Systemic absorption of estrogen from premarin vaginal cream. In I. D. Cooke (ed.), *The Role of Estrogen/Progestogen in the Management of the Menopause*, pp. 63–71. (Lancaster: MTP Press)

10. Rigg, L. A., Milanes, B., Villanueva, B. and Yen, S. S. C. (1977). Efficacy of intravaginal and intranasal administration of micronized estradiol-17β. *J. Clin. Endocrinol. Metab.*, 45, 1261

11. Spona, J. and Schneider, W. H. F. (1977). Bioavailability of natural estrogens in young females with secondary amenorrhea. *Acta Obstet. Gynecol. Scand.*, **Suppl.** 65, 33

4
Progestogen Modification of Estrogen-induced Endometrial Proliferation in Climacteric Women

M. I. WHITEHEAD, J. McQUEEN, J. MINARDI
and S. CAMPBELL

INTRODUCTION

Few topics provoke more discussion than the relationship between exogenous estrogens and endometrial carcinoma, and the recent publication in America of retrospective studies reporting an increase in the risk ratio for cancer following prolonged estrogen therapy[1-6] has further fuelled this controversy. The statistical, clinical and pathological biases and inadequacies of this type of investigation have been discussed extensively[7-11], but it is highly unlikely that the reported relationship is spurious[12].

A direct drug effect is strongly suggested by the observed increase in risk ratio with greater dosage of estrogen, with increased duration of usage and probably with administration in a continuous manner. As these associations were strongest for the early less-invasive cancers (Stage 1) and weakest for the more invasive (Stages 2–4), the implication is that the etiology of the more advanced lesions may be largely unaccounted for by estrogen use[12]. Also, although all the studies were flawed to a varying extent and the elements of bias in each were different, all reached the same conclusion. The available evidence therefore suggests a true link between exogenous estrogen and the early forms of endometrial carcinoma.

The exact increase in the risk for carcinoma following estrogen therapy has still to be defined. Various biases operating in the studies, especially the over-diagnosis of endometrial hyperplasia as neoplasia[13], may have falsely increased the magnitude of that reported. It is important that this risk be put into proper perspective. In untreated postmenopausal women there is a probability that one per 1000 per annum will develop endometrial carcinoma[14]. The *highest* reported risk ratio with exogenous estrogen was 8:1[4], and this, if correct, indicates that eight women per 1000 per annum will develop neoplasia: *the other 992 will not*. The incidence of estrogen-related endometrial carcinoma therefore is likely to be very small. However, the size of the population at risk – and there are over 200000 women in the United Kingdom receiving some form of 'estrogen replacement therapy' at present – will necessarily result in an appreciable number of cases, approximately 140 in the first year. Furthermore, it is unclear at present whether the association between increase in risk and duration of usage is linear or exponential as both types of regression curve can be fitted equally well to the available evidence. In a linear relationship the increase in risk rises by a factor of approximately one per annum; in the exponential model the risk remains relatively small for the first 3 or 4 years of estrogen usage but thereafter doubles every 3 years[12].

All iatrogenic disease should be prevented as far as is possible. Therefore methods of modifying estrogen-induced endometrial proliferation in climacteric women are currently being investigated. There is good biochemical and clinical evidence that in the premenopausal woman progestins modify endometrial estrogen metabolism. For example, progesterone lowers the endometrial concentration of estrogen receptor[15], thus depressing estrogenic stimulation which is receptor-mediated; and induces the activity for formation of the enzyme estradiol 17β-dehydrogenase[16, 17], which 'detoxifies' the potent intracellular estrogen, estradiol, into the less potent estrone. Clinically, combined estrogen–progestogen therapy, as prescribed in oral contraception, has not resulted in an epidemic of endometrial cancer or pre-malignant endometrial hyperplasia.

In 1973, before the publication of the American retrospective studies, we began monitoring the endometrial response to unopposed cyclical estrogen therapy and sequential estrogen–progestogen therapy – outpatient biopsy being performed serially at 6–15-month intervals with the Vabra aspirator[18]. Our aims were to quantify both the endometrial response to estrogen and the modifying effect, if any, of progestogens on this response. During therapy the nature of uterine bleeding was correlated with the endometrial histology and thus its reliability as an indicator of underlying endometrial pathology has been determined. These results are now presented and their significance is discussed. The methodology has been detailed elsewhere[19, 20] and is only summarized here.

METHODOLOGY

One hundred and eighty-two patients were recruited between 1973 and 1978. When the study commenced, curettage was only performed before therapy was started if specifically indicated. To establish baseline endometrial values this policy was later changed and thereafter a pretreatment biopsy was obtained from every patient.

One hundred and eight patients, not one of whom had previously experienced abnormal vaginal bleeding, commenced clinic therapy without a pretreatment curettage. Seventy-four patients, all with normal endometrium at pretreatment curettage, were also admitted to the study. Normal endometrium was defined as either proliferative, secretory, menstrual or atrophic endometrium, benign polypi or 'no curettings'. One hundred and sixteen patients (63.7%), with a mean age of 54.1 years, were postmenopausal (i.e. no spontaneous menstruation in the previous 12 months); and 66 patients (36.3%), with a mean age of 50.8 years, were perimenopausal (i.e. spontaneous menstruation within the previous 12 months but with at least 3 months between menses).

All symptomatic patients were prescribed either cyclical or sequential therapy. With both therapies 'natural' estrogens, i.e. compounds which after administration give rise in the plasma to estrogens similar to those produced endogenously[21], were used exclusively and at dosages recommended by the manufacturers.

Cyclical therapy

The estrogen was given daily in 3-week cycles with one intervening treatment-free week. Patients received one of three estrogen preparations and high- and low-dose regimens of each were prescribed depending upon the severity of symptomatology. High-dose regimens were: Premarin (conjugated estrogens: Ayerst Laboratories) 1.25 mg daily; Harmogen (piperazine estrone sulphate: Abbott Laboratories) 3 mg daily; and Progynova (estradiol valerate: Schering Chemicals) 2 mg daily. Low-dose regimens were the above halved.

Sequential therapy

The estrogen preparations and dosages prescribed were as for cyclical therapy and one of two progestogens was added for either 5 or 7 days each month. The progestogens were: norethisterone (Primolut N: Schering Chemicals) or medroxyprogesterone acetate (Provera: Upjohn Ltd). The dosages of progestogens were 5 mg daily with a high-dose estrogen regimen, and 2.5 mg daily with a low-dose regimen.

In addition, a small number of patients received Cyclo-Progynova (estradiol valerate 2 mg for 21 days, with DL-norgestrel 0.5 mg added from the 12th to 21st day).

Patterns of vaginal bleeding

During cyclical therapy withdrawal bleeding was defined as bleeding occurring in the treatment-free week between each 3-week treatment cycle; and during sequential therapy as bleeding occurring in the 7-day period following ingestion of the progestogen. Light bleeding of up to 2–3 days duration which was continuous with the withdrawal bleed was also classified as such, but with both types of therapy unscheduled bleeding occurring at any other time was classified as breakthrough bleeding.

RESULTS

Endometrial histology related to type of therapy (Table 4.1)

Cyclical therapy

This ranged from 2 to 47 months (mean duration 15.8 months). With high-dose estrogen, cystic glandular hyperplasia was diagnosed in 16 patients (23%) and atypical hyperplasia in six patients (9%); with low-dose regimens cystic glandular hyperplasia was diagnosed in four patients (11%) and atypical hyperplasia in two patients (5%).

Table 4.1 Endometrial histology related to type of therapy

Type of therapy	Total number of patients	Number of patients with normal endometrium	Number of patients with cystic glandular hyperplasia	Number of patients with atypical hyperplasia
Cyclical high-dose	69	47	16 (23%)	6 (9%)
Cyclical low-dose	37	31	4 (11%)	2 (5%)
Sequential high-dose	47	44	1 (2%)	2 (4%)
Sequential low-dose	29	28	—	1 (3%)

Total number of patients: 182
Percentages are in parentheses
The observed incidences of hyperplasia during cyclical and sequential high- and low-dose therapy were significantly different from the expected (chi-squared = 17.853: 3 degrees of freedom: $p < 0.001$). Reproduced, with permission of the Editor, from Whitehead, M. I. (19/8). The effects of oestrogens and progestogens on the post-menopausal endometrium. *Maturitas*, 1, 87–98

Sequential therapy

This ranged from 2 to 50 months (mean duration 16.2 months). With high-dose regimens one patient (2%) was found to have cystic glandular hyperplasia and two patients (4%) atypical hyperplasia; with low-doses, atypical hyperplasia was diagnosed in one patient (3%).

The observed incidences of hyperplasia during high- and low-dose cyclical therapy and high- and low-dose sequential therapy were significantly different from the expected (chi-squared = 17.853: 3 degrees of freedom: $p < 0.001$).

It was not always possible to time exactly the onset of hyperplasia as curettage was not performed on all patients at regular intervals. With cyclical therapy hyperplasia was diagnosed as early as 2 months, or as long as 35 months, after treatment started. The condition was found in 11 patients in the first 12 treatment months; in 12 patients between the 13th and 24th treatment months; and in five patients receiving therapy for more than 25 months. In 11 of the 28 patients normal endometrium had been obtained at first curettage and hyperplasia was found at second or subsequent curettage.

One of the three patients in whom hyperplasia was found during sequential high-dose therapy had received treatment for 17 months and the other two patients had been on therapy for only 3 months. In one, atypical hyperplasia had been diagnosed 13 years previously following abnormal vaginal bleeding. A pretreatment curettage had been performed and it is probable that this patient had a predisposition towards hyperplasia. During sequential low-dose therapy, atypical hyperplasia was diagnosed in one patient at fourth curettage after 50 months of treatment.

Follow-up of patients with endometrial hyperplasia

Twenty of the 28 patients in whom endometrial hyperplasia was diagnosed during cyclical therapy subsequently received sequential regimens. In all cases but one, normal endometrium was obtained at repeat curettage. Two of the four patients in whom hyperplasia was diagnosed during sequential therapy subsequently received a combined estrogen–progestogen regimen (norethisterone 2.5 mg given in combination with the estrogen daily), and in both cases normal endometrium was obtained at repeat curettage.

Patterns of vaginal bleeding (Table 4.2)

The bleeding patterns are shown with respect to the histology of the endometrium.

Table 4.2   The patterns of vaginal bleeding in patients with normal and hyperplastic endometrium during cyclical and sequential therapy

Type of therapy	Endometrial histology	Number of patients with withdrawal bleeding	Number of patients with breakthrough bleeding	Number of patients with no vaginal bleeding
Cyclical high-dose	Normal endometrium	14 (64%)	11 (69%)	22 (71%)
	Endometrial hyperplasia	8 (36%)	5 (31%)	9 (29%)
Cyclical low-dose	Normal endometrium	3 (75%)	5 (56%)	23 (96%)
	Endometrial hyperplasia	1 (25%)	4 (44%)	1 (4%)
Sequential high-dose	Normal endometrium	42 (98%)	2 (50%)	—
	Endometrial hyperplasia	1 (2%)	2 (50%)	—
Sequential low-dose	Normal endometrium	23 (96%)	3	2
	Endometrial hyperplasia	1 (4%)	—	—

Percentages are in parentheses

Reproduced with permission of the Editor, from Whitehead, M. I. (1978). The effects of oestrogens and progestogens on the post-menopausal endometrium. *Maturitas*, 1, 87–98

Cyclical high-dose therapy

Of the 22 patients with scheduled withdrawal bleeding, 14 (64%) were found to have normal endometrium and hyperplasia was diagnosed in the remaining eight (36%) patients. Eleven (69%) of the 16 patients with unscheduled break-through bleeding had normal endometrium and hyperplasia was diagnosed in the other five patients (31%). Twenty-two (71%) of the 31 patients who had no vaginal bleeding were found to have normal endometrium and the remaining nine (29%) had hyperplasia.

Cyclical low-dose therapy

Endometrial hyperplasia was diagnosed in one of the four patients with scheduled withdrawal bleeding; in four (44%) of the nine patients experiencing unscheduled breakthrough bleeding; and in one (4%) of the 24 patients who had no vaginal bleeding.

Sequential high-dose therapy

All patients experienced vaginal bleeding. Endometrial hyperplasia was found in one (2%) of the 43 patients with withdrawal bleeding. Four patients had unscheduled breakthrough bleeding, of whom two had normal endometrium and two had endometrial hyperplasia.

Sequential low-dose therapy

Normal endometrium was diagnosed in 23 (96%) of 24 patients with scheduled withdrawal bleeding; in all three patients with breakthrough bleeding and in both patients who had no vaginal bleeding.

DISCUSSION

The study presented here has shown that cyclical regimens of unopposed estrogens are associated with the development of both cystic glandular and atypical hyperplasia. After a mean treatment period of 16 months the incidence of hyperplasia with high-dose regimens was 32% (22 of 69 patients) and with low-dose regimens 16% (6 of 37 patients) and this suggests a dose-dependent relationship.

The association between spontaneously arising hyperplasia and endometrial cancer is well founded upon extensive documentation and the literature has been reviewed[22]. Estimates of the risk of the subsequent development of carcinoma range from 1% with cystic glandular hyperplasia[23] to 45% with severe atypical hyperplasia[24]; the best-designed study reported a cumulative risk of 30% at 10 years over controls[25]. As the estrogen-induced and spontaneously arising hyperplasias are indistinguishable histologically, we believe it would be unwise to regard the induced condition as carrying a lesser risk of subsequent malignancy unless shown conclusively from long-term studies.

The development of hyperplasia during therapy is to be expected, however, as there is good evidence that the estrogenic stimulus being applied to the endometrium is potent. First, we have reported previously[20] that during treatment the 24-hour urinary 'total' estrogen excretion is not only within and above the range associated with the premenopausal, mid-cycle ovulatory peak – the 3-day period of maximal estrogen production in the non-pregnant female – but also the range associated with the development of hyperplasia in anovulatory women[26]. Thus the term 'hormone *replacement* therapy' is a misnomer. Urinary estrogen concentrations, however, cannot be *directly* related to the degree of endometrial stimulation as much of the measured steroid is in the 'bound', and therefore physiologically inactive, form. The biological response of the endometrium depends much more on the mass of non-bound or 'free' estrogen available in the plasma. Although data are sparse, Lebech observed free estradiol levels within, and free estrone levels somewhat higher than, the pre-menopausal mid-cycle range following oral administration of 2 mg estradiol[27]. In addition, measurement of soluble progesterone receptor concentrations (which are an index of estrogen stimulation) in endometrial samples from some of our patients gave values again within the pre-menopausal proliferative phase range[28].

At present there are no means available for predicting, before treatment starts, those patients likely to develop hyperplasia with unopposed estrogens. Also, with cyclical regimens, vaginal bleeding failed to act as a reliable indicator of underlying endometrial pathology. For example, during high-dose therapy unscheduled breakthrough bleeding was associated more often with the finding of normal endometrium than hyperplasia. Scheduled withdrawal bleeding could not be considered a reassuring sign, hyperplasia being found in eight (36%) patients with this pattern. The absence of bleeding was no guarantee that underlying hyperplasia did not exist as nine (29%) of the patients who failed to experience bleeding had this condition. Similarly, during cyclical low-dose therapy normal endometrium and hyperplasia were both associated with scheduled, unscheduled and no vaginal bleeding.

As continued unopposed estrogens subsequent to the development of hyperplasia cannot be justified, it must be concluded that curettage is required on every patient during cyclical high- and low-dose therapy *irrespective of the bleeding pattern*. Furthermore, as after treatment starts the development of hyperplasia can be either rapid, within 2 months, or can be delayed for as long as 35 months, and as the finding of a normal endometrium on one occasion does not exclude the subsequent development of hyperplasia, we believe that endometrial biopsy should be performed approximately every 6 months for as long as cyclical treatment is continued.

During sequential therapy the incidence of hyperplasia was significantly lower than that with cyclical therapy (Table 4.1), with both high- and low-dose regimens. Therefore our dosages of progestogens – given for 5 or 7 days each calendar month – were not totally effective in preventing endometrial hyperstimulation. It has been reported that no case of hyperplasia arose amongst 102 women taking regimens incorporating 10 to 13 days of progestogen each calendar month[29]. However, the mean duration of therapy in this study – 9.7 months – may have been insufficient for the cumulative effect of estrogens to become apparent.

The protective effect of progestogen also extended to patients with estrogen-related hyperplasia, subsequent sequential regimens causing a return to normal endometrium in 19 of 20 patients (95%). We have reported elsewhere on their ability to reverse hyperplasia arising spontaneously in untreated women[30, 31] and Gambrell also observed a return to normal endometrium in 133 of 139 patients (95.7%), the majority with spontaneously arising hyperplasia, following therapy with norethisterone acetate, medroxyprogesterone acetate or a combination of ethinyl estradiol and norgestrel[12]. Logically, prevention of hyperplasia, whether estrogen-induced or spontaneously arising, will reduce the risk of subsequent carcinoma and Gambrell has reported cancer incidence rates (per 1000 women per annum) of 4.7 with unopposed estrogen therapy; 2.0 in an untreated population and 0.8 with estrogen–progestogen therapy[32].

The beneficial effects of progestogens are probably exerted in at least two ways. Biochemically, norethisterone, in endometRial samples from some of our patients, decreased the concentrations of nuclear estrogen and soluble progesterone receptor, and induced the production of estradiol 17β-dehydrogenase – thereby reproducing some of the depressant actions on cell biosynthesis of progesterone[28]. Also, by provoking regular endometrial shedding, manifest as a withdrawal bleed, progestogens prevent the prolonged stimulation of an otherwise retained endometrium. The re-establishment of vaginal bleeding, contrary to expectation, was associated with a high patient compliance, 90% of women preferring the monthly 'menstruation' to symptoms[20].

Endometrial hyperplasia was diagnosed in 3% of patients (two of 67 patients: Table 4.2) with scheduled withdrawal bleeding, and therefore regular endometrial biopsy is required even with this pattern of bleeding. However, because of the low incidence of hyperplasia, we believe that on present evidence curettage need be performed only at intervals of 12–15 months when using sequential therapy. Two of the seven patients experiencing breakthrough bleeding during sequential therapy were found to have hyperplasia and therefore unscheduled bleeding demands investigation. However, the low incidence of breakthrough bleeding with sequential high- and low-dose regimens (9%; seven of 76 patients: Table 4.2) reduces the number of patients in whom curettage is indicated. Furthermore, discontinuation of treatment because of persistent and erratic vaginal bleeding is likely to be less during sequential therapy than during cyclical therapy when the incidence of breakthrough bleeding was 24% (25 of 106 patients: Table 4.2).

CONCLUSIONS

The undoubted benefits of unopposed exogenous estrogens, given cyclically, can be achieved only at a risk of excessive stimulation of the endometrium in an unacceptably high number of patients. As, at present, there is no simple test which will accurately predict those patients who will develop endometrial hyperplasia, and as vaginal bleeding is unreliable as an indicator of those patients who have developed this condition as a result of exogenous estrogens, serial endometrial biopsy is required at intervals of 6 months on every patient for as long as cyclical therapy is prescribed.

The addition of a progestogen for 5 or 7 days each calendar month is protective to the endometrium. The incidence of hyperplasia is significantly reduced and estrogen-related hyperplasia can be reversed to normal endometrium. However, these regimens of progestogens were not totally protective and serial endometrial biopsy is still required at intervals of 12–15 months in patients experiencing scheduled withdrawal bleeding. Breakthrough bleeding demands immediate investigation.

It remains to be determined whether greater endometrial protection which results in a complete suppression of hyperplasia can be achieved by increasing the dose or duration of progestogen therapy.

Acknowledgements

We thank Drs H. Ferreira and J. Pryse-Davies for reporting the endometrial histology; and Dr A. P. Roberts, Department of Medicine, Charing Cross Hospital Medical School, for statistical advice.

This work was funded by Ayerst Laboratories.

This paper was first given at an earlier date and was previously published by MTP Press Limited in *The Role of Estrogen/Progestogen in the Management of the Menopause*, edited by I. D. Cooke.

References

1. Quint, B. C. (1975). Changing patterns in endometrial adenocarcinoma. *Am. J. Obstet. Gynecol.*, **122**, 498
2. Smith, D. C., Prentice, R., Thompson, D. and Herrman, W. (1975). Association of exogenous estrogens and endometrial carcinoma. *N. Engl. J. Med.*, **293**, 1164
3. Ziel, H. and Finkle, W. (1975). Increased risk of endometrial carcinoma among users of conjugated estrogens. *N. Engl. J. Med.*, **293**, 1167
4. Mack, T., Pike, M., Henderson, B., Pfeffer, R., Gerkins, V., Arthur, M. and Brown, S. (1976). Estrogens and endometrial cancer in a retirement community. *N. Engl. J. Med.*, **294**, 1262

5. Gray, L. A. Sr., Christopherson, W. M. and Hoover, R. N. (1977). Estrogens and endometrial carcinoma. *Obstet. Gynecol.*, **49**, 385

6. McDonald, T. W., Annegers, J. F., O'Fallan, W. M., Dockerty, M. B., Malkasian, G. D. and Kurland, L. T. (1977). Exogenous estrogen and endometrial carcinoma: case-control and incidence study. *Am. J. Obstet. Gynecol.*, **127**, 572

7. Cooke, I. D. (1976). Oestrogens as a cause of endometrial carcinoma. *Br. Med. J.*, **1**, 1209

8. Feinstein, A. R. and Horwitz, R. I. (1977). An analytic critique of five studies investigating the relationship of estrogens and endometrial cancer. Presented to the American Society for Clinical Investigation, 1 May, Washington DC, USA

9. Gordan, G. S. and Greenberg, B. G. (1976). Exogenous estrogens and endometrial cancer. *Postgrad. Med.*, **59**, 66

10. Greenwald, P., Caputo, T. A. and Wolfgand, P. E. (1977). Endometrial cancer after menopausal use of estrogens. *Obstet. Gynecol.*, **50**, 239

11. Berger, G. S. and Fowler, W. C. (1977). Exogenous estrogens and endometrial carcinoma: review and comments for the clinician. *J. Reprod. Med.*, **18**, 177

12. Campbell, S. and Whitehead, M. I. (1978). The endometrium in the menopause. In P. A. van Keep, D. M. Serr and R. B. Greenblatt (eds), *Female and Male Climacteric*, pp. 111–120. (Lancaster: MTP)

13. Szekely, D. R., Weiss, N. S. and Schweld, A. I. (1978). Incidence of endometrial carcinoma in King County, Washington: a standardized histological review. *J. Natl. Cancer Inst.*, **60**, 985

14. Weiss, N. S. (1975). Risks and benefits of estrogen use. *N. Engl. J. Med.*, **293**, 1200

15. Flickinger, G. L., Elsner, C., Illingworth, D. V., Muechler, E. K. and Mikhail, G. (1977). Estrogen and progesterone receptors in the female genital tract of humans and monkeys. *Ann. N.Y. Acad. Sci.*, **286**, 180

16. Pollow, K., Bognoi, E., Lubbert, H. and Pollow, B. (1975). The effect of gestagen therapy on 17-hydroxy steroid dehydrogenase in human endometrial adenocarcinoma. *J. Endocrinol.*, **67**, 131

17. Gurpide, E., Gusberg, S. B. and Tseng, L. (1976). Estradiol binding and metabolism in human endometrial hyperplasia and adenocarcinoma. *J. Steroid Biochem.*, **7**, 891

18. Holt, E. M. (1970). Out-patient and diagnostic curettage. *J. Obstet. Gynaecol. Br. Commonw.*, **77**, 1043

19. Campbell, S., McQueen, J., Minardi, Jane and Whitehead, M. I. (1978). The modifying effect of progestogen on the response of the post-menopausal endometrium to exogenous oestrogens. *Postgrad. Med. J.*, **54** (Suppl. 2), 59

20. Whitehead, M. I., McQueen, J., Minardi, Jane and Campbell, S. (1978). Clinical considerations in the management of the menopause: the endometrium. *Postgrad. Med. J.*, **54** (Suppl. 2), 69

21. Fotherby, K. (1976). Pharmacology of natural and synthetic estrogens. In S. Campbell (ed.), *The Management of the Menopause and Post-Menopausal Years*, p. 87 (Lancaster: MTP Press)

22. Gusberg, S. B. (1976). The individual at high risk for endometrial carcinoma. *Am. J. Obstet. Gynecol.*, **126**, 535

23. McBride, J. M. (1959). Pre-menopausal cystic hyperplasia and endometrial carcinoma. *J. Obstet. Gynaecol. Br. Emp.*, **66**, 288

24. Campbell, P. E. and Barter, G. A. (1961). The significance of atypical hyperplasia. *J. Obstet. Gynaecol. Br. Commonw.*, **68**, 668

25. Gusberg, S. B. and Kaplan, A. (1963). Precursors of corpus carcinoma. IV. Adenomatous hyperplasia as Stage O carcinoma of the endometrium. *Am. J. Obstet. Gynecol.*, **87**, 662

26. Brown, J., Kellar, R. and Matthew, G. (1959). Preliminary observations on urinary oestrogen excretion in certain gynaecological disorders. *J. Obstet. Gynaecol. Br. Commonw.*, **66**, 177

27. Lebech, P. (1974). In R. B. Greenblatt, V. B. Mahesh and P. McDonaugh (eds), *The Menopausal Syndrome*, p. 199 (New York: Madison Press)

28. King, R. J. B., Whitehead, M. I., Campbell, S. and Minardi, Jane (1978). Effects of estrogens and progestogens on the biochemistry of the post-menopausal endometrium. In I. D. Cooke (ed.), *The Role of Estrogen/Progestogen in the Management of the Menopause*, p. 111 (Lancaster: MTP Press)

29. Sturdee, D. W., Wade-Evans, T., Paterson, M. E. L., Thom, M. and Studd, J. W. W. (1978). Relations between bleeding pattern, endometrial histology and estrogen treatment in menopausal women. *Br. Med. J.*, **1**, 1575

30. Whitehead, M. I., McQueen, J., Beard, R. J., Minardi, Jane and Campbell, S. (1977). The effects of cyclical oestrogen therapy and sequential oestrogen/progestogen therapy on the endometrium of post-menopausal women. *Acta Obstet. Gynecol. Scand.*, Suppl. **65**, 91

31. Whitehead, M. I. and Campbell, S. (1978). Endometrial histology, uterine bleeding and oestrogen levels in menopausal women receiving oestrogen therapy and oestrogen/progestogen therapy. In M. J. Brush, R. W. Taylor and R. J. King (eds), *Proceedings of the Second International Meeting on Endometrial Cancer and Allied Topics*, pp. 65–80. (London: Ballière Tindall)

32. Gambrell, R. D. Jr. (1977). Estrogens, progestogens and endometrial cancer. *J. Reprod. Med.*, **18**, 301

5
New Concepts of Estrogenic Activity: the Role of Metabolites in the Expression of Hormone Action

J. FISHMAN and C. P. MARTUCCI

The most striking and possibly the most significant hormonal change associated with the menopause is the cessation of estrogen secretion by the ovaries. The resultant sharp decrease in circulating estrogens has been presumed to be causally related to many of the physical and behavioral symptoms which are frequently associated with the climacteric. It is axiomatic that to comprehend the deficits which result from the decrease in circulating estrogens it is necessary to understand the nature of the action of the female sex hormone on its various target sites. The purpose of this contribution is to describe studies which have been directed to the concept that modulation of the activity of estradiol both in quantitative and qualitative terms is achieved by its metabolism either peripherally or in the target tissues.

The biological actions of estradiol consist of a spectrum of morphological and physiological changes in a large number of target tissues. This diversity of changes elicited by a single substance can be rationalized as being due to its metabolism, in that the different metabolites originating from estradiol could be responsible for some of the different specific effects ascribed to the parent hormone. These biotransformations can take place in the liver to provide metabolites which can act systemically, or they can occur *in situ* in specific target tissues. In the latter instance the activity of the metabolite formed at the site of action may be responsible for the tissue specificity associated with some of the actions of estradiol.

The metabolism of estradiol in the human involves an initial massive and rapid oxidation to estrone[1] (Figure 5.1). The reaction is reversible, but the reduction of estrone to estradiol is a much slower process so that estrone predominates in this equilibrium and is therefore the central compound in estradiol metabolism. The further irreversible transformations of estrone proceed largely via two separate pathways[2] involving hydroxylation at positions 16 or at 2. The former leads via 16α-hydroxyestrone to estriol, one of

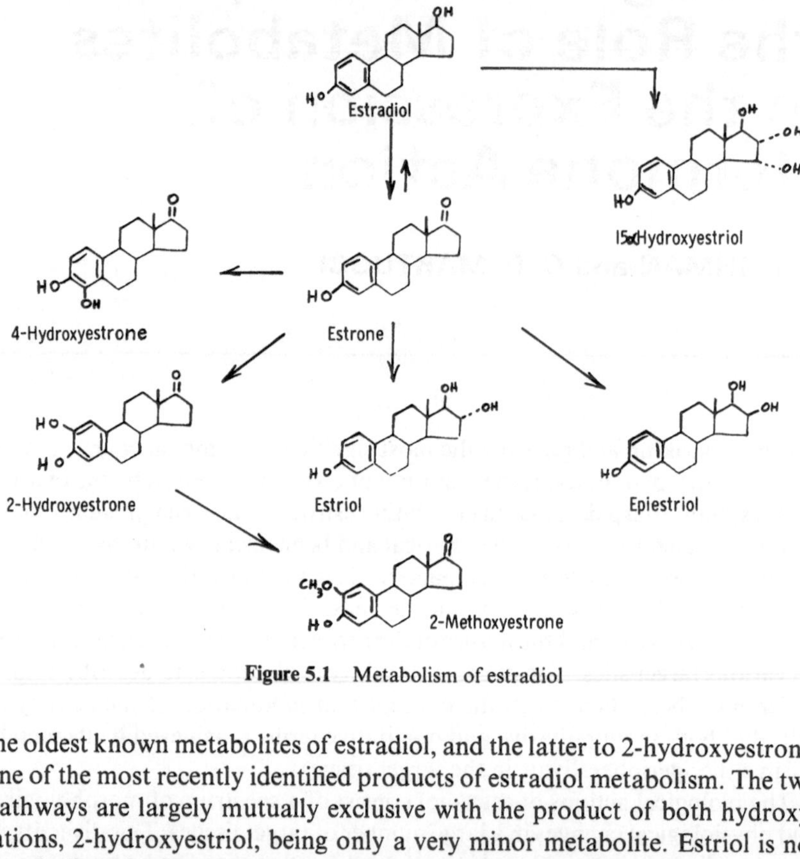

Figure 5.1 Metabolism of estradiol

the oldest known metabolites of estradiol, and the latter to 2-hydroxyestrone, one of the most recently identified products of estradiol metabolism. The two pathways are largely mutually exclusive with the product of both hydroxylations, 2-hydroxyestriol, being only a very minor metabolite. Estriol is not metabolized further except for conjugation, but 2-hydroxyestrone is partially transformed by O-methylation to 2-methoxyestrone. In addition to these major metabolic pathways, the biotransformations of the female hormone produce a number of other compounds of lesser quantitative importance. Among the substances of particular interest are 4-hydroxyestrone[3] and 15α-hydroxyestriol or estetrol[4]. Even though a relatively minor product, 4-hydroxyestrone is, like 2-hydroxyestrone, a catechol estrogen, but its biological activity is quite different from that of the isomeric 2-hydroxy-estrone, and it is therefore important to stress that the term catechol estrogen encompasses two different categories of substances with quite different properties and it should therefore be used with appropriate modification. Estetrol is the major metabolite of estradiol in the human fetus and neonate, but it virtually disappears after the first 10 days of life. Its function, and indeed its biological activity, have been, and are, still largely unknown.

For the past 30 years studies of the female sex hormone have focused on the biological activity of the three so-called primary natural estrogens, the hormone estradiol and its two metabolites, estrone and estriol. Estrone was judged to be an active estrogen whose activity, although less potent than that of estradiol, was qualitatively equivalent to that of the parent substance. Indeed, all the biological activity of estrone may derive from its conversion to estradiol *in vivo*. Estriol, however, on the basis of its pharmacology, was considered to be an impeded estrogen[5], in that its administration induced a partial rather than the full uterotropic response obtained with estradiol. Under the test conditions used it did not induce cancer in rodents and in fact appeared to block the oncogenic properties of estradiol so that it acquired a reputation as a 'safe' estrogen. It is only quite recently that it has been demonstrated that these concepts of estriol action were incorrect because they were based on the response to a single injection of the substance. Because the nuclear estriol-receptor complex is short-lived a single dose of estriol fails to provide the necessary duration of stimulation to elicit the full estrogenic response[6]. When, however, estriol is administered continuously, the response obtained is indistinguishable from that produced by estradiol[7]. Under this schedule of administration estriol, like estradiol, also induces cancer in susceptible rodents[8]. Endogenous estriol is secreted continuously and therefore the current pharmacological information requires that under physiological circumstances estriol must be considered an active estrogen with a biological profile similar to that of estradiol and estrone. The observation that a natural estrogen exhibited quite different activities, depending on whether it was administered acutely or continuously, required that the testing of the activity of other endogenous estrogens must also be carried out under chronic administration conditions to approximate more closely the situation *in vivo*.

The biological role of 2-hydroxyestrone, the product of the competing estradiol metabolic pathway, was essentially unexplored until quite recently. The reasons for this neglect was twofold. First, the substance is exceptionally labile and difficult to work with and, secondly, the quantitative significance of the catechol estrogens was not appreciated. The use of improved analytical procedures have now confirmed the original observation that the major catechol estrogen, 2-hydroxyestrone, is quantitatively the largest estradiol metabolite excreted in the urine of women and men[9, 10, 11] and that it is also a major factor in the plasma estrogen content[12, 13]. In view of this new role as the principal metabolite of the female sex hormone, its biological activity becomes of vital importance to our understanding of the physiology of estradiol. Initial tests[14, 15] suggested that both 2-hydroxyestrone and its 17β-hydroxy derivative, 2-hydroxyestradiol, were largely ineffective uterotropic agents, but these studies were conducted using the single injection modality and could fail to reflect the *in vivo* role of these metabolites. We sought to investigate the activity of these estrogens in terms of receptor binding and uterotropic criteria. Affinity for the uterine cytosolic estradiol receptor is a prerequisite for uterotropic action and we examined the binding to the receptor of the various natural estrogens by means of their ability to displace radiolabelled estradiol[16]. The results which are listed in Table 5.1 show that both 2-hydroxy-estradiol and 2-hydroxyestrone bound to the receptor with the former exhibiting an affinity more than double that of estriol. The affinity of the 2-hydroxyestrogens for the receptor was exceeded considerably by the

Table 5.1   Relative binding affinities (RBA) of various estrogens for rat uterine cytosol receptor*

Compound	RBA	SD or range	n
Estradiol-17β	100		
4-Hydroxyestradiol-17β	45	± 12	5
2-Hydroxyestradiol-17β	24	± 7	7
Estrone	11	± 8	5
4-Hydroxyestrone	11	± 4	3
Estriol	10	± 4	5
Estradiol-17α	4.2	± 0.8	2
2-Hydroxyestrone	1.9	± 0.8	3
4-Methoxyestradiol-17β	1.3	± 0.2	2
4-Hydroxyestradiol-3-methyl ether	0.6	± 0.3	2
15α-Hydroxyestriol (estetrol)	0.5	± 0.2	3
4-Methoxyestrone	0.13	± 0.04	2
2-Methoxyestradiol-17β	0.05	± 0.04	2
2-Methoxyestrone	0.01	± 0.00	2
2-Methoxyestradiol-3-methyl ether	0.01	± 0.00	2

* The data were obtaied by the methods described in Martucci and Fishman[17].

corresponding isomeric 4-hydroxyestrogens, the quantitatively less significant catechol estrogens. The methylated derivatives of the catechol estrogens have drastically reduced affinities for the uterine receptor. Interestingly, the fetal metabolite, estetrol, had only minimal ability to bind to the receptor and thus would qualify better than estriol as the protective estrogen of pregnancy, since it presumably is an ineffective estrogen. Binding of a substance to the cytosolic estradiol receptor is required for uterotropic activity, but it does not necessarily assure it and the uterotropic effect of these metabolites was studied under conditions of continuous administration. The test estrogens were administered at the rate of 1 μg/h from osmotic pumps subcutaneously implanted in either oophorectomized or immature rats and their uterotropic effect was measured by means of the increase in uterine weight every 24 h for up to 72 h (Table 5.2).

Estradiol was found to be the most effective uterotropic agent with the uterine weight showing progressive increases over the entire test period. At the dose level employed estriol fully equalled the estradiol effect. The 4-hydroxy-estrogens and even their 4-O-methylated metabolites also exhibited very considerable uterotropic activity. 2-Hydroxyestradiol provided anomalous results, producing weight increases for 48 h and then failing to provide further stimulation, a result reminiscent of the synthetic anti-estrogens such as tamox-ifen[17]. The only natural estrogens which showed essentially no uterotropic activity were 2-hydroxyestrone and its metabolic product, 2-methoxyestrone.

Table 5.2   Effect of continuous estrogen on wet uterine weights (% of control)

	Hours after implantation		
	24	48	72
Estradiol	177	374	506
Estriol	160	352	468
4-Hydroxyestrone	192	315	351
2-Hydroxyestradiol	233	288	285
4-Methoxyestradiol	139	194	260
4-Methoxyestrone	127	225	338
2-Hydroxyestrone	98	124	130
2-Methoxyestradiol	109	118	101

Rats were implanted with osmotic pumps containing propylene glycol with 1 mg/ml ascorbic acid and 1 mg/ml of the various estrogens tested (1 µg/h). Groups of animals were sacrificed at the indicated time intervals. Uteri were removed, blotted, and weighed. Each value is the mean of four animals per time point. The standard errors of the mean were 10% or less.

The absence of any uterotropic action by 2-hydroxyestrone in conjunction with its binding to the receptor suggested that the substance might act as an endogenous anti-estrogen by occupying the receptor without expressing any activity. However, when 2-hydroxyestrone was administered together with estradiol or estriol, it failed to reduce the effect of these estrogens, indicating that when present in equivalent quantitites this catechol estrogen does not function as an anti-estrogen[18]. The lack of uterotropic activity by 2-hydroxy-estrone and the estrogenic character of estriol have important consequences, since they imply that the direction of the metabolism of estradiol serves as a control of the expression of its biological activity. Metabolism directed to hydroxylation at C-16 and estriol formation serves to perpetuate the periph-eral activity of the hormone while the competing 2-hydroxylation terminates it. Thus, distortion of the metabolism of estradiol in either one or the other direction can have hyper- or hypo-estrogenic consequences.

There have now been identified a number of pathological situations in man which are associated precisely with such alterations in the metabolism of estradiol. Hyperthyroidism, whether endogenous or drug induced, is invariably reflected in a decrease in 16α-hydroxylation and a concomitant increase in 2-hydroxylation of estradiol, while hypothyroid individuals metabolize the hormone predominantly in the direction of estriol at the expense of the 2-hydroxyestrogens[19]. The reproductive disorders encountered frequently in women with dysthyroidism could therefore result from the hyper- or hypo-estrogenic impact of the alteration in estradiol metabolism in

Table 5.3 **Effect of body weight in estradiol metabolism**

Age	Estrone	Estradiol	Estriol	2-Hydroxyestrone
Anorexia nervosa subjects				
19	7.8	5.9	12.6	32.7
22	22.2	8.4	11.8	22.9
23	12.9	3.3	8.4	18.9
17	10.9	3.6	6.1	28.6
21	14.2	4.6	12.2	35.9
17	16.1	7.4	17.4	24.8
16	16.5	8.2	19.9	20.1
Mean	14.1	5.9*	12.6*	26.3†
±SD	4.5	2.1	4.8	6.4
Control subjects				
17	14.8	10.7	37.8	6.3
15	17.1	4.3	37.1	12.1
26	18.4	7.4	15.6	14.1
13	22.4	10.5	24.2	8.2
16	11.6	5.6	33.3	7.4
13	14.9	10.6	6.5	10.6
19	16.8	3.8	8.8	21.0
18	11.6	5.2	15.5	14.6
Mean	15.0	7.3	22.4	11.8
±SD	3.7	3.0	12.6	4.8
Obese subjects				
27	23.0	9.0	20.0	8.3
28	22.5	16.4	26.2	4.1
14	8.8	8.4	31.0	5.5
21	8.0	6.2	36.0	1.4
Mean	15.6	10.0	28.3	4.8‡
±SD	8.3	1.7	6.8	2.9

* Significantly lower than obese $p < 0.1$
† Significantly higher than control or obese $p < 0.01$
‡ Significantly lower than control $p \sim 0.02$

hypo- and hyperthyroid individuals respectively. Men with breast cancer, and to a lesser degree women with this disease, exhibit a preferential metabolism of estradiol in the direction of estriol[20, 21]. This is not in agreement with the concept that estriol is an estrogen which protects from the disease[22], but the results do conform to the new status of estriol as a fully active potent estrogen. Metabolism of estradiol in subjects with alcoholic cirrhosis is distinguished by an increase in 16α-hydroxylation and a decrease in 2-hydroxylation[23]. This alteration in estradiol metabolism in the direction of continuing estrogenicity may be responsible for the gynecomastia frequently associated with this disease in men. The effect of body weight or body composition on estradiol metabolism is of particular interest. Young women with anorexia nervosa metabolize estradiol predominantly to 2-hydroxyestrone, while in obese women metabolism of the hormone is mainly in the direction of estriol (Table 5.3)[24]. The consequence of these changes could be responsible for the amenorrhea which accompanies drastic decreases in body weight.

The above examples of distortion of estradiol metabolism and its possible consequences suggest that pathological conditions which exhibit symptoms associated with the action of the female sex hormone should be examined for possible involvement of such metabolic changes.

The large number of biological actions of estradiol can be broadly categorized as being either peripheral or central in nature. The former are expressed at the recognized estrogen target sites, such as the uterus, while the central activities incorporate the regulation of pituitary hormone release and control of behavior. Based on abundant analogies in other systems, such as the androgens[25] and vitamin D^{26}, where metabolism at the target site generates the active hormone specific for that tissue, we conceived the possibility that the central actions of estradiol are due to a biotransformation of the hormone in the brain. The catechol estrogens, because of their structural similarity to the catecholamine neurotransmitters, appeared to be particularly attractive candidates for products of such a transformation. This hypothesis was borne out when incubations of rat brain homogenates with estradiol showed the existence of the biotransformation to 2-hydroxyestrogens, localized predominantly in the hypothalamic area[27]. Subsequently, the conversion of estradiol to 2-hydroxyestrone was also demonstrated in human fetal brain[28]. The 2-hydroxylation of estradiol in brain tissues has now been confirmed by a number of other investigators[29, 30]. The formation of these catechol estrogens in central sites assumes additional significance from the demonstration that these estrogen derivatives are potent inhibitors of the O-methylation of catecholamines by the catechol-O-methyl transferase enzyme[31]. More recently it was reported that the catechol estrogens function also as inhibitors of tyrosine hydroxylase, the rate-determining enzyme of catecholamine biosynthesis[32]. These biochemical links between estradiol and the catecholamine neurotransmitters, implicated in both behavior and in pituitary gonadotropin release and also the binding of the catechol estrogens to the brain estrogen receptors[33], offered several possible mechanisms by which these substances may be responsible for some of the central actions of estradiol. Confirmation of such central actions of the 2-hydroxyestrogens was obtained when injection of large doses of 2-hydroxyestrone resulted in a surge of LH in both male[34] and female rats[35]. In ovariectomized rats exposed to continuous administration of various natural estradiol metabolites, 2-hydroxyestrone was the only substance that produced an increase in plasma LH concentration (Table 5.4). All the other estrogen metabolites, including the 4-hydroxyestrogens, produced the suppression of LH release expected from active estrogens. These results indicate that 2-hydroxyestrone is the first estrogen, either natural or synthetic, which exhibits a separation of central from peripheral estrogenic activity. The compound is ineffective as a uterotropic agent but is capable of positive feedback on LH release. Its formation in the brain may be responsible for the preovulatory LH surge and may help to explain the puzzle of the dual, positive and negative feedbacks of estradiol on gonadotropin secretion. The activity of the 2-hydroxyestrogens in the human has not yet been reported in any published work. It is, however, under intense study in a number of clinics and unpublished information indicates that 2-hydroxyestrone also exhibits central activity in the human.

Table 5.4 Effect of continuous estrogen in ovariectomized rats on serum LH (% of control)

	Hours after implantation		
	24	48	72
2-Hydroxyestrone	110	134	142
4-Methoxyestrone	88	65	92
4-Hydroxyestrone	21	28	50
Estradiol	12	12	19

Animals were implanted as described in the legend of Table 5.2. Groups of 3–4 animals were decapitated and trunk blood was collected at the indicated time intervals. LH was determined by RIA on the serum. The values given are the mean of the separate determinations with the standard error of the mean less than 20%

Much additional investigation is necessary before all of the roles of the catechol estrogens in estrogen physiology are elucidated. A particular problem in these studies is the concern whether the peripherally administered 2-hydroxyestrone can reproduce the actions of the same material biosynthesized in the brain, and it is also possible that the catechol estrogens may exhibit specific properties distinct from estradiol in other sites besides the brain. It is, however, already clear that it is inappropriate to determine and define estrogenic activity solely in terms of uterotropic action. It is also apparent that different natural estrogens can exhibit distinct biological activities. An understanding of these functions may make it possible that the deficits associated with the decrease in estradiol secretion in the menopause may be compensated more selectively, in that only those estrogens are used in replacement therapy which relieve the most relevant symptoms without introducing any undesirable hazards or side-effects.

Acknowledgment

This work was supported by grant CA 22795 from the National Cancer Institute and grant RF 70095 from The Rockefeller Foundation.

References

1. Fishman, J., Bradlow, H. L. and Gallagher, T. F. (1960). Oxidative metabolism of estradiol. *J. Biol. Chem.*, **235**, 3104
2. Dorfman, R. I. and Ungar, F. (1965). *Metabolism of Steroid Hormones*, p. 534. (New York: Academic Press)
3. Williams, J. G., Longcope, C. and Williams, K. I. H. (1974). 4-Hydroxyestrone: a new metabolite of estradiol 17β in humans. *Steroids*, **24**, 687
4. Gurpide, E., Schwers, J., Welch, M. T. and Lieberman, S. (1966). Fetal and maternal metabolism of estradiol during pregnancy. *J. Clin. Endocrinol. Metab.*, **26**, 1355
5. Huggins, C. and Jensen, E. (1955). The depression of estrone-induced uterine growth by phenolic estrogens with oxygenated functions at positions 6 or 16: the impeded estrogens. *J. Exp. Med.*, **102**, 335
6. Anderson, J. N., Clark, J. H. and Peck, E. J. (1972). The relationship between nuclear receptor estrogen binding and uterotropic responses. *Biochem. Biophys. Res. Commun.*, **48**, 1460
7. Clark, J. H., Paszko, Z. and Peck, E. J. (1977). Nuclear binding and retention of the receptor estrogen complex: relation to the agonistic and antagonistic properties of estriol. *Endocrinology*, **100**, 91
8. Rudali, G., Apiou, F. and Muel, B. (1975). Mammary cancer produced in mice with estriol. *Eur. J. Cancer*, **11**, 39
9. Ball, P., Gelbke, H. P. and Knuppen, R. (1975). The excretion of 2-hydroxyestrone during the menstrual cycle. *J. Clin. Endocrinol. Metab.*, **40**, 406
10. Chattoraj, S. C., Farous, A. S., Cecchini, D. and Lowe, E. (1978). A radioimmunoassay method for urinary catechol estrogens. *Steroids*, **31**, 375
11. Ball, P., Reu, G., Schwab, J. and Knuppen, R. (1979). Radioimmunoassay of 2-hydroxyestrone and 2-methoxyestrone in human urine. *Steroids*, **33**, 563
12. Yoshizawa, I. and Fishman, J. (1971). Radioimmunoassay of 2-hydroxyestrone in human plasma. *J. Clin. Endocrinol. Metab.*, **32**, 3
13. Ball, P., Emons, G., Haupt, O., Hoppen, H.-O. and Knuppen, R. (1978). Radioimmunoassay of 2-hydroxyestrone. *Steroids*, **31**, 249
14. Gordon, S., Cantrall, E. W., Cekleniak, W. P., Albers, H. J., Mauer, S., Stolar, S. M. and Bernstein, S. (1964). Steroid and lipid metabolism. The hypocholesteremic effect of estrogen metabolites. *Steroids*, **4**, 267
15. Hilgar, A. G. and Plamore, J. (1968). Uterotropic evaluation of steroids and other compounds. In A. G. Hilgar and L. C. Trench (eds.). *Uterotropic Endocrine Bioassay Data*, p. 58. (National Cancer Institute)
16. Martucci, C. and Fishman, J. (1976). Uterine estrogen receptor binding of catechol estrogens and estetrol. *Steroids*, **27**, 325
17. Koseki, Y., Zava, D. T., Chamness, G. C. and McGuire, W. L. (1977). Estrogen receptor translocation and replenishment by the antiestrogen tamoxifen. *Endocrinology*, **101**, 1104
18. Martucci, C. and Fishman, J. (1977). Direction of estradiol metabolism as a control of its hormonal action – uterotropic activity of estradiol metabolites. *Endocrinology*, **101**, 1709
19. Fishman, J., Hellman, L., Zumoff, B. and Gallagher, T. F. (1965). Effect of thyroid on hydroxylation of estrogen in man. *J. Clin. Endocrinol. Metab.*, **25**, 365
20. Zumoff, B., Fishman, J., Cassouto, J., Hellman, L. and Gallagher, T. F. (1966). Estradiol transformation in men with breast cancer. *J. Clin. Endocrinol. Metab.*, **26**, 960
21. Hellman, L., Zumoff, B., Fishman, J. and Gallagher, T. F. (1971). Peripheral metabolism of ³H-estradiol and the excretion of endogenous estrone and estriol glucosiduronate in women with breast cancer. *J. Clin. Endocrinol. Metab.*, **33**, 138
22. Cole, P. and MacMahon, B. (1969). Estrogen fractions during early reproductive life in the etiology of breast cancer. *Lancet*, **1**, 604

23. Zumoff, B., Fishman, J., Gallagher, T. F. and Hellman, L. (1968). Estradiol metabolism in cirrhosis. *J. Clin. Invest.*, **47**, 20

24. Fishman, J., Boyar, B. and Hellman, L. (1975). Influence of body weight on estradiol metabolism in young women. *J. Clin. Endocrinol. Metab.*, **41**, 989

25. King, R. J. B. and Mainwaring, W. I. P. (1974). *Steroid Cell Interactions*, p. 41. (Baltimore: University Park Press)

26. DeLuca, H. F. and Schnoes, H. K. (1976). Metabolism and mechanism of action of vitamin D. *Annu. Rev. Biochem.*, **45**, 631

27. Fishman, J. and Norton, B. (1975). Catechol estrogen formation in the central nervous system of the rat. *Endocrinology*, **96**, 1054

28. Fishman, J., Naftolin, F., Davies, T. J., Ryan, K. J. and Petro, Z. (1976). Catechol estrogen formation by the human fetal brain and pituitary. *J. Clin. Endocrinol. Metab.*, **42**, 177

29. Paul, S. M. and Axelrod, J. (1977). Catechol estrogens: presence in brain and endocrine tissues. *Science*, **197**, 657

30. Ball, P. and Knuppen, R. (1978). Formation of 2- and 4-hydroxyestrogens by brain, pituitary and liver of the human fetus. *J. Clin. Endocrinol. Metab.*, **47**, 732

31. Ball, P., Knuppen, R., Haupt, M. and Breuer, H. (1972). Interactions between estrogens and catechol amines. III. Studies of the methylation of catechol estrogens, catechol amines and other catechols by the catechol-*O*-methyltransferase of human liver. *J. Clin. Endocrinol. Metab.*, **34**, 736

32. Lloyd, T. and Weisz, J. (1978). Direct inhibition of tyrosine hydroxylase activity by catechol estrogens. *J. Biol. Chem.*, **253**, 4841

33. Davies, I. J., Naftolin, F., Ryan, K. J., Fishman, J. and Siu, J. (1975). The affinity of catechol estrogens for estrogen receptors in the pituitary and anterior hypothalamus of the rat. *Endocrinology*, **97**, 554

34. Naftolin, F., Morishita, H., Davies, I. J., Todd, R., Ryan, K. J. and Fishman, J. (1975). 2-Hydroxyestrone induced rise in serum luteinizing hormone in the immature male rat. *Biochem. Biophys. Res. Commun.*, **64**, 905

35. Gethmann, U. and Knuppen, R. (1976). Effect of 2-hydroxyestrone on LH and FSH secretion in the ovariectomized primed rat. *Hoppe-Seyler's Z. Physiol. Chem.*, **357**, 1011

Section II
Clinical Update

6
Hormonal Influences on α-Adrenoreceptors: Preliminary Results

K. WOOD and A. COPPEN

INTRODUCTION

The menopause and the corresponding decline in circulating estrogens has been implicated as a possible contributory factor in the onset of depressive illnesses which characteristically arise in later life. Noradrenaline has been implicated in the aetiology of this illness[1] and a study of the interaction between estrogens and progestogens with noradrenaline might prove a useful focus in the study of depressive illnesses.

Noradrenaline initiates its biological response by first interacting with discrete sites (receptors) on the cell membrane and the response is proportional to the number of receptors occupied. Since these responses can be divided into two distinct groups which are based on the order of potency of the agonists in eliciting responses, it has been concluded that two types of receptors (α and β) exist on the membranes of responsive cells.

One method of studying the activity of α-receptors is the introduction of an indirectly acting sympathomimetic amine such as tyramine, which is actively accumulated by the adrenergic neurones and releases noradrenaline from intraneuronal stores to produce its action on the receptor. Amongst the various pharmacological effects of noradrenaline, the blood pressure response is relatively easy to measure and gives a reliable, although indirect, index of tyramine's action and the sensitivity of the receptor. Noradrenaline and phenylephrine pressor tests have also been used in these studies.

Since the results of the tyramine test may be due not only to a change in adrenergic receptor sensitivity but also to (a) a change in monoamine oxidase activity, (b) a change in the accumulation of tyramine by noradrenaline-containing neurones, or (c) a change in the stores of noradrenaline and/or change in the release of noradrenaline, the assay is not specific.

Another approach to the study of adrenergic receptors has been the use of radioactive ligands as probes to directly identify and quantitate α-adrenergic receptors[2]. We have used this direct approach to study the hormonal influences on adrenergic receptors present on the membranes of blood platelets by [³H]dihydroergocryptine binding assays.

METHODS

Depressed patients

Male and female patients diagnosed to be suffering from primary depressive illness[3] were studied, and although many of these patients had more than one episode of depression, none had a history of mania. Our investigations were performed on inpatients in a clinical investigation ward under careful medical and nursing supervision. All patients remained drug-free for 7–12 days and during this period they were treated with placebo tablets and supportive psychotherapy. The severity of depression was assessed by the Hamilton Rating Scale[4] (HRS) and only patients with HRS scores of 16 or more on the first 16 items of the scale at the end of the drug-free period were studied.

Control subjects

Men and women who volunteered to act as control subjects had no known history of psychiatric disorder nor had taken any medication 7–10 days prior to testing. Women were asked whether they were taking any hormonal preparations and the date of the last menstrual period of premenopausal controls was noted.

Tyramine-dose pressor response test

The tyramine-dose pressor response test was carried out and the amount of tyramine required to increase the systolic blood pressure by 30 mmHg was determined[5].

Noradrenaline-dose pressor response test

Noradrenaline-dose pressor response curves were determined as described previously[6]. The amount of noradrenaline (μg/min) required to increase the systolic blood pressure by 30 mmHg was determined from the dose response curves.

Phenylephrine-dose pressor response test

Phenylephrine is a direct α-adrenoreceptor agonist[7] that has no significant effect on re-uptake mechanisms. An initial dose of 50 μg of phenylephrine in 2 ml of normal saline was slowly injected intravenously over a period of 1 min. Blood pressure was measured after the injection and thereafter at intervals of 30 s for 5 min. The next dose of phenylephrine was injected after 5–6 min or when the blood pressure returned to basal level, and the procedure was repeated to obtain an increase of 30 mmHg.

[³H]Dihydroergocryptine binding assay

Blood (20 ml) was collected from controls after overnight fasting into 3.2% (w/v) sodium citrate. The blood was centrifuged at 380 g for 10 min and the resulting platelet-rich plasma was centrifuged at 2000 g for 15 min at 22°C. The resulting platelet pellet was resuspended in 0.05 mol/l Tris-HCl buffer, 0.15 mol/l NaCl and 0.02 mol/l EDTA, pH 7.45, and centrifuged at 2000 g for 15 min, resuspended in the buffer, recentrifuged and resuspended in the buffer for the binding assay. Aliquots (25 μl) of the platelet suspension were diluted with 5 ml of Lempbert–Kristenson's staining solution and the cells were counted in an aliquot of this mixture using an Improved Neubauer Haemo-cytometer.

[³H]Dihydroergocryptine (range 0.5–18 nmol/l; The Radiochemical Centre, Amersham, Bucks., UK) and intact platelets were incubated at 37°C with shaking for 50 min in a total volume of 150 μl. In competition experiments, varying concentrations of estrone 3-sulfate, β-estradiol and progesterone (Sigma Chemical Co. Ltd., Poole, Dorset, UK) were added to the incubation as indicated. Incubations were terminated by rapidly diluting the total volume with 6 ml of buffer containing 10 μmol/l phentolamine[8] at 37°C, followed by rapid filtration through Whatman GF/C glassfibre filters using a Millipore Sampling Manifold (Millipore (UK) Ltd, London NW10). The tubes were washed out with 6 ml of buffer and the filters rapidly washed with 3 × 6 ml of buffer. After drying, the filters were counted for radioactivity in NE262 scintillation mixture (Nuclear Enterprises, Sighthill, Edinburgh).

Non-specific binding was determined by incubating platelets with 10 μmol/l phentolamine and [³H]dihydroergocryptine. Specific binding, i.e. binding to the receptor, is defined as total binding minus non-specific binding and was generally 60–70% of the total binding. This data was subjected to Scatchard plot analysis and the values of the dissociation constant, K_d, and the number of binding sites, B_{max}, were calculated[9].

RESULTS

Pressor tests

The results of the dose pressor response tests are shown in Table 6.1. Female controls required less tyramine and phenylephrine than male controls to increase their blood pressure by 30 mmHg. Male patients required less tyramine and noradrenaline than their respective controls and female patients required less tyramine, noradrenaline and phenylephrine than their respective controls to elevate their blood pressure by 30 mmHg.

Table 6.1 Tyramine, noradrenaline and phenylephrine-dose pressor response tests in untreated depressed patients and control subjects

		Tyramine		*Noradrenaline*		*Phenylephrine*
	n	mg, mean ± SE	*n*	µg/min, mean ± SE	*n*	µg/min, mean ± SE
Male						
Control subjects	13	6.62* ± 0.54	14	15.54 ± 1.76	14	183.9* ± 14.0
Depressed patients	18	4.00† ± 0.31	11	9.96† ± 1.53	7	126.4 ± 31.0
Female						
Control subjects	23	5.22 ± 0.29	22	12.93 ± 1.40	20	143.8 ± 12.3
Depressed patients	42	3.75‡ ± 0.26	22	6.73‡ ± 0.74	21	97.6‡ ± 10.9

* Male *vs.* female controls, $p < 0.05$ ‡ Female controls *vs.* female depressives, $p < 0.01$
† Male controls *vs.* male depressives, $p < 0.05$

The tyramine-dose pressor response test was also carried out on depressive patients at the end of 6 weeks medication during two treatment phases (placebo and estrogen) (Table 6.2)[10]. There was an increased tyramine requirement in each patient during estrogen therapy when compared to the placebo treatment period. The mean tyramine requirement during the placebo period was 3.3 mg, which is similar to the mean tyramine requirement of depressed patients (see Table 6.1). Estrogen therapy increased this mean tyramine requirement to 5.0 mg, which is similar to the mean amount required by normal control subjects.

Table 6.2 Tyramine required to increase the systolic BP by 30 mmHg during two treatment phases. From ref. 10

Patient's age (y)	*Tyramine requirement* (mg) *during:*	
	Placebo phase	*Estrogen phase*
64	1.5	2.5
47	5.0	7.5
48	3.5	5.0

There is a greater tyramine requirement during the perimenstrual period of female control subjects (Table 6.3).

[³H]Dihydroergocryptine binding assays

The binding characteristics (K_d, the dissociation constant, and B_{max}, the number of binding sites per blood platelet) in controls and depressed patients

Table 6.3   Change in tyramine-dose pressor response test during different phases of the menstrual cycle. From ref. 10

		Tyramine (mg)			
Female subjects Age (y)	*Menstrual cycle* (days)	*Week 1 (0–5 days after)*	*Week 2*	*Week 3*	*Week 4 Pre-menstrual phase (5–0 days prior)*
1.	44	30 ± 2	5.0	6.0	6.0	4.0
2.	35	28 ± 1	2.5	5.5	7.0	4.5
3.	23	28 ± 2	3.5	5.0	5.0	5.0
4.	26	33 ± 2	3.5	4.5	6.0	4.5
5.	22	28 ± 2	2.5	3.5	4.0	3.5
		mean	3.4	4.9	5.6	4.3
		SE	0.46	0.43	0.51	0.25

Week 4 vs. week 1, NS
Week 4 vs. week 2, NS
Week 4 vs. week 3, $t = 2.83$, $p < 0.05$
Week 1 vs. week 3, $t = 3.52$, $p < 0.05$

are shown in Table 6.4. There is a trend toward higher values of K_d in the premenopausal controls when compared to the older postmenopausal controls and depressed patients. There were significantly fewer α-receptors on the platelets of depressed patients when compared to the pre- and post-menopausal controls (Table 6.4).

Table 6.4   [³H]Dihydroergocryotine binding characteristics (K_d and B_{max}) in pre- and post-menopausal controls and female depressed patients. Results presented as means ± SEM

	n	Age	K_d (nmol/l)	B_{max} (receptors/cell)
Premenopausal controls	8	34.0 ± 3.1	3.43 ± 0.25	336.2 ± 40.7
Postmenopausal controls	5	59.8 ± 2.5	2.80 ± 0.21	299.1 ± 18.6
Depressed patients	7	58.4 ± 3.0	2.99 ± 0.18	208.9* ± 24.4

* Significantly lower than pre- and postmenopausal controls, $p < 0.05$

Estrone-3-sulfate, β-estradiol and progesterone (10^{-4}–10^{-8} mol/l) did not inhibit the binding of [³H]dihydroergocryptine to intact platelets of control subjects.

DISCUSSION

The tyramine, noradrenaline and phenylephrine pressor tests all show a result that is consistent with increased sensitivity of the peripheral α-adreno-receptors in females and especially in depressed patients. Supersensitivity of α-receptors is usually related to a decreased concentration of α-adrenergic agonists. We have, however, failed to confirm any decrease in the urinary excretion of MHPG (an important metabolite of noradrenaline) by depressed patients[11]. It is interesting to note, however, that female controls excrete significantly less MHPG than do male controls.

It is also possible that estrogens affect the sensitivity of α-adrenoreceptors *in vivo*, since females are most sensitive to tyramine during the part of the menstrual period when estrogen secretion is low, and we have also found that estrogen therapy decreases this supersensitivity in depressive patients. There is also evidence that depressive patients excrete significantly less estrogens than control subjects[12].

The sensitivity of the α-adrenoreceptors on the blood platelet can be monitored by measuring K_d and B_{max}. A low value of K_d and a relatively high value of B_{max} indicates supersensitivity of the receptors. In contrast to the pressor tests, [³H]dihydroergocryptine binding assays have demonstrated subsensitivity of the platelet α-adrenoreceptors of depressed patients. It is interesting to note, however, that the picture of reduced numbers of binding sites with no change in the values of the dissociation constant (K_d) is similar to the results obtained with estrogen and progesterone effects on rabbit uteri[13].

Estrogen and progesterone dominance were induced in immature rabbits and [³H]dihydroergocryptine binding was assayed in membrane preparations from these primed uteri[13]. The mean K_d of [³H]dihydroergocryptine for the binding sites in the estrogen-primed uterine membranes was not statistically different from that in the progesterone-primed membranes. However, the mean number of binding sites (B_{max}) was significantly lower in the pro-gesterone-primed uteri than in the estrogen-primed uteri.

The influences of progesterone and estrogen may be responsible for the abnormal number of platelet binding sites in depressed patients. The mechanism of these effects on receptor sensitivity is unknown, and although both the pressor tests and the platelet binding assays are peripheral mechanisms, the data about the sensitivity of the α-adrenoreceptors in depression are conflicting. These observations, therefore, merit further experimentation.

References

1. Schildkraut, J. J. (1965). The catecholamine hypothesis of affective disorders: a review of supporting evidence. *Am. J. Psychiatry*, **122**, 509
2. Newman, K. D., Williams, L. T., Bishopric, N. H. and Lefkowitz, R. J. (1978). Identification of α-adrenergic receptors in human platelets by [³H]dihydroergocryptine binding. *J. Clin. Invest.*, **61**, 395
3. Medical Research Council Clinical Psychiatry Committee (1965). Medical Research Council trial of the treatment of depressive illness. *Br. Med. J.*, **1**, 881
4. Hamilton, M. (1960). A rating scale for depression. *J. Neurol. Neurosurg. Psychiatry*, **23**, 56
5. Ghose, K., Turner, P. and Coppen, A. (1975). Intravenous tyramine pressor response in depression. *Lancet*, **i**, 1317

6. Ghose, K., Gupta, R., Coppen, A. and Lund, J. (1977). Antidepressant evaluation and the pharmacological actions of FG4963 in depressive patients. *Eur. J. Pharmacol.*, **42**, 31

7. Innes, I. R. and Nickerson, M. (1965). Drugs acting on postganglionic adrenergic nerve endings and structures innervated by them (sympathomimetic drugs). *In:* L. S. Goodman and A. Gilman (eds.). *The Pharmacological Basis of Therapeutics*, 4th edn., pp. 478–523. (New York: MacMillan)

8. Insell, P. A., Nirenberg, P., Turnbull, J. and Shattil, S. J. (1978). Relationships between membrane cholesterol, α-adrenergic receptors and platelet function. *Biochemistry*, **17**, 5269

9. Bennett, J. P. (1978). Methods in binding studies. *In:* H. I. Yamamura, S. J. Enna and M. J. Kuhar (eds.). *Neurotransmitter Receptor Binding*, pp. 57–90. (New York: Raven Press)

10. Wood, K. and Coppen, A. (1978). The effect of estrogens on plasma tryptophan and adrenergic function in patients treated with lithium. In I. D. Cooke (ed.). *The Role of Estrogen/Progestogen in the Management of the Menopause*, pp. 29–37. (Lancaster: MTP Press)

11. Coppen, A., Rao, V. A. R., Sandler, M., Ruthven, C. R. J., Goodwin, B. L. and Reynolds, G. P. (1979). Urinary excretion of 3-methoxy-4-hydroxyphenylglycol in depressive illness and response to amitriptyline. *Psychopharmacologia* (in press)

12. Coppen, A., Julian, T., Fry, D. E. and Marks, V. (1967). Body build and urinary steroid excretion in mental illness. *Br. J. Psychiatry*, **113**, 269

13. Williams, L. T. and Lefkowitz, R. J. (1977). Regulation of rabbit myometrial alpha-adrenergic receptors by estrogen and progesterone. *J. Clin. Invest.*, **60**, 815

7
'Psychotherapeutic Effects' of Estrogen Substitution during the Climacteric Period

J. M. WENDERLEIN

In the future, physicians will to a greater extent weigh the advantages and disadvantages of hormone replacement therapy in the climacteric. They must consider not only the risks of endometrial neoplasm with long-term estrogen therapy, but also the more critical and inquiring attitudes of women patients. The patient's basic medical knowledge, experience with medical errors, expectations of the physician and her state of health at the time must all be considered in order for the physician to fully explain estrogen replacement therapy.

The consultation will be more effective if empirically secured knowledge is disclosed to the patients. Does estrogen replacement therapy merely eliminate unpleasant manifestations of the menopause, such as hot flushes and sweats, or is much more taking place? Is it possible in a psychometrically objective manner to clearly and frequently

eliminate depressive moods,
alleviate states of anxiety,
promote extroverted personality traits and emotional stability, and
generally reduce psychovegetative disorders?

Can one frequently expect such far-reaching, psychotherapeutic effects? To examine these questions by sociological methods was one of the objectives of this investigation.

METHODS

Female patients in our polyclinic aged between 40 and 60 with amenorrhea for at least 6 months and with other menopausal symptoms (mainly hot flushes and sweating attacks) and who were not using hormone replacement therapy were given a questionnaire to collect simple biographical and gynecological data. The poll was directed at 16 complaints that may be caused by lack of estrogen, based on a scale (frequently/rarely/not at all) with 2, 1 and 0 points, which were added up (see Table 7.1). A standardized history was taken with respect to contra-indications of estrogen replacement[17, 18, 19, 25, 33].

Table 7.1 Women of the polyclinic aged 40 to 60 with amenorrhoea at least 6 months (not due to pregnancy) were asked to check off their present complaints with respect to frequency

Are you presently suffering or have you for the last few months suffered from any of the following complaints:

	Frequently	*Rarely*	*Not at all*
1. Hot flushes	...	...	...
2. Sweating attacks/perspiration	...	...	...
3. Feelings of dizziness	...	...	...
4. Heart-hurry/palpitation	...	...	...
5. Excitability	...	...	...
6. Anxiety	...	...	...
7. Sleep disorders/insomnia	...	...	...
8. Depressions/feeling down	...	...	...
9. Headaches	...	...	...
10. Disorders of memory/concentration	...	...	...
11. Getting tired quickly	...	...	...
12. Moodiness/lability of mood	...	...	...
13. Irritability	...	...	...
14. Nervousness	...	...	...
15. Susceptibility to illness	...	...	...
16. Muscle, joint or bone pains	...	...	...

Following the gynecological examination, the possibility of estrogen replacement therapy was explained and discussed according to individual needs with each patient. Estrogen replacement therapy was considered only in cases of significant menopausal complaints, since serious objections exist against routine estrogen prophylaxis[10].

Among the total of 455 women, 161 decided on starting a substitution therapy. Before this therapy was started, we first collected psychometrically the following data:

(1) Personality dimensions in extro/introversions (MPI)
(2) Emotional stability/lability (MPI)[4]
(3) Anxiety scale (EAS)[6]
(4) Depression scale (EDS)[27]

(5) Scale of physical well-being (BS)[38]
(6) List of complaints (BL)[39]
(7) Summation of climacteric complaints according to frequency.

This self-evaluation was subsequently carried out during estrogen replacement therapy after 6 weeks, 3 months and 6 months. The following procedures were used.

The investigation was limited to 1 year. During the first weeks, substitution was carried out only with conjugated estrogens (1.25 mg daily – 3 weeks/ 1 week pause); thereafter alternating with estriol succinate 4 mg, 2 × 1 tablet without pause (uneven–even years of birth). The conjugated estrogens were thus dosed as recommended on the instruction slip enclosed with the drug; the dosing of estriol succinate was increased to twice the recommended dose. Since the difference between the results obtained in both groups by the above-stated test method is statistically insignificant (results checked by χ^2-method), we combined these results.

After 6 months it was recommended to all women to make a longer pause (1–2 months) in the estrogen therapy; thereafter, they were asked to decide whether they wanted to continue the substitution with lower doses and an addition of gestagen[2, 7, 14, 23].

RESULTS

Of the 161 women who had started the estrogen replacement therapy, 122 visited our polyclinic after 6 weeks for their first follow-up examinations. After 3 and 6 months, 99 and 64 women, respectively, appeared for their examinations. Not all women were able to come on the dates scheduled for the last two control check-ups because the first substitution was not started until 6 weeks prior to the end of the investigation. The drop-out rate in connection with the last two follow-up examinations amounted to 13–17 women. The drop-outs were rather heterogeneous and it was almost impossible to establish the reasons. The method of selection is presented in the discussion.

(1) *Personality dimension: extro/introversion (MPI)*. In the course of estrogen replacement therapy, we noticed a tendency towards polarization: both extroverted and introverted personality traits were encountered more frequently than before therapy. See Table 7.2.

(2) *Emotional stability/lability (MPI–N)*. The group of women without any neurotic tendencies (according to MPI) was twice as large after at least 3 months of estrogen substitution (42%) than before hormone therapy (20%). See Table 7.3. The proportion of women with neurotic personality characteristics remained about the same before and after hormone substitution. The third group in-between decreased as the duration of substitution increased.

(3) *Anxiety (EAS)*. Twenty per cent of the women complained about pronounced anxiety before estrogen replacement therapy. After only 6 weeks of hormone therapy, only 13% of the same group showed great anxiety.

Table 7.2 The frequency both of introverted and extroverted tendencies in the personality structure increased under estrogen replacement therapy

Personality dimension according to MPI-E	Estrogen replacement			
	before	for 6 weeks	for 3 months	for 6 months
Introversion 0–3 P	21%	25%	25%	28%
Neither–nor 4–9 P	65%	60%	52%	52%
Extroversion 10–12 P	14%	15%	23%	20%
No. of patients	100% (122)	100% (122)	100% (99)	100% (64)

P = number of points in the short form of the MPI (Maudsley Personality Inventory – Eysenck)

Table 7.3 After at least 3 months of estrogen replacement therapy for climacteric complaints, lowest test values (0–3 P) could be proved on the neuroticism scale twice as often (42%) as before therapy (20%). The frequency of clearly neurotic tendencies (10–12 P) remained unchanged

Personality characteristic: Neuroticism according to MPI-N	Estrogen replacement			
	before	for 6 weeks	for 3 months	for 6 months
without neurotic tendencies 0–3 P	20%	35%	42%	42%
neither–nor 4–9 P	67%	46%	45%	45%
with neurotic tendencies 10–12 P	13%	19%	13%	13%
No. of patients	100% (122)	100% (122)	100% (99)	100% (64)

P = number of points in the short form of the MPI (Maudsley Personality Inventory – Eysenck)

Table 7.4 With estrogen replacement therapy the lowest values on the anxiety scale (0–5 P) were obtained three times as frequently as before therapy. Conversely, in women treated for 6 months, high anxiety was shown in only 1% of the patients, whereas before therapy, anxiety was shown in 20% of the patients

Anxiety: Psychometric determination based on anxiety scale	Estrogen replacement			
	before	for 6 weeks	for 3 months	for 6 months
'none' 0–5 P	15%	41%	50%	47%
6–10 P	36%	34%	33%	44%
11–15 P	29%	12%	10%	8%
'high' in excess of 15 P	20%	13%	7%	1%
No. of patients	100% (122)	100% (122)	100% (99)	100% (64)

The group without any symptoms of anxiety was three times larger (47%) after estrogen replacement than before (15%). See Table 7.4.

(4) *Depressive moods (EDS)*. Among the women who had been on estrogen replacement therapy for 6 months, only 9% suffered from pronounced moods of depression (in excess of 15 points on the EDS). After only 6 weeks of hormone therapy, high depression values occurred only half as often (15% instead of 29%). See Table 7.5.

Table 7.5   After 6 months of estrogen replacement therapy, clearly depressive tendencies (in excess of 15 P of the EDS) were seen in 9% of the patients, whereas before therapy 29% showed these tendencies

Depression: determined with the EDS depression scale	Estrogen replacement			
	before	for 6 weeks	for 3 months	for 6 months
0–5 P	27%	45%	48%	48%
6–10 P	27%	20%	21%	30%
11–15 P	17%	20%	15%	13%
in excess of 15 P	29%	15%	16%	9%
	100%	100%	100%	100%
No. of patients	(122)	(122)	(99)	(64)

P = number of points on the Erlanger Depression Scale (EDS) – Lehrl

(5) *Impairment of well-being (BS)*. Within the groups with 3-month and 6-month estrogen replacement therapy a clearly noticed impairment of the state of well-being occurred in only 6% of the patients (in excess of 20 points on the BS-scale). Before estrogen substitution, such impairment applied to every fourth woman. See Table 7.6.

Table 7.6   Before estrogen replacement, feelings of impaired well-being were present in one out of every four patients, whereas after 3 months of therapy, only one out of every 15 women showed impairment

Well-being scale: BS	Estrogen replacement			
	before	for 6 weeks	for 3 months	for 6 months
0–10 P 'feeling well'	34%	49%	60%	58%
11–20 P 'neither–nor'	41%	34%	33%	36%
in excess of 20 P 'feeling poorly'	25%	17%	7%	6%
	100%	100%	100%	100%
No. of patients	(122)	(122)	(99)	(64)

P = number of points on the 'state of physical well-being' scale according to Zerssen

(6) *Psychovegetative disorders (BL)*. Before estrogen replacement therapy, 22% of the patients complained of many psychovegetative disorders (in

excess of 40 points on the list); after 6 weeks of therapy, the percentage was reduced to 16%; and after 6 months, to 8%. See Table 7.7.

Table 7.7   Before estrogen replacement, four times as many women suffered from considerable psychosomatic disorders (32%) than after 6-month therapy (8%)

List of complaints: BL	Estrogen replacement			
	before	for 6 weeks	for 3 months	for 6 months
0–20 P	9%	23%	34%	25%
no psychovegetative disorders				
21–30 P	34%	29%	23%	33%
31–40 P	25%	32%	26%	34%
over 40 P	32%	16%	17%	8%
many psychovegetative disorders				
No. of patients	100% (122)	100% (122)	100% (99)	100% (64)

P = number of points in the list of complaints by Zerssen

Table 7.8   16 subjective complaints which may be caused by lack of estrogen, were documented with respect to frequency on a three-stage scale

Summation of climacteric complaints based on three-stage scale with 16 elimacteric symptoms	Estrogen replacement			
	before	for 6 weeks	for 3 months	for 6 months
0–10 P	8%	25%	29%	28%
11–15 P	16%	25%	23%	24%
16–20 P	25%	23%	29%	31%
in excess of 20 P	51%	27%	19%	17%
No. of patients	100% (122)	100% (122)	100% (99)	100% (64)

One rating was used: frequent = 2 points; rarely = 1 point; none at all = 0 points. These points were added up for each patient; the maximum number of points achievable was 48. Prior to the estrogen therapy, half of the women reached more than 20 points; after 3 months therapy, only one out of every five women reached more than 20 points on the complaint scale

(7) *Summation of 16 possible complaints caused by the climacteric (according to frequency of occurrence)*. Many of the complaints, which may be caused by lack of estrogen, can be reduced according to the following rough quantification and rating (frequently = 2/rarely = 1/not at all = 0) by two-thirds (from 51% to 17%) after estrogen replacement therapy. See Table 7.8.

DISCUSSION

The positive psychotropic effect of estrogen replacement therapy in the climacteric period cannot be doubted[1, 3, 5, 9, 16, 19, 22, 29, 34, 36]. The psycho-social advantage resulting from hormone substitution is of more interest than placebo tests. Medical action has always been governed by the weighing of advantages and risks which to be useful must be based on empirically secured knowledge. If medical decisions can be accepted by the patient, the relation of mutual trust will benefit. What help can a woman with menopausal symptoms expect from estrogen replacement therapy beyond the elimination of manifestations of deficiency?

(1) Extroversion–introversion

The number of introverted, i.e. calm, shy and rather reserved and distant, women increased in the course of substitution. This tendency is not based on selections in the comparison before and after 6 weeks of estrogen substitution, because the comparison involved the same group. Estrogen administration could cause the promotion of introverted personality traits which may have been present before eliminating conditions of excitement and disorder in the life style due to manifestations of climacteric deficiency.

We must expect that introverted women have a positive experience of these psychotropic effects. These women are more likely to stay longer with their decision to accept estrogen substitution, a decision most of them made carefully and not out of a sudden impulse. This observation was made in individual discussions with introverted women. The number of extroverted women, i.e. sociable, spontaneous and rather impulsive personalities, did not increase after 6 weeks of estrogen substitution. The revival of such personality traits after longer hormone therapy is presumably connected with a more pronounced elimination of psychovegetative disorders. The slight decline in extroversion after 6 months of therapy could be interpreted in the light of the following observations: some extroverted women, after 3 months of estrogen replacement therapy, showed a tendency towards impatience, combined with aggressive tendencies, if not all expected improvements occurred. Some women discontinued the therapy for that reason; their further development was not observed in the present study.

(2) Emotional stability/lability

The emotional stability present before the occurrence of climacteric symptoms can often be restored by estrogen replacement therapy alone. The group with the lowest neuroticism score doubled within 3 months (from 20% to 42%). This increase is more than just a trend and should be considered in the discussion of the disadvantageous effects of estrogen substitution.

Naturally, as this study confirmed, estrogen replacement therapy does not alter pronounced neurotic personality structures. A methodical aspect is of interest in this connection. The constant percentage of neurotic women before and after 6 months of estrogen substitution (13% in each case) can be interpreted to mean that the drop-out is caused less by negative personality traits than by external factors, such as place of residence too far from clinic for short-term check-ups (control examinations). These factors were more of scientific than clinical interest. The hormone therapy was observed further by the patient's private physician or gynecologist.

(3) Reduction of anxiety

The anxiety scale used in the present investigation recorded transitory and habitual anxiety and situational anxiety without investigating their quality in depth. In gynecological practice, what matters is whether reactions of anxiety in the climacteric period can be reduced by estrogen replacement therapy either on the subjectively verbal, motor-behavioral or physiological plane. This could be confirmed with the self-evaluation scale ETS, which measures subjectively verbal reactions of anxiety. The fact that the group *without* symptoms of anxiety is three times as large after estrogen replacement than before is important for providing orientation in practical life.

(4) Moods of depression

Symptoms of depressions, which are attendant conditions widely found in all kinds of illness, are found to be more or less severe in almost one-third of the women in the climacteric, as indicated by the self-evaluation scale used in the present study. After only 6 weeks of estrogen replacement therapy, such symptoms were observed in only half as many cases. The fact that only one in every ten women reaches more than 15 points on the depression scale after 6 months of hormone therapy justifies the primary omission of antidepressive drugs. Psychopharmaceutical drugs should be used in the climacteric only if estrogen action is not sufficiently antidepressive. This excludes, of course, psychoses and endogenous depressions and cases with absolute contra-indications to estrogen replacement therapy.

(5) Change in well-being

The physical well-being was considerably impaired (more than 20 points on the scale) in 25% of the patients before estrogen replacement therapy and after 3 months of estrogen replacement therapy in only 6% of the patients. The psychohygenic benefit of this reduction needs no further discussion. Well-being (up to 10 points on the scale) found in one-third of the women prior to estrogen substitution and in more than half of the women after estrogen substitution should be of politico–economical interest to working women. Performance aspects are of secondary interest in medical consultation; however, it should be remembered that the experience of professional efficiency and success is as important in feelings of self-appreciation and self-worth of women as of men.

(6) Elimination of psychovegetative disorders

The frequency of pronounced psychovegetative lability (more than 40 points on the list of complaints) was reduced from 32% to 8%, an achievement which hardly requires discussion. Many of these women spontaneously reported less susceptibility to illness with positive effects on the psychosocial level.

(7) Chronological development of the alleviation of complaints

Climacteric complaints (in this test, 16 different complaints summed up according to frequency) were reduced most noticeably during the first 6 weeks of estrogen substitution. A further reduction was achieved after another 6 weeks. This makes it clear to the patient and physician relatively quickly what improvement in the quality of life can be expected from estrogen replacement therapy. With the exception of a few complaints, the patient should be counseled after 3 months to counteract exaggerated and unrealistic expectations, which might lead to disappointments and impair the relation between physician and patient.

On the whole, the psychotropic effects of estrogen replacement therapy – reduction of anxiety, antidepressive effects, emotional stability – are closely akin to the objectives of psychotherapy. The objective of psychotherapy is to act on the behavior of the patient seeking help so that an improvement of the physical state of well-being and of the psychic and social efficiency (capabilities) is achieved. More consciously experienced and more clearly planned interactions on all levels of life can be expected only, of course, in cases of less serious behavioral disorders which coincide with the climacteric complaints and did not exist before. Ego-invigoration as a result of the effects of estrogen replacement therapy in cases of climacteric complaints is, in this phase of life, not only more economical than psychotherapy but also less problematic than long-term use of psychopharmaceutical drugs.

The advantages of estrogen substitution must be weighed against disadvantages caused by bleeding in the menopause. In order to obtain histological clarification, it was necessary to perform endometrial assessment in one out of every ten women in this study. This was done either in the hospital or on an out-patient basis. Such procedures create feelings of uncertainty and stress for the patient, requiring a minimum of psychotherapeutic skills on the part of the physician.

SUMMARY

Psychosocial aspects of estrogen replacement therapy for climacteric deficiencies were investigated in 161 women using psychometric methods before therapy and after 6 weeks, 3 months and 6 months of estrogen therapy.

(1) *The personality dimension extro/introversion* (MPI-I) indicated a tendency towards polarization in the course of estrogen replacement therapy.

(2) *Emotional stability* (MPI-N) was found to exist twice as often after 3 months of estrogen therapy as before therapy.

(3) *No anxiety symptoms* (EAS) were found during the estrogen replacement in three times as many women as before the therapy.

(4) Clearly *depressive moods* (EDS) occurred after 6 weeks of estrogen replacement therapy in only half as many cases.

(5) *Impairment of well-being* (BS) was observed in 25% of the patients before estrogen replacement therapy; but during therapy it was noted in only 6% of the patients.

(6) *Psychovegetative disorders* (BL = list of complaints) were reduced after 6 weeks from 32% to 16%, and to 8% after 6 months of estrogen replacement therapy.

Such results, based on psychometric test methods, should be seriously considered in any discussion of estrogen replacement therapy in the climacteric period.

References

1. Artner, J. (1961). 'Psychosomatik' der klimakterischen Störungen. *Wien Klin., Wochenschr.*, **73**, 565
2. Baumann, R. and Taubert, H.-D. (1979). Das klimakterische Syndrom: Substitutionstherapie mit Östrogenen *and* Pathogenese, Symptomatik und Diagnose. *Dtsch. Ärzteblatt*, **76**, 572
3. Erkath, F.-A. (1969). Der Einfluss des Klimakterium auf den betrieblichen Krankenstand. *Zeutralbl. Gynäkol.*, **91**, 607
4. Eysenck, H. J. (1959). *Das 'Maudsley Personality Inventory' (MPI)*. (Göttingen: Verlag für Psychologie)
5. Fedor-Freybergh, P. (1977). The influence of oestrogens on the wellbeing and mental performance in climacteric and postmenopausal women. *Acta Obstet. Gynecol. Scand.*, **Suppl. 64**
6. Galster, J. V. and Spörl, G. (1979). Entwicklung einer Skala zur Quantifizierung transitorischer und habitueller Angstzustände. *Neurol. Psychiatr.*, **5**, 223
7. Gambrell, R. D. Jr. (1978). The role of hormones in endometrial cancer. *South. Med. J.*, **71**, 1280
8. Gordan, G. S. (1976). Exogene Östrogene und Endometrium-Karzinom. *Postgrad. Med.*, **59**, 66
9. Herrmann, W. M. and Beach, R. C. (1978). The psychotropic properties of estrogens. *Pharmakopsychiatry*, **11**, 164
10. Holzmann, K. (1977). Sexualhormone im Klimakterium. *Ärztl. Praxis*, **29**, 3696
11. Hoover, R., Gray, L. A., Cole, Ph. and MacMahon, B. (1976). Menopausal estrogens and breast cancer. *N. Engl. J. Med.*, **295**, 401
12. Jick, H., Watkins, R. N., Hunter, J. R. *et al.* (1979). Replacement estrogens and endometrial cancer. *N. Engl. J. Med.*, **300**, 218

13. Judd, H. L., Lucas, W. E. and Yen, S. S. C. (1976). Serum 17β-estradiol and estrone levels in postmenopausal women with and without endometrial cancer. *J. Clin. Endocrinol. Metab.*, **43**, 272
14. Kaiser, R. (1973). *Gestagenanwendung bei Genital- und Mammatumoren.* (Stuttgart: Thieme)
15. Kaiser, R. (1978). Östrogentherapie im Klimakterium. *Dtsch. Med. Wochenschr.*, **103**, 1059
16. Kantor, H. I., Milton, L. J. and Ernst, M. L. (1978). Comparative psychologic effects of estrogen administration on institutional and non-institutional elderly women. *J. Am. Geriatr. Soc.*, **26**, 9
17. van Keep, P. A. and Haspels, A. A. (1977). *Östrogene in der Perimenopause.* (Amsterdam: Excerpta Medica)
18. van Keep, P. A. and Lauritzen, Ch. (1973). *Älter werden und Östrogene.* (Berlin: Karger)
19. van Keep, P. A. and Lauritzen, Ch. (1975). *Östrogene in der Postmenopause.* (Berlin: Karger)
20. van Keep, P. A., Greenblatt, R. B. and Albeaux-Fernet, M. (Hrsg.) (1977). *Die Menopause.* (Lancaster: MTP)
21. Kistner, R. W. (1976). Estrogens and endometrial cancer. *Obstet. Gynecol.*, **48**, 479
22. Krüskemper, G., Török, M. and Riedel, H. (1977). Die Wechseljahre. *Med. Monatschr.*, **31**, 108
23. Lauritzen, Ch. (1977). Östrogen-Therapie in der Praxis. *Fortschr. Med.*, **95**, 1132
24. Lauritzen, Ch. (1976). Östrogentherapie und Korpuskarzinom: Gibt es einen Zusammenhang? *Med. Trib.* 1977, Nr. 41, *Sexualmedizin*, **5**, 624
25. Lauritzen, Ch. (1975). Erfolge der hormonalen Therapie klimakterischer Beschwerden. *Dtsch. Ärzteblatt*, **72**, 9
26. Lauritzen, Ch. (1978). Östrogene und Endometriumkarzinom. *Fortschr. Med.*, **96**, 2293
27. Lehrl, S. and Gallwitz, A. (1977). *Erlanger Depressions-Skala EDS.* Reiher Psychopathometrie, Erlangen
28. Plotz (1978). Ist die Ostrogenbehandlung mit einem erhöhten Krebsrisiko verbunden? *42. Verhanglg. d. Dtsch. Ges. Für Gynäkologie*, München
29. Schellen, A. M. C. A., Declercq, J. A. *et al.* (1978). Eine vergleichende klinische Doppelblind-Untersuchung von tierischen Östrogenen (Stuten), Äthinyl-Östradiol und Placebo bei Frauen nach der Menopause. *Acta Ther.*, **4**, 133
30. Smith, D. C., Prentice, R., Thompson, D. C. and Herrmann, W. L. (1975). Association of exogenous estrogen and endometrial carcinoma. *N. Engl. J. Med.*, **293**, 1164
31. Stead, W. W. (1978). *J. Am. Med. Assoc.*, **240**, 2544
32. Stolley, P. D. *et al.* (1979). *N. Engl. J. Med.*, **300**, 9
33. Schneider, H. P. G. (1978). Endokrine Veränderungen und diagnostische Möglichkeiten im weiblichen Klimakterium. *Euromed.*, **18**, 690
34. Thomson, J. (1977). Double blind study on the effect of oestrogen on sleep, anxiety and depression in perimenopausal women: preliminary results. *Br. Med. J.*, **6090**, 1317
35. Völker, W., Kannengiesser, U., Majewski, A. and Vasterling, H. W. (1978). Östrogentherapie und Endometriumkarzinom. *Geburtsh. Frauenhk.*, **38**, 735
36. Wortmann, W. K.-H. (1977). Östrogene und Schmerz. *Therapiewoche*, **27**, 1822
37. Zander, J. (1979). Östrogene und Endometriumkarzinom. *Münch. Med. Wochenschr.*, **121**, 443
38. von Zerssen, D. and Koeller, D.-M. (1970). Die Befindlichkeits-Skala (D-S) – ein einfaches Instrument zur Objektivierung von Befindlichkeitsstörungen, insbesondere im Rahmen von Längsschnittuntersuchungen. *Arzneim. Forsch.*, **20**, 915
39. von Zerssen, D. (1971). Die Beschwerden-Liste als Test. *Therapiewoche*, **21**, 1908
40. Ziel, H. K. and Finkle, W. D. (1975). Increased risk of endometrial carcinoma among users of conjugated estrogens. *N. Engl. J. Med.*, **293**, 1167

8
Double-blind Studies on the Effects of Natural Estrogens on Postmenopausal Women: A Follow-up Report

P. T. TOWNSEND, M. I. WHITEHEAD, J. McQUEEN, J. MINARDI and S. CAMPBELL

INTRODUCTION

Within the last 7 years five placebo-controlled trials have attempted to determine the true effects of estrogen therapy in the treatment of climacteric symptoms. Utian[1, 2] in well-documented studies demonstrated that estrogens control vasomotor instability and the symptoms of vaginal atrophy and in addition observed a 'mental tonic' effect. His assessments were single-blind (i.e. he was aware of which type of therapy was being administered) and a truly sensitive method of symptom evaluation was not used.

In a 6-month, double-blind, cross-over study Coope[3] observed a similar response to conjugated estrogens or placebo when given as the first course of treatment. Only after the cross-over at 3 months did the gross disparity between the treatments become obvious – the group then receiving placebo experiencing a recurrence of vasomotor symptoms. For ethical reasons patients had been informed that they were to receive a placebo at some stage in the study. The author commented that this information may have influenced the objectivity of the assessments as with the return of hot flushes patients knew that they were taking an inert preparation.

Campbell[4] and Campbell and Whitehead[5] reported two randomized, double-blind, cross-over studies, the first of 4 and the second of 12 months' duration. To avoid the problems encountered by Coope all patients were told that they were to receive tablets of different strengths. Patients with severe symptoms were allocated to the short-term 4-month study in which conjugated estrogens (Premarin) 1.25 mg daily and placebo were each given cyclically for 2 months. Using a Graphic Rating Scale system of assessment (visual analogues) a statistically significant improvement was observed with Premarin over placebo in not only vasomotor instability and vaginal dryness but also in 10 other physical and psychological scores. A comparison of the results of the patients with and without vasomotor symptoms suggested that the improvement in the 10 additional symptoms resulted in part from the relief of hot flushes, i.e. a domino effect was operating. However, the patients without vasomotor symptoms exhibited an improvement in memory and a reduction in anxiety which suggested that conjugated estrogens have a direct effect on the mental status which is independent of vasomotor symptoms. The earlier observations of Utian[1, 2] were thus confirmed. Patients with less severe symptoms were allocated to the long-term, 12-month study and received 6 months' Premarin and 6 months' placebo in a manner identical to the shorter study. Graphic Rating Scales were completed at 2-monthly intervals and the mean score of the three assessments obtained in each 6-month treatment period was used for statistical analyses. Significant improvements with Premarin over placebo were observed in five physical and psychological scores, including relief of hot flushes and vaginal dryness and improvement in memory. Despite the lessening of the domino effect there was a non-significant improvement with Premarin over placebo in 15 of the remaining 16 symptoms and it was thought probable that the cumulative effect of these small improvements would result in an overall enhancement of patient well-being.

The validity of the design and analyses of the latter two studies, although in our opinion scientifically correct, has been challenged. Firstly, it has been claimed that the effects of estrogen therapy may persist and are 'carried over' after the cross-over to placebo. Thus the initial assessments made during the latter treatment period may have been influenced by previous estrogen administration. We consider this unlikely, however, as there were no statistical differences in the scores obtained from the first and second courses of treatment no matter which tablet was being taken. This suggests that the effect of placebo administration was similar whether ingested before or after Premarin. Secondly, it has been proposed that certain tissues and organs derive benefit from estrogen therapy but that this response becomes apparent only after several months of treatment. The design of our studies, whereby comparisons were made either after 2 months' therapy or in which the aggregate score obtained during a 6-month treatment period was used for analysis, may have failed to detect subtle changes in these less responsive tissues.

To investigate these claims we have re-analyzed the data from our long-term 12-month study. We have compared the baseline scores with those obtained in the fifth and sixth months of estrogen therapy and with those recorded during the fifth and sixth months of placebo administration. Thus we believe we have minimized any possible 'carry-over' effect of estrogen therapy and have determined whether long-term treatment modifies symptoms unaffected by short-term therapy. These data are now presented and their significance is discussed.

In addition to the physical and psychological assessments plasma and urinary calcium concentrations were also measured at 2-monthly intervals during the 12-month study. These data are now presented. Osteoporosis and bone fractures are a major cause of mortality and morbidity in post-menopausal women. For example, the wrist fracture rate rises about 10-fold between the fourth and seventh decades of life[6]. After the age of 60 years the risk of femoral neck fracture doubles every 5 years and 15% of all patients with this fracture die within 3 months of the event[7]. Although estrogens have been shown to conserve bone mass[8, 9], the mechanism of action remains unknown. Plasma calcium concentration and urinary calcium excretion are elevated in postmenopausal and oophorectomized women[10, 11] and have been reported as being lowered during estrogen therapy[10, 12].

PATIENTS AND METHODS

Full details of the patients studied and the methodology employed have been published elsewhere[4, 5] and are only summarized here. Although the majority of the patients in the 12-month study experienced vasomotor symptoms, for most this was not the presenting complaint. For 6 months each patient received conjugated equine estrogens (Premarin: Ayerst International) 1.25 mg daily in 3-weekly courses with one treatment-free week between each course. An identical placebo tablet was also taken for 6 months in the same manner. Patients were randomly allocated to commence treatment with Premarin or placebo. Twenty-seven patients received Premarin first and 29 initially took placebo.

Self-assessment of the physical and psychological status was made with Graphic Rating Scales which are a sensitive method of measuring sympto-matic and emotional change[13]. To obtain baseline values each patient was assessed prior to admission to the study and then reassessed after 6 months of Premarin therapy and after 6 months of placebo. These latter scores represented the physical and emotional state in the fifth and sixth months of tablet ingestion. Statistical comparisons were made with Student's t test.

Venepuncture, which was always undertaken at the same time of day, was performed pretreatment and then at 2-monthly intervals during Premarin and placebo therapy. Urine was collected for 24 hours at the same intervals. Patients were given a list of calcium foods and for 2 days prior to and on the day of collection avoided taking these foods.

RESULTS AND DISCUSSION

The Graphic Rating Scale scores obtained when Premarin was the first course of treatment were compared with those recorded when Premarin was given as the second course of treatment. There were no significant differences. Similarly, comparison of the scores obtained after 6 months of placebo administration showed no significant differences irrespective of whether placebo had been given as the first or second course of treatment. Therefore the placebo effect was similar whether administered before or after Premarin thus indicating, in our opinion, that the 'carry-over' effects of estrogen were nil.

Changes in the Graphic Rating Scale scores on placebo relative to baseline and Premarin relative to placebo are presented in Figure 8.1. Premarin exerted beneficial effects over placebo on hot flushes, vaginal dryness, insomnia and irritability, thus confirming our earlier reports[4, 5]. In addition, we observed for the first time significant improvements in coital satisfaction, frequency of orgasm and backache. Thus longer-term estrogen administration exerted beneficial effects not demonstrated by short-term therapy. It is possible that the improvement in sexual satisfaction and response is either a direct estrogen effect or is secondary to a reduction in vaginal dryness. As there is no evidence of a direct effect on the patients' libido, as reflected by masturbation and frequency of intercourse, we conclude that estrogen acts indirectly and the improvement is qualitative rather than quantitative.

The improvement in backache was an unexpected finding and the mechanism of action is unclear. Estrogen prevents against loss of bone mass in the vertebral bodies, and using serial radiological assessments Lindsay (personal communication) has shown that following the menopause or oophorectomy the vertebrae lose bone substance much earlier than was believed previously. The subtle compression of the vertebral bodies which results is possibly the cause of the backache experienced by so many postmenopausal women.

The continuing importance of the response to placebo even after 6 months' therapy is illustrated by the significant, beneficial, placebo effect on hot flushes, masturbation, activity, optimism, worry about self and worry about age. These responses are inexplicable except as part of the general psychological uplift which all patients experience when attending a clinic and receiving sympathy and attention. The improvement in optimism, worry about self and worry about age with placebo in this group of patients with moderate climacteric symptoms is in sharp contrast to the responses observed in patients with severe climacteric disturbances[4, 5]. In the latter group these three symptoms of psychological retardation were not altered by placebo but were significantly improved by estrogen therapy. The most likely explanation for the observed differences is that attendance at a clinic is of psychological

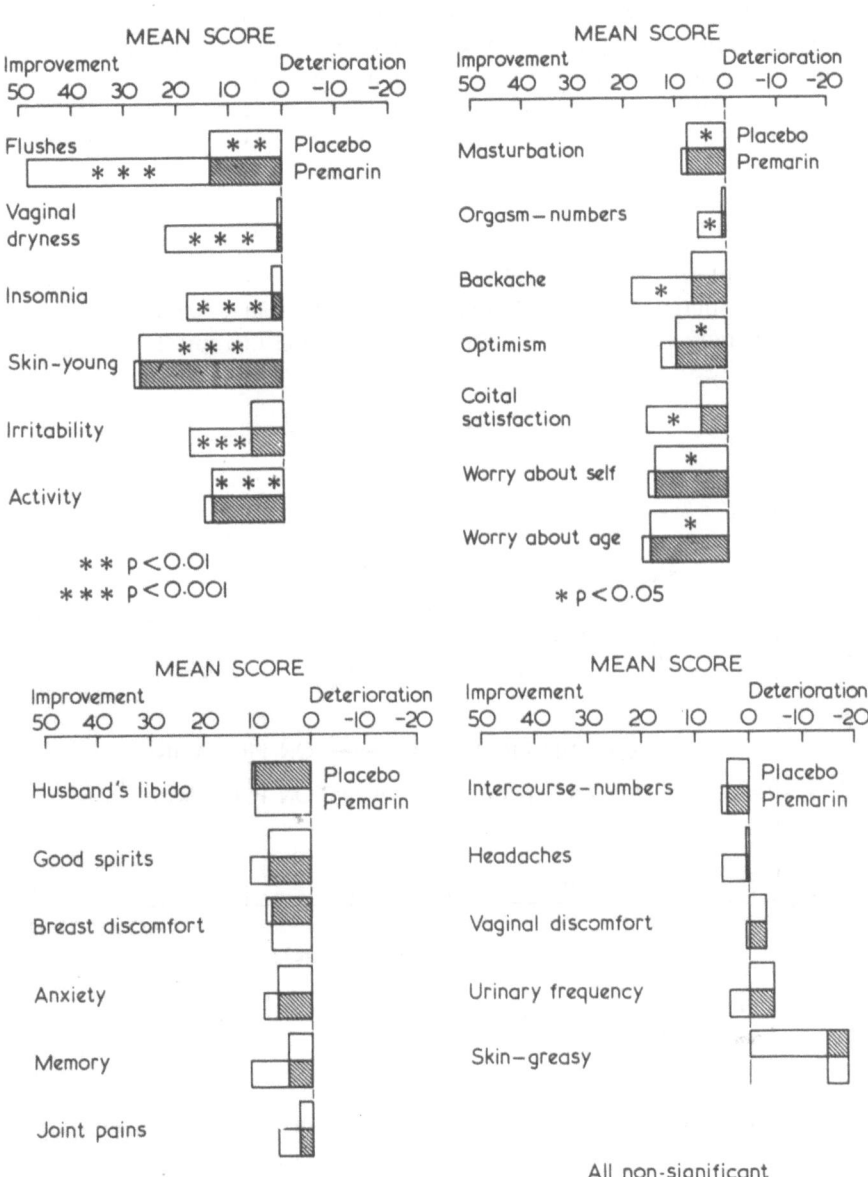

Figure 8.1 Differences in the Graphic Rating Scale scores between the pretreatment assessments and after 6 months of Premarin or placebo therapy

benefit to patients with less severe symptoms in whom the domino effect of estrogen is presumably less marked. Conversely, patients with severe symptoms derive no psychological benefit from merely attending a clinic and need estrogen to improve their emotional state. The significant placebo effect on 'youthful skin' may help explain the continuing success of beauty parlours.

Plasma calcium

The mean plasma calcium levels are shown in Figure 8.2. The mean calcium value for patients receiving Premarin for the first course of treatment was reduced within 2 months of commencing therapy. Following the

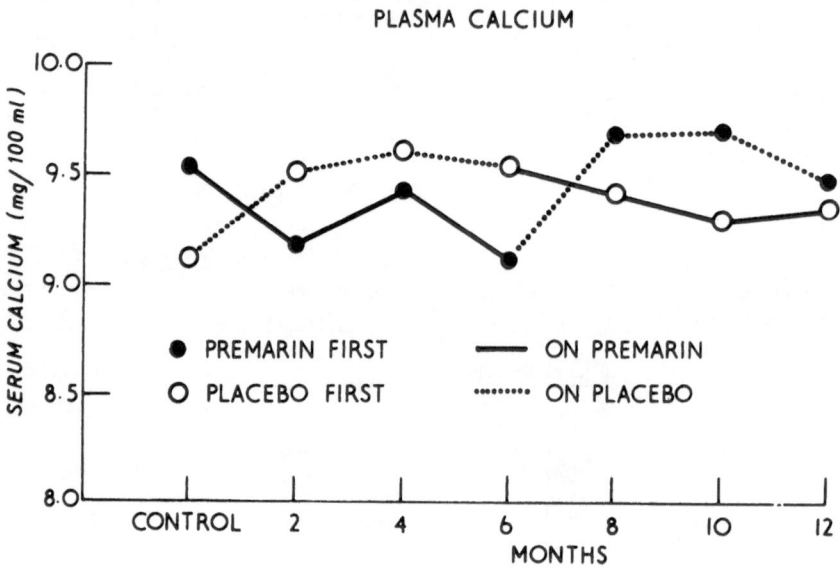

Figure 8.2 Mean plasma calcium levels; pretreatment and then at 2-monthly intervals during Premarin and placebo therapy

change from Premarin to placebo at 6 months the mean plasma calcium value returned to the pretreatment range within 2 months. Patients receiving Premarin as the second course of treatment demonstrated a similar reduction in mean plasma calcium when taking estrogen. The mean plasma calcium of all patients during placebo administration, whether given as the first or second course of treatment, was 9.57 mg/100 ml; and during Premarin therapy, again irrespective of being given as the first or second course of treatment, was 9.30 mg/100 ml. The original observations of Gallagher and Nordin[10] and Aitken et al.[12] are thus confirmed but caution is required in the interpretation of all such results. Firstly, the majority of the measured calcium mass is physiologically inactive as it is in the un-ionized form. Only measurements of ionized calcium accurately reflect bioavailability. Secondly, estrogens are known to increase the plasma volume and thus it is possible that the reduction in plasma calcium concentration during estrogen therapy is not a primary effect but occurs secondary to hemodilution.

Urinary calcium excretion

The mean 24-hour urinary calcium excretion is shown in Figure 8.3. A reduction in mean daily urinary calcium excretion is demonstrated during

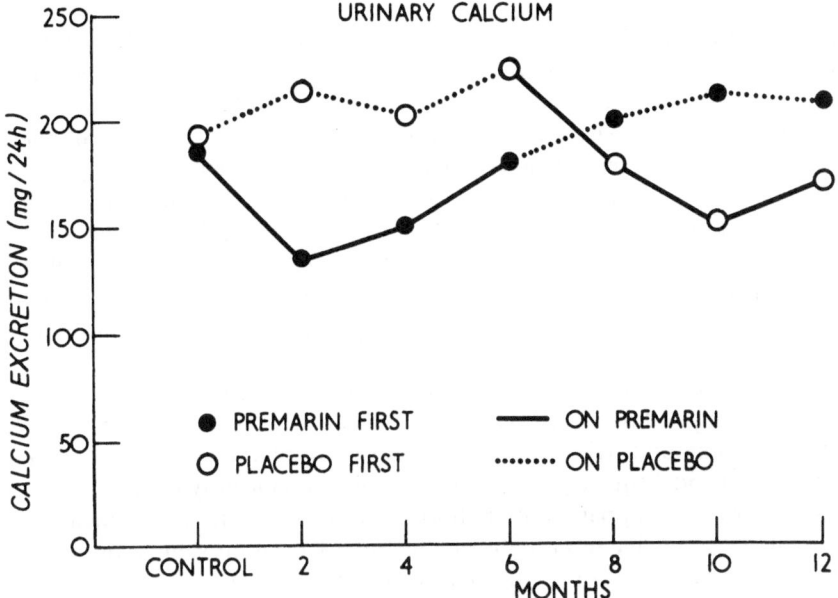

Figure 8.3 Mean 24-hour urinary calcium excretion; pretreatment and then at 2-monthly intervals during Premarin and placebo therapy

Premarin therapy whether given as the first or second course of treatment. As with the reduction in plasma calcium this was evident within 2 months of the commencement of estrogen treatment and a similar cross-over effect is clearly shown. The original observations of Gallagher and Nordin[10] and Aitken *et al.*[12] are confirmed. The mean 24-hour urinary calcium excretion of all patients during placebo administration was 210 mg/24 hours, and during Premarin therapy was 161 mg/24 hours. Therefore Premarin 1.25 mg daily, cyclically, caused a reduction in mean daily urinary calcium loss of 49 mg. A daily loss of 30 mg calcium is equivalent to a reduction in bone mineral content of 1% per annum. Bone loss exceeding 0.6% of the skeletal mass per annum has been associated with increased susceptibility to osteoporosis.

The daily reduction in calcium excretion was maintained for the 6-month period during which Premarin was prescribed. As there is no rise in fecal calcium excretion during estrogen therapy[10] the fall in urinary calcium loss represents a true, calcium-sparing effect and results in an improvement in calcium balance[14]. When maintained over a period of years with long-term estrogen therapy the cumulative effect upon the skeleton is considerable and is associated with a conservation of bone mass[9].

SUMMARY

A 12-month, double-blind, cross-over, placebo-controlled study was performed with Premarin (conjugated equine estrogen) 1.25 mg daily cyclically on climacteric women with moderate symptoms. As the effects of estrogen therapy possibly persist for 2 or 3 months after treatment is discontinued patients were assessed using Graphic Rating Scales before therapy commenced and again in the fifth and sixth months of Premarin or placebo administration. The risk of previous estrogen therapy influencing scores obtained during placebo ingestion was evaluated and found to be nil. In addition, from a comparison with results previously obtained it has been possible to determine whether long-term therapy modifies symptoms unaffected by short-term treatment.

Premarin exerted significant, beneficial effects over placebo in seven physical and psychological assessments. Vasomotor instability, vaginal dryness, insomnia and irritability were significantly relieved. Backache, coital satisfaction and frequency of orgasm were also significantly improved, these benefits not being apparent after short-term therapy. The latter benefits are more likely to be due to an indirect effect of estrogen on vaginal dryness as there was no evidence of a direct effect, the libidos of the patients and their husbands being unaltered by treatment.

The mechanism whereby backache was relieved by estrogen therapy requires elucidation. As compared to placebo there was a reduction in both the plasma calcium concentration and urinary calcium excretion during Premarin therapy. Whilst the former results must be interpreted with caution as they may result from hemodilution, the reduction in urinary calcium loss is likely to be representative of a highly beneficial calcium-sparing effect.

Even after 6 months' therapy there was a significant, beneficial, placebo effect on seven physical and psychological symptoms. These benefits most probably resulted from the feeling of well-being which is experienced by patients with moderate symptoms attending a menopause clinic and receiving sympathy and attention. The degree of psychological uplift that is generated by clinic attendance may be determined by the severity of initial symptomatology as patients with severe climacteric disturbances are not placebo responsive and only estrogen therapy significantly relieves their symptoms.

Acknowledgments

We thank the Consultant Gynaecologists at the Chelsea Hospital for Women, especially Professor Sir John Dewhurst, for allowing us to study their patients, and Dr I. D. Hill and Miss S. MacDermott, Division of Medical Computing, Clinical Research Centre, for their help and advice. This work was funded by Ayerst Laboratories.

References

1. Utian, W. H. (1972). The mental tonic effect of oestrogens administered to oophorectomized females. *S. Afr. Med. J.*, **46**, 1079

2. Utian, W. H. (1975). Definitive symptoms of post-menopause incorporating use of vaginal para-basal cell index. In: P. A. van Keep and C. Lauritzen (eds.), *Frontiers in Hormone Research: Vol. 3 Estrogens in the Post-menopause*, pp. 74–93 (Basel: S. Karger)

3. Coope, J. (1976). Double blind, cross over study of oestrogen replacement therapy. In: S. Campbell (ed.), *The Management of the Menopause and Post-menopausal Years*, pp. 159–168 (Lancaster: MTP Press)

4. Campbell, S. (1976). Double-blind psychometric studies on the effects of natural oestrogens on post-menopausal women. In: S. Campbell (ed.), *The Management of the Menopause and Post-menopausal Years*, pp. 149–158 (Lancaster: MTP Press)

5. Campbell, S. and Whitehead, M. I. (1977). Oestrogen therapy and the menopausal syndrome. In: R. B. Greenblatt and J. W. W. Studd (eds.), *Clinics in Obstetrics and Gynaecology, Vol. 4, No. 1. The Menopause*, pp. 31–47 (London and Ontario: W. B. Saunders Company Ltd)

6. Knowelden, J., Buhr, A. J. and Dunbar, O. (1964). Incidence of fracture rates in persons over 35 years of age. A report to the Medical Research Council working party on fractures in the elderly. *Br. J. Prevent. Soc. Med.*, **18**, 130

7. Alffram, P. S. (1964). An epidemiological study of cervical and trochanteric fractures of the femur in an urban population. *Acta Orthopaed. Scand. Suppl.* **65**, 1

8. Aitken, J. M. (1976) Osteoporosis and its relation to oestrogen deficiency. In: S. Campbell (ed.), *The Management of the Menopause and Post-menopausal Years*, pp. 225–236 (Lancaster: MTP Press)

9. Lindsay, R., Aitken, J. M., Anderson, J. B., Hart, D. M., MacDonald, E. B. and Clarke, A. C. (1976). Long-term prevention of post-menopausal osteoporosis by oestrogen. *Lancet*, **1**, 1038

10. Gallagher, J. C. and Nordin, B. E. C. (1973). Oestrogens and calcium metabolism. In: P. A. van Keep and C. Lauritzen (eds.), *Frontiers in Hormone Research. Vol. 2. Ageing and Oestrogens*, pp. 98–110 (Basel: S. Karger)

11. Young, M. M. and Nordin, B. E. C. (1967). Effects of natural and artificial menopause on plasma and urinary calcium and phosphorus. *Lancet*, **3**, 118

12. Aitken, J. M., Hart, D. M. and Lindsay, R. (1973). Oestrogen replacement therapy for prevention of osteoporosis after oophorectomy. *Br. Med. J.*, **3**, 515

13. Lader, M. H. and Wing, L. (1966). Physiological measures, sedative drugs and morbid anxiety. *Institute of Psychiatry Maudsley Monographs*. (Oxford: Oxford University Press)

14. Gallagher, J. C. and Nordin, B. E. C. (1975). Effect of oestrogen and progestogen therapy on calcium metabolism in post-menopausal women. In: P. A. van Keep and C. Lauritzen (eds.), *Frontiers in Hormone Research. Vol. 3. Estrogens in the Post-menopause*, pp. 150–170 (Basel: S. Karger)

9
Considerations concerning the Clinical Treatment of the Principal Micturitional Disturbances of the Post-menopause

M. MANESCHI, S. M. RUBINO and V. MESSANA

The modifications directly caused by estrogen loss in the menopause or by the phenomena of aging which the menopause accelerates also include hyper-dystrophy of the tissues and urethrovesical support structures. If these modifications reach considerable proportions, find any constitutional predisposition or build upon previous lesions in the urethrovesical area, then they cause micturitional disturbances which in the main take the form of postmenopausal cystic conditions and stress incontinence, and some 20% of menopausal women suffer from these symptoms.

POSTMENOPAUSAL CYSTIC CONDITIONS

The phrase *postmenopausal cystic conditions* is understood to cover all recurrent micturitional disturbances with symptoms similar to cystitis common after the menopause. On one hand, estrogen deficiency associated with the menopause leads to some lowering of resilience in the utero-urethrovesical support structures; on the other hand, dystrophic modifications take place in the vaginal–urethrovesical epithelium and these compromise the tissue defence mechanisms[1].

Estrogen loss, affecting urethrovesical support structures in subjects show-ing any signs of weakness, either by constitution or from traumatic lesions due to previous childbearing, accelerates the appearance of a cystocele or aggravates the condition.

The cystocele inevitably brings about urinary stagnation, with decompo-sition of the urine and irritation of urethrovesical mucosa; the tissue defences are notably reduced by dystrophic modifications consequent on estrogen loss and so in turn provide an ideal ground for bacterial development. Thus post-menopausal cystic conditions often come to be labelled dystrophic cystitis. This is to oversimplify, since in reality the clinical picture is more complicated and relates more particularly to three factors, namely dystrophy, cystocele and infection[2].

That dystrophy cannot be the only pathogenetic factor in postmenopausal cystic conditions is apparent also from the fact that about 80% of post-menopausal women present an atrophic-type urologic picture[3], the propor-tion of which is far higher than that for women with postmenopausal cystic conditions.

Table 9.1

	Postmenopausal cystic disease %	Control %
Dystrophy	86.7	76.7
Cystocele	93.3	13.3
Infection	40	0

Again, a report by the present authors[4] concerning 60 patients with postmenopausal cystic conditions makes it apparent that the pathogenesis of this syndrome includes many factors (Table 9.1).

STRESS INCONTINENCE

For about 15% of women, the advent of the menopause brings stress incontinence or aggravates the condition.

Stress incontinence, a symptom that may arise from diverse etiological origins; during the menopause, it is mainly due to sphincter deficiency[5]. Estrogens influence some of the diverse mechanisms governing urinary con-tinence; when the effects of estrogen deficiency act on structures constitution-ally defective or weakened by previous traumatic events, sphincter activity can lose its effectiveness and incontinence results.

In Table 9.2, the principal mechanisms are indicated by means of which estrogen loss impinges at various levels in determining or aggravating stress incontinence through sphincter deficiency. Current research by the present

Table 9.2

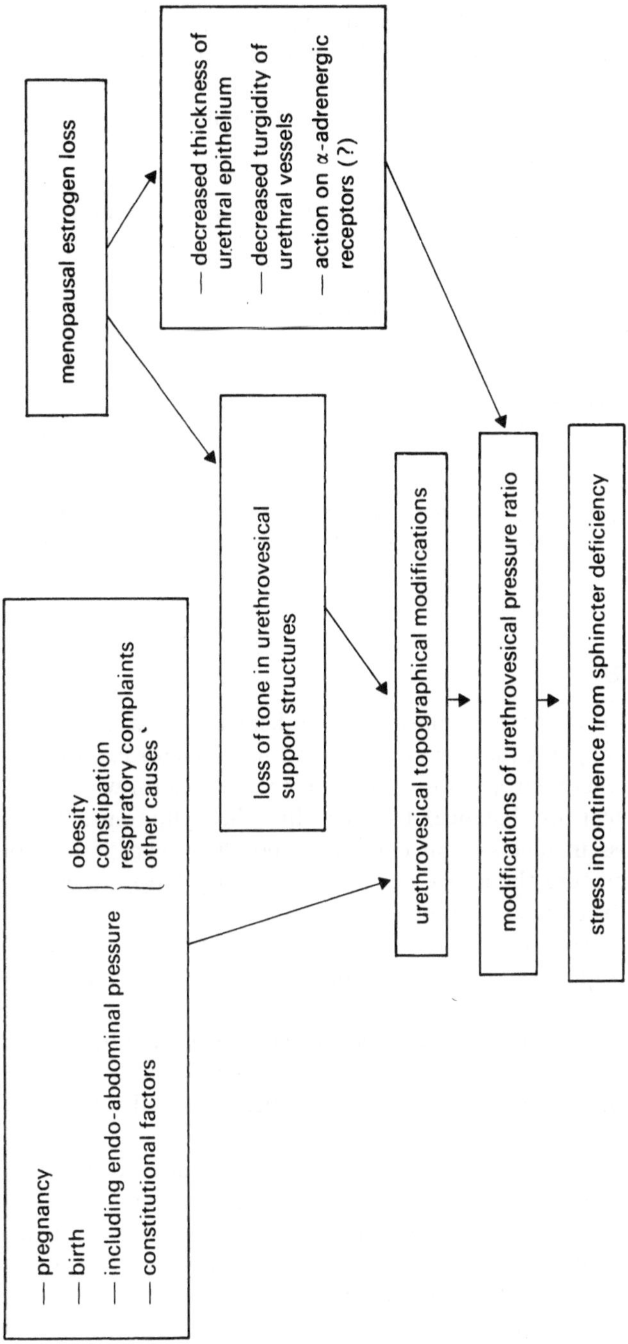

— pregnancy
— birth
— including endo-abdominal pressure
— constitutional factors

— obesity
— constipation
— respiratory complaints
— other causes

menopausal estrogen loss

— decreased thickness of urethral epithelium
— decreased turgidity of urethral vessels
— action on α-adrenergic receptors (?)

loss of tone in urethrovesical support structures

urethrovesical topographical modifications

modifications of urethrovesical pressure ratio

stress incontinence from sphincter deficiency

authors is tending to show that many women can reach the menopause in a condition that may be defined as one of *potential sphincter deficiency*, that is to say in a state in which, although topographical urethrovesical alterations are in evidence, compensating mechanisms come into play which despite the abnormal topographical situation succeed in maintaining the normal urethrovesical pressure ratio[6].

Table 9.3   Urethrocystograph on 60 women continent premenopause

	1-2 years postmenopause			
	Incontinent		Continent	
	No.	%	No.	%
Abnormal—42	31	51.7	11	18.3
Normal—18	1	1.7	17	28.3

In a high percentage of these patients the effects of estrogen loss during the menopause upset this precarious balance, from which incontinence results (Table 9.3).

REMARKS

Considerations of the two most frequent disturbances which arise or worsen after the menopause make it evident that a multi-factor pathogenesis is to be envisaged, where estrogen loss represents that last factor which may upset an already precarious balance, thus causing the symptoms. The effects of estrogen loss in fact seldom determine, on their own, lesions on a scale sufficient to cause the above syndrome, but they have a participating role which may be defined as complementary.

Therefore, sole blame for the clinical picture arising must never be attributed to the age at the appearance of the symptoms, that is to say the menopause; the presence must be sought and the scale evaluated of other lesions in which the lesions due to deficient estrogen stimulus begin and grow. Only thus can choice of treatment be made to correspond with the entity of each single factor and the course of treatment planned which may be most appropriate to it.

For example, in a case of postmenopausal cystic disease, the topographical change is slight, therefore the urinary residue is minimal but the hormone deficiency is clear; and in this instance hormone replacement therapy will often be enough to remedy the topographical change, associated with perineal exercises. If, on the other hand, the topographical change is marked and the urinary residue conspicuous, then besides hormone therapy, corrective surgery will be required; or if there is infection, evaluation will have to be made of the pathogenetic importance of the other factors after a suitable course of corrective treatment.

It may seem that the usefulness of estrogen therapy is being underplayed in relation to these disturbances; in reality it needs stressing that the positive effects of estrogen therapy achieve maximum results when other basic lesions are also cared for.

SUMMARY

Micturitional disturbances which arise or become more pronounced after the menopause almost always have a multi-factor origin where estrogen loss represents that last factor which, by upsetting an already precarious balance, makes the symptoms appear.

Postmenopausal cystic disease and stress incontinence from sphincter deficiency, which are the most frequent micturitional disturbances of the post-menopause, may thus be adequately treated and cared for, with this proviso: that after careful assessment of the patient, other pre-existing lesions are also treated and cared for, it being on these that lesions from failed estrogen stimulus arise and enlarge.

References

1. Hafez, E. S. E. (1976). Aging and reproductive physiology. *Ann. Arbor Sci.*, Vol. 2
2. Rubino, S. M. and Messana, V. (1978). *Note di Urologia Ginecologica*, p. 81. (Palermo: Libreria Clemenza ed.)
3. Lencioni, I. (1975). *L'Urocytogramme*, p. 132. (Maloine, S. A. (ed.))
4. Rubino, S. M., Messana, V. and Di Pasquale, D. (1979). Cistopatia post-menopausale. (In press)
5. Arnold, E. P., Webster, J. R., Loose, H., Brown, A. D. G., Turner-Warwick, R. T., Whiteside, C. G. and Jequier, A. M. (1973). Urodynamics of female incontinence: factors influencing the results of surgery. *Am. J. Obstet. Gynecol.*, **117**, 805
6. Rubino, S. M. (1979). Significato delle alterazioni uretrocistografiche in donne continenti. 1st National Congress on *Gli Apparati della Continenza*, Rome, 1979

10
The Urethral Syndrome –
Role of Estrogens in the
Therapy

P. SMITH

INTRODUCTION

Episodes of frequency, urgency and dysuria are common complaints of many women and may arise at any stage of their life. In physiological terms this life can be divided into premenstrual, reproductive and postmenopausal phases, all of which relate to natural variations in hormone activity, particularly estrogen. The clinical significance of these symptoms will vary in relation to the phase of life in which they arise (Figure 10.1).

It is clearly recognized that such lower urinary tract symptoms in a child require urgent investigation to exclude active urinary infection and upper tract disease, particularly reflux nephropathy.

Symptoms arising in the young woman during the reproductive phase of life are rarely related to any significant disease in the urinary tract, but nonetheless require treatment due to their recurrent and demoralizing nature. This group of women in the reproductive phase of life is by far the largest section of patients with such symptoms.

There remains, however, a third and significant group of women who first experience these lower urinary tract symptoms after the menopause. As with women in the reproductive age group, mid-stream urine culture will be positive in approximately only half of these patients. Those with positive culture, invariably enterococci, are labelled urinary tract infection, those with similar symptoms but without significant bacteriuria are termed urethral syndrome. Much time and effort has been expended in trying to differentiate between these two groups, but for practical purposes they are the same and for pedantic reasons could all be described as urethral syndrome, since by definition a syndrome is a collection of symptoms alone. What is certain is that many patients will derive temporary relief of their symptoms following antibiotic therapy whether or not the urine is subsequently shown to contain a significant bacteriuria. It seems likely, therefore, that in all women with lower urinary tract symptoms bacterial contamination of the urethra and subsequently the bladder is an important factor in the causation of symptoms. These organisms would appear to reach the lower urinary tract by way of the urethra. In the reproductive age the onset of sexual activity and, at a later stage, childbirth and pelvic surgical insults may interfere with urethral function and encourage this bacterial contamination. Women in the postmenopausal group have already gone through this reproductive phase of their life without significant urinary tract problems, so it would seem that some other factor may be involved at this phase of their life.

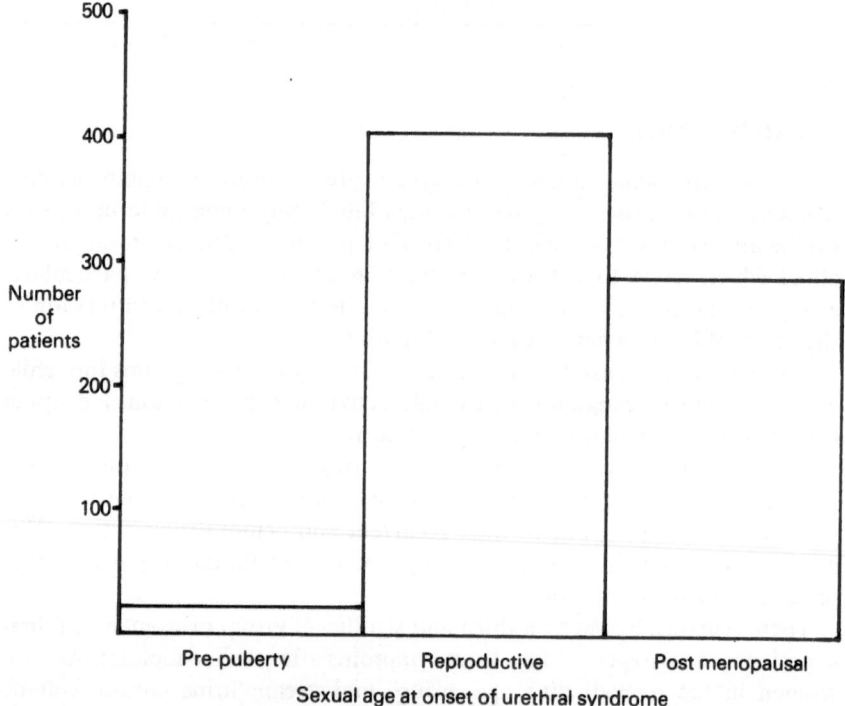

Figure 10.1   Physiological age distribution of 792 females presenting with the urethral syndrome

It is now many years since Everett[1] pointed out the associated atrophic vaginitis that many of these women suffered from concurrently with their urinary symptoms. He first proposed that the urinary symptoms were due to atrophic changes in the urethra similar to those in the vagina. Before going on to test this hypothesis it is important first to mention some basic facts about the development, structure and function of the female urethra.

The downgrowing urorectal septum divides the cloaca into anterior urogenital and posterior rectal compartments. In association with the allantois or primitive bladder the proximal segment of the urethra arises to communicate with the cloaca. At the same time the fused müllerian ducts project into the urogenital sinus to form the müllerian tubercle (Figure 10.2). Further differentiation of these tissues gives rise to the vagina and distal urethra. This is only a very brief description of a complicated process but serves to underline the fact that the female urethra develops in two quite distinct parts – a proximal segment derived from the allantois and a distal segment derived from the urogenital sinus in conjunction with the vagina.

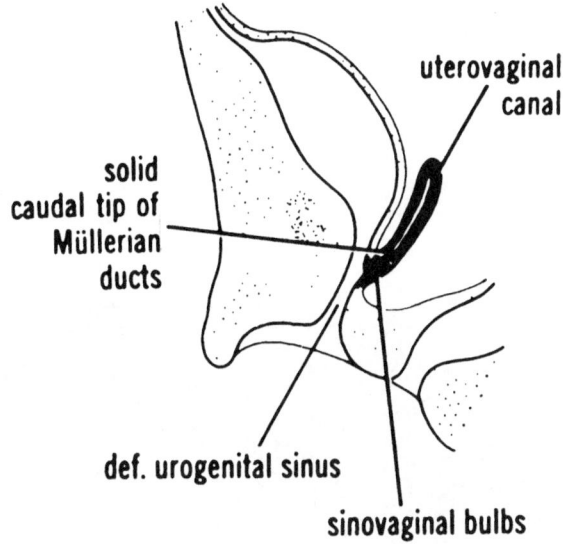

Figure 10.2 Diagrammatic representation of development of the urethra showing development of the distal segment from the urogenital sinus

The anatomy of the mature urethra reflects these developmental differences. The proximal urethra is composed of muscle and glandular tissue and covered by a transitional epithelium continuous with that of the bladder. The distal urethra is a much simpler structure containing virtually no muscle elements and most significantly being covered by a stratified squamous epithelium, similar to that covering the vagina. The transition from transitional to squamous epithelium is abrupt (Figure 10.3, a and b), the junction usually lying at the mid-point of the urethra. Functionally these anatomical features can be seen to relate to, firstly, a primary sphincteric component occupying the proximal urethra which is concerned with urinary continence and, secondly, an apparently simple urinary conduit occupying the distal component of the urethra (Figure 10.4). In some ways the distal urethra can be seen as a vaginal diverticulum rather than a urinary organ. Thus there could

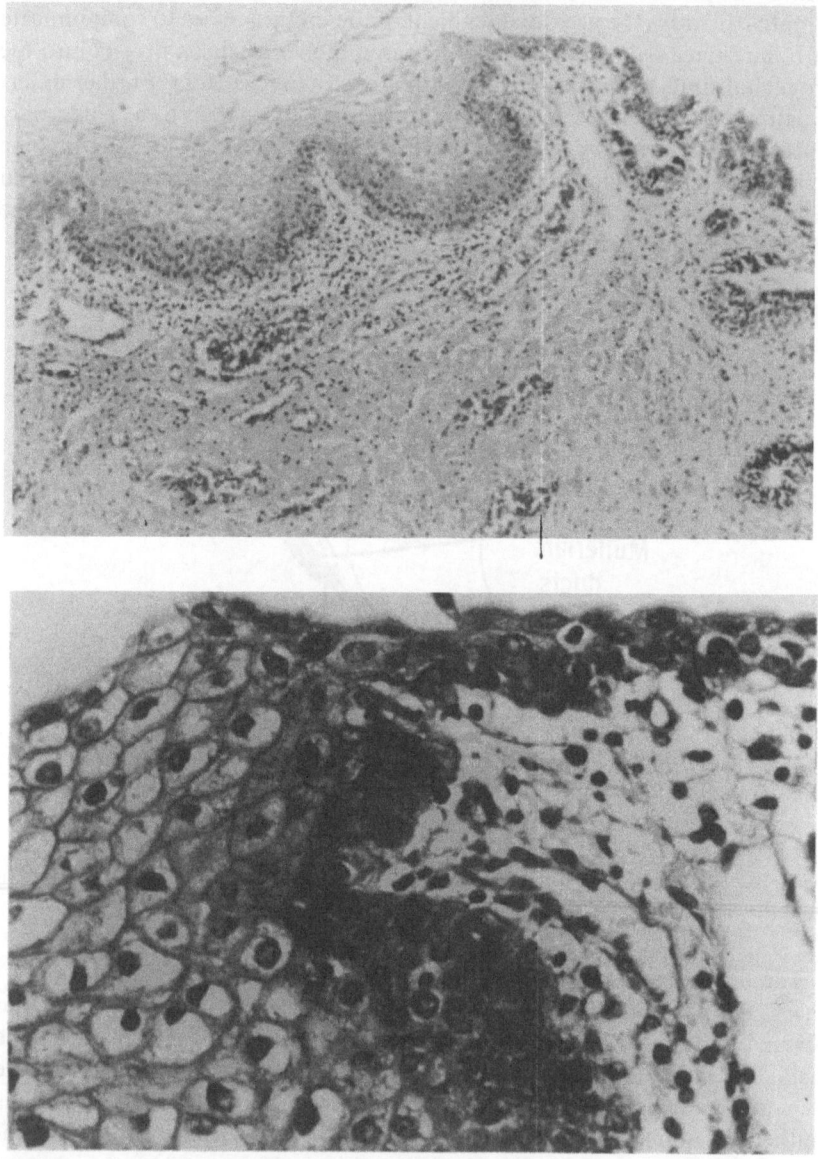

Figure 10.3 Longitudinal section of female urethra showing abrupt transition of proximal transitional epithelium to distal squamous epithelium: a (upper) low-power view; b (lower) high-power view

be an additional hazard for the urethra of the postmenopausal woman in the possibility of estrogen deficiency producing atrophic changes in the distal urethra.

Previous animal studies by Parkes and Zuckerman[2] support this concept. They commented on the close relationship between structure and development of the urethra and vagina in the female and noted an increase in the stratification of the squamous epithelium of female monkeys in both genital and extragenital tissues after the administration of large doses of estrogen. This extragenital estrogen sensitivity was found to be most marked in those structures claiming origin from the urogenital sinus, in particular the distal urethra, where it was manifest by the maturation of its squamous epithelium.

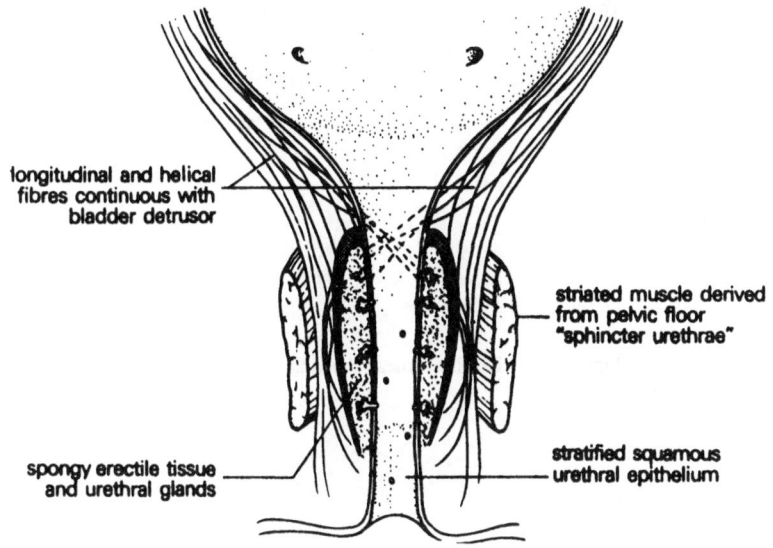

longitudinal and helical fibres continuous with bladder detrusor

striated muscle derived from pelvic floor "sphincter urethrae"

spongy erectile tissue and urethral glands

stratified squamous urethral epithelium

Figure 10.4 Diagrammatic representation of anatomical features of the urethra showing proximal sphincter component and distal 'vaginal' component

A prospective study has been carried out to see if a similar hormone sensitivity is present in the human female urethra[3]. The method used to study estrogen sensitivity was that of cytohormonal analysis of the epithelium of the distal urethra, which is based on the maturation effect of estrogen on this squamous epithelium. Any squamous epithelium consists of three well-defined layers derived from a basal germinal layer. The first layer consists of round, plump, so-called para-basal cells. The next cell layer consists of intermediate cells which are flat and irregular with eccentrically placed vesicular nuclei. Finally, above this layer come the superficial cells which are thin and irregular with pyknotic nuclei. In an estrogen-sensitive tissue the maturation of these cells from the para-basal through the intermediate to the superficial cell is dependent upon an adequate level of circulating estrogen. By sampling the type of cell occupying the topmost layer of the squamous epithelium in the distal urethra it is possible to estimate the degree of estrogen activity. Thus a urethral smear consisting of predominantly para-basal cells (Figure 10.5) will

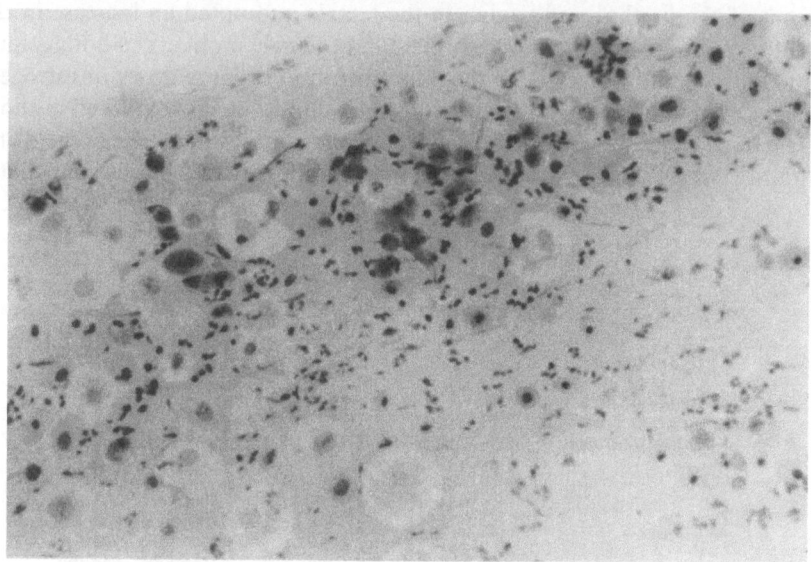

Figure 10.5   Urethral smear showing para-basal cells

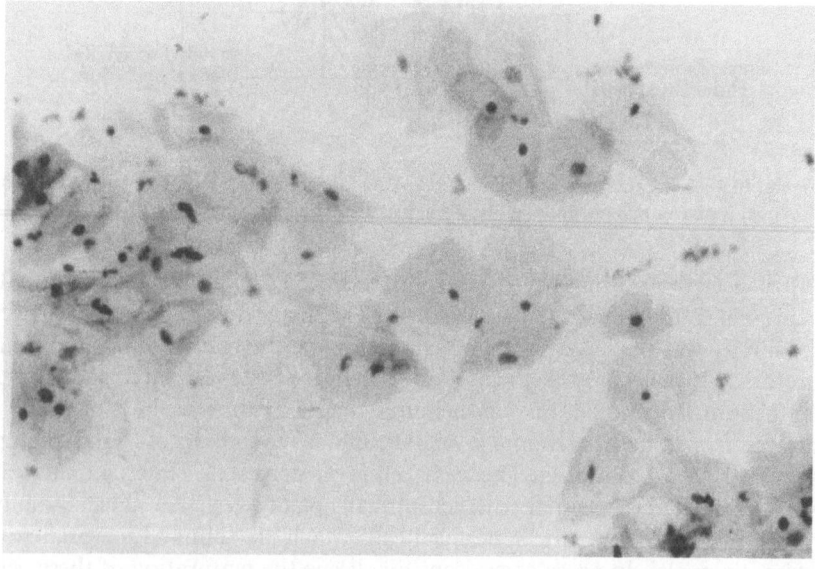

Figure 10.6   Urethral smears showing intermediate cells

reflect low estrogen activity (Figure 10.6), whilst cells of the superficial variety indicate adequate levels of estrogen activity (Figure 10.7).

A total of 402 females were studied by means of urethral cytology to see if estrogen changes could be detected in the squamous epithelium of their distal urethras at the different physiological stages of life. Of the 18 children examined, 16 demonstrated typical atrophic changes in the urethral smear, indicating premenstrual low estrogen activity. In two there was evidence of some estrogen activity and both girls commenced menstruation within 3 months of the examination. Two hundred and sixty women were in the reproductive phase of life and all had evidence of estrogen activity in the urethral smear, varying from the fully mature appearances associated with full estrogen activity immediately prior to ovulation to a less mature smear associated with decline of estrogen activity in the postovulatory phase of the cycle. The urethral smears in these two groups were therefore accurate indices of estrogen activity.

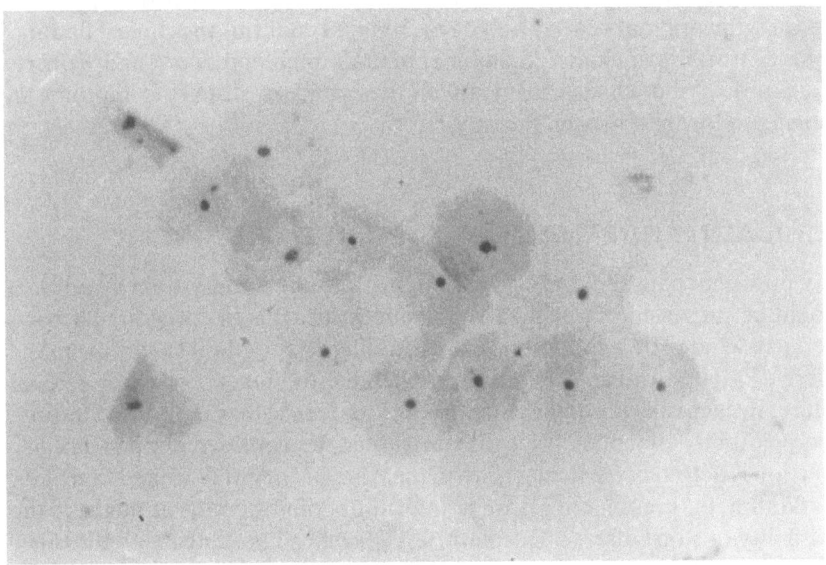

Figure 10.7 Urethral smears showing superficial cells

The urethral smear patterns of the 123 postmenopausal women showed three different patterns. Fifteen women had smears containing mature cells indicating the normal cyclic activity associated with full estrogen activity. In 85 patients there was evidence of a decline in estrogen activity, as shown by a crowded pattern of para-basal and intermediate cells. In only 23 cases was there a true atrophic smear showing only para-basal cells and indicating a severe depression of estrogen activity.

This distribution of urethral smears in these postmenopausal women indicates varying levels of estrogen activity and is in accordance with the vaginal cytohormonal studies of Meisel[4]. They clearly demonstrate that abrupt atrophic changes in the urethra do not immediately follow the onset of the menopause and that many postmenopausal women continue to have an estrogen-stimulated urethral epithelium to an advanced age. In all the females studied vaginal cytology taken concurrently showed a similar pattern to urethral smear, with the same variations under the differing estrogen environments associated with the varying age groups. This study, therefore, clearly demonstrated that there is a natural ageing change in the female urethra associated with the variable but inevitable physiological decline in estrogen activity that follows the menopause.

Thus the same atrophic changes that give rise to the thin, rigid and often ulcerating epithelium of the vagina will also occur in the distal urethra. These atrophic changes arising in the epithelium of the distal urethra may give rise to lower urinary tract symptoms and will respond to estrogen therapy. This supports the original observation of Everett and confirms the clinical findings of other workers, including Salmon et al.[5], Youngblood et al.[6] and Roberts and Smith[7], who all described an improvement in urinary symptoms in patients following estrogen therapy.

CLINICAL MANAGEMENT OF ATROPHIC URETHRITIS

Any postmenopausal patient presenting with lower urinary tract symptoms should be suspected of having atrophic urethritis. It is essential firstly, however, to exclude other conditions masquerading as a urethral syndrome in the elderly. Polyuria causing frequency can be due to diabetes or chronic renal failure; in each case the diagnosis can readily be made on simple urine testing. The possibility of upper tract disease should be considered when urinary infection is detected, particularly when there is a history of fever and loin pain. In addition, the presence of a proteus infection should alert the urologist to the possibility of stone disease. Haematuria, even when associated with the other urinary symptoms, requires full investigation to exclude the presence of a tumor in the urinary tract.

Physical examination of women with lower urinary tract symptoms is usually directed towards abdominal palpation to exclude renal swellings or bladder enlargement. In all women with lower urinary tract symptoms it is equally important to examine the urethra, introitus and vagina. In the elderly female, evidence of acute or chronic atrophic changes in the introitus and vagina are readily identified. Though, apart from its meatus, the distal urethral cannot be visualized directly, it can be assumed that changes in the epithelium of the vagina will be reflected by similar changes in the squamous epithelium of the distal urethra. If necessary, vaginal cytology, a simple investigation, can be used to confirm the presence of atrophic changes in the urethra, since there is an absolute correlation with urethral cytology.

In practice, though, the macroscopic changes are easily recognized and cytology is rarely required. Thus, an acute generalized atrophic change will reveal a sore, tender, thin, reddened epithelium involving the urethral meatus, introitus and vagina (Figure 10.8); in more chronic cases the inflammatory

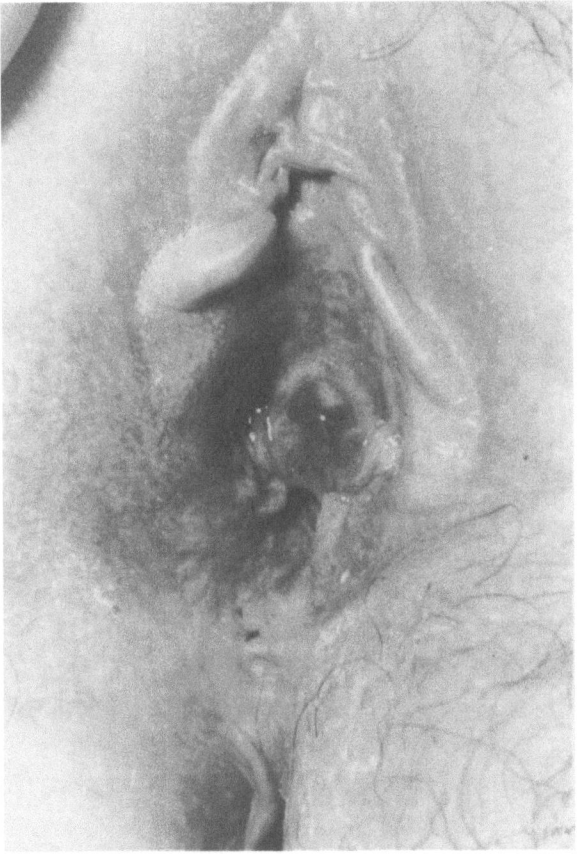

Figure 10.8   Acute atrophic changes in urethra, introitus and vagina

changes can be most marked in the urethral meatus (Figure 10.9). Finally, in some women there is a generalized stenosis of the introitus, vagina and urethral meatus, due to long standing atrophic changes (Figure 10.10). Urine examination and blood picture are routine studies in these patients. Excretion urography is only required for those patients with upper tract symptoms, haematuria or persistent bacteriuria. Cystoscopy is required for those patients with haematuria, to exclude bladder tumor. Occasionally, also, cystoscopy will reveal trabeculation and a raised residual urine, again indicating the possibility of obstructive disease, associated with distal atrophic urethritis. Urethroscopy will demonstrate these atrophic changes (Figure 10.11) but is rarely required as these can be deduced, as mentioned above, from clinical appearances of the superficial tissues.

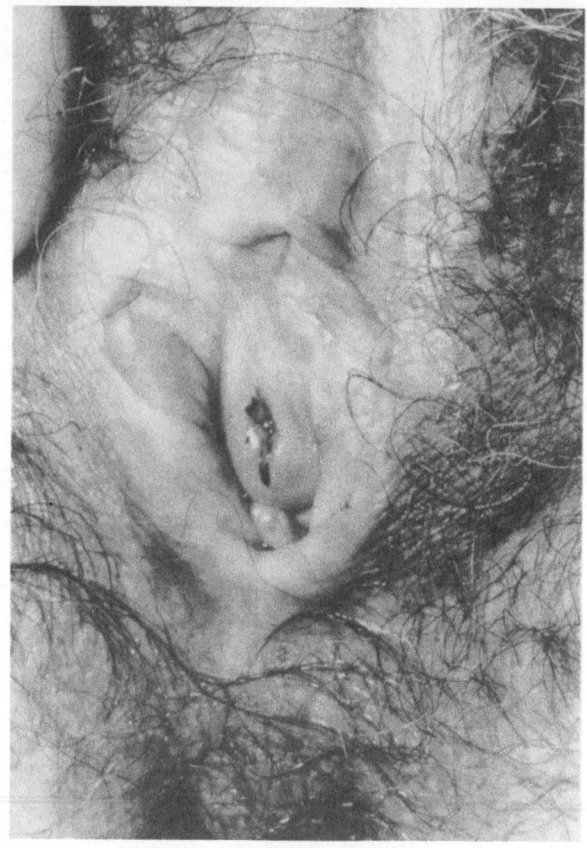

Figure 10.9 Chronic atrophic changes in introitus and vagina with acute atrophic changes at external urethral meatus

It now seems that there are two basic types of presentation in post-menopausal atrophic urethritis[8]. Those women presenting with acute symptoms and a short history of usually less than 6 months will have associated acute atrophic changes in the introitus and vagina. Such patients respond rapidly to estrogen therapy. A 3-month course of continuous low-dose hormone therapy is indicated using Premarin 0.625 mg daily for 3 weeks. The fourth week may be left without any treatment or advantage can be taken to provide a 1-week challenge of progestogen. This type of therapy is available in the form of Prempak. When present, secondary urinary infection should be treated by the appropriate antibiotic.

In patients presenting with a longer history, usually more than 6 months, there may be secondary changes in the wall of the urethra in association with

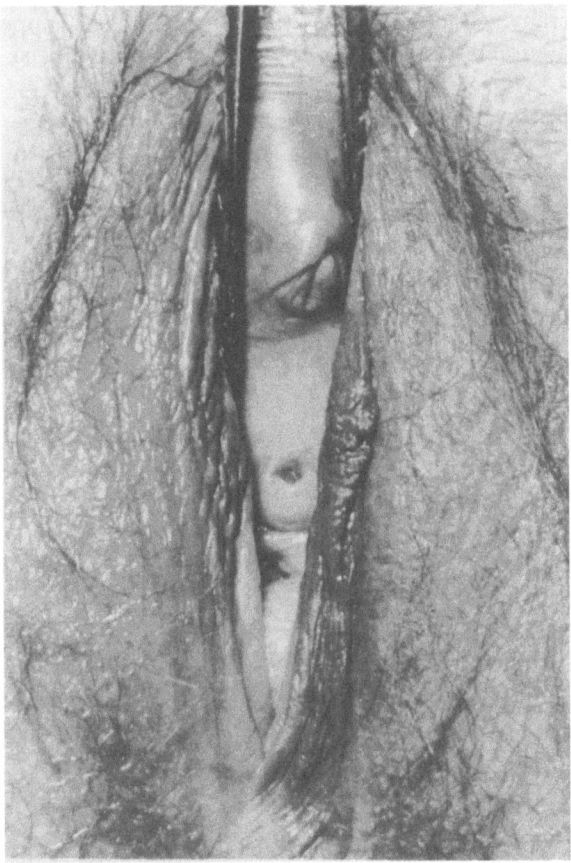

Figure 10.10   Generalized chronic atrophic changes with urethral stenosis

the atrophic changes in the epithelium. Such patients, often without acute changes in the vagina, are likely to have a urethral stenosis in association with a low grade urethritis. In practice it is easy to see such a urethral stenosis, since it occupies the distal segment and usually involves the external urethral meatus. These patients may admit to longstanding hesitancy, slow stream and nocturia in addition to their acute symptoms. In these patients hormone replacement therapy and, where necessary, antibiotics are insufficient to eradicate the symptoms completely. The acute phase may well be relieved by this therapy, but recurrent symptoms are inevitable due to the persistent urethral stenosis. In these patients a wide uretheral dilatation should be performed. Dilatation using graduated urethral sounds can be a traumatic process and a better way to dilate the distal urethra is to use the Otis urethrotome without the blade (Figure 10.12). The instrument should be expanded slowly to a diameter of 35 Charriere. Again a 3-month course of Premarin therapy, either alone or with a progestogen support, is given following dilatation both to promote healing and reduce the risk of recurrent stenosis.

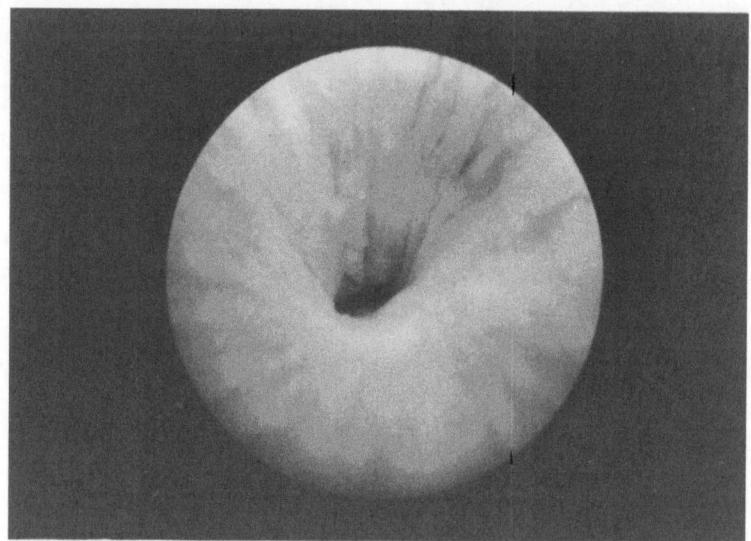

a

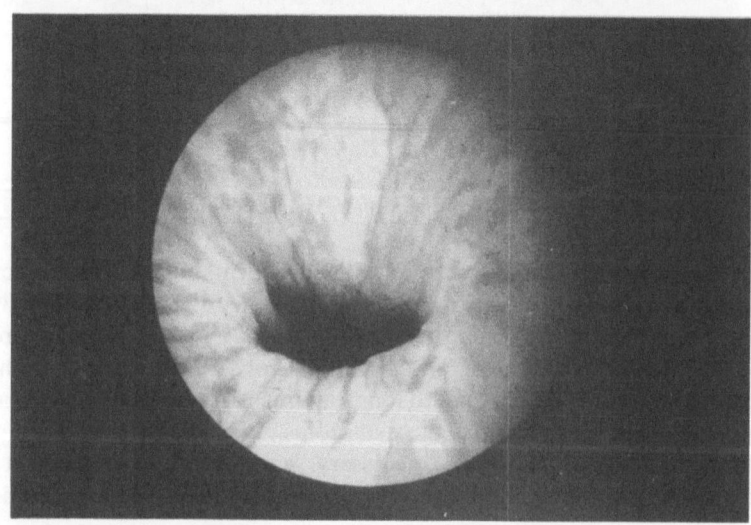

b

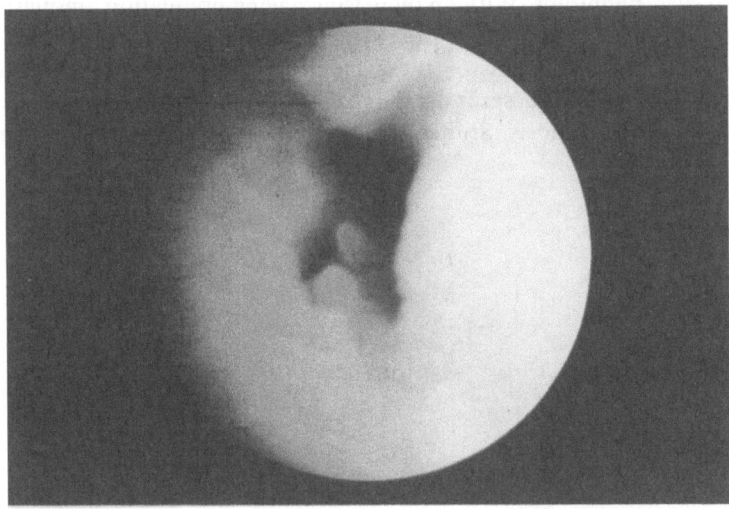

c

Figure 10.11 Urethroscopy – a: normal urethra; b: acute atrophic urethritis; c: chronic urethral stenosis

At the moment hormone replacement therapy is given over a 3-month period. Should symptoms recur following this, further 3-month courses of hormone therapy may be indicated. Prolonged hormone therapy is rarely required as most patients are unlikely to continue on treatment once their symptoms have settled. Some patients are unable to tolerate the hormone therapy by mouth, even in the very low dose prescribed. In these patients topical applications of hormone cream can be employed. Again Premarin 2–4 g omne nocte instilled into the vagina is an adequate alternative.

In both groups of patients treated with Premarin in this way it is important to remember that the hormone does not appear to affect the bladder function directly, its therapeutic effect being entirely due to the improvement in the tissues of the distal urethral segment. It will, therefore, take some time for the symptoms to settle and patients should be warned not to expect a rapid response, it sometimes taking 2–4 weeks before any real improvement is noted. This is despite the fact that the stratified squamous epithelium in the distal urethra may well revert to a normal pattern within days of hormone stimulation. This is understandable, as relief of what is effectively an inflammatory and obstructing lesion of the lower urinary tract will take time, as any patient undergoing prostatectomy will vouch.

CONCLUSION

Whilst its precise role in the causation of lower urinary tract symptoms remains unclear, there is no doubting the significance of the urethra in women with such symptoms. With an increasing ageing population amongst women the problem of lower urinary tract symptoms arising in the elderly will become more significant. Many of these elderly patients will have an atrophic urethritis, often with secondary infection and occasionally with secondary distal urethral stenosis. Studies have conclusively shown that these atrophic

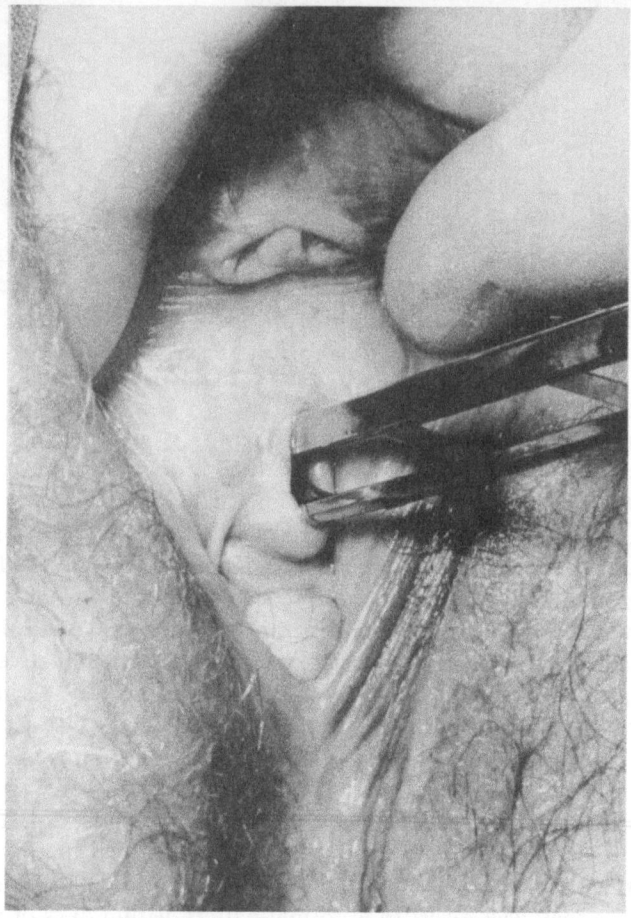

Figure 10.12   Dilatation of distal urethra using Otis urethrotome

changes are part of a physiological ageing pattern which can be rapidly reversed by estrogen therapy, combined, when necessary, with antibiotic treatment and, where stenosis is present, with a wide.urethral dilatation. These simple measures will result in a considerable improvement in symptoms for these patients and relieve them of much urinary misery. In the same way as improvements in prostatic surgery have enabled the elderly male to relax and enjoy life, so it would seem that a proper awareness of the management of atrophic urethritis in the elderly female may enable her to join him dancing in the street.

References

1. Everett, H. S. (1941). Urology in the female. *Am. J. Surg.*, **52**, 521
2. Parkes, A. S. and Zuckerman, S. (1931). The menstrual cycle of the primates. II. Some effects of oestrin on baboons and macaques. *J. Anat.*, **65**, 272
3. Smith, P. (1972). Age changes in the female urethra. *Br. J. Urol.*, **44**, 667
4. Meisel, A. (1966). The menopause. A cytohormonal study. *Acta Cytol.*, **10**, 49
5. Salmon, U. J., Walter, R. and Geist, S. H. (1941). The use of oestrogens in the treatment of dysuria and incontinence in post-menopausal women. *Am. J. Obstet. Gynecol.*, **42**, 845
6. Youngblood, V. H., Tomlin, E. M., Williams, J. O. and Kimmelsteil, P. (1958). Exfoliative cytology of the senile female urethra. *J. Urol.*, **79**, 110
7. Roberts, M. and Smith, P. (1968). Non-malignant obstruction of the female urethra. *Br. J. Urol.*, **40**, 694
8. Smith, P. (1977). The menopause and the lower urinary tract. Another case for hormone replacement therapy. *Practitioner*, **218**, 97

11
Relationships of Ovary, Endometrium and Vagina to Estrogen Therapy in the Postmenopause

S. CIANCI and P. BOEMI

Relationships are known to exist between the ovary with its hormonal secretion on the one hand and on the other hand the main peripheral receptors, endometrium and vagina; also known is the multiple variety of aspects of the ovary, endometrium and vagina in the pre- and postmenopause, both from the microscopic and macroscopic standpoint, together with the polymorphism of clinical symptomatology associated mainly with hormonal variations consequent upon ovarian senescence, which remains the focal point in periclimacteric physiopathology. Successive stages – first, failure of ovulation, then failure of follicular maturation whence failure of follicles – make the ovary represented eventually by a cortical part having stromal cells, atresic follicles, whitish and vitreous bodies and by a medullary part with clear signs of vasal sclero-ialinosis deteriorating in the course of time.

The functional result is that ovarian progesterone will be the first hormone to become deficient; progressively, at differing rates, the ovarian estrogens will then diminish.

Amenorrhoea will set in at some stage, because the flow rate of estrogens falls below the threshold of endometrial receptivity. All organs and organic systems influenced by the estrogens (uterus, vagina, mammae, uterine tubes, external genitalia, skin, bladder, bones, muscles, vessels, intermediate metabolism, psyche, etc.) will inevitably lose that impetus of estrogen-linked eutrophic stimulus.

Histological studies, both histoenzymological and ultra-structural, have clearly demonstrated the presence in the post-menopausal ovary of steroido-genic cells in stroma and hilum.

Research with incubation and dosage levels of plasmatic steroids, both in peripheral venous blood and ovarian vein blood, has shown that the normally steroidogenic activity of this ovary is quite capable of producing androgens (androstenedione and testosterone), whereas estrogen production is very low or absent through enzymatic deficiency.

Upsetting hypophyseal hypothalamic cortical activity, given the failed ovarian response, with hyperproduction of FSH and especially LH, stimulates the ovarian stroma and hilum further; because of their mesenchymal nature, evolving in several ways, they can increase androgen production or resume steroidogenic activities already abandoned.

The suprarenal gland also produces androstenedione and testosterone, besides dehydroepiandrosterone, and of these estrogens especially E_1. These androgens are then converted peripherally, especially at subcutaneous level, to E_1 with activity rates double or triple those of premenopausal women.

The relationship E_1/E_2 always shifts, therefore, more in E_1's favour and maintains itself above par. Tseng and Gurpide[1] have suggested, in this regard, that E_1 may be transformed into E_2 directly in the endometrium, triggering in certain cases the chain of proliferative processes from which endometrial pathology can ensue. The endometrium, in any case, is a faithful mirror of ovarian changes; usually, after the menopause, the simple atrophy of the latter is progressive and achieves stabilization over an average 2-year span.

In thickness on the thin side, usually reducing progressively from the tubo-uterine angles and from the base towards the isthmus, the epithelium follows suit, progressively decreasing in size from cylindrical–cubic to cubic with small cells, scarce cytoplasm and evident nuclei without or with rare mitoses; then it decreases further still until it even flattens with endothelial-like aspects; sometimes, through strangling the glandular outlets, secretion material accumulates inside the lumen which dilates the gland, conferring an atrophic cystic aspect on the endometrium; the stroma becomes denser with small round cells; vascularization is scarce and arterio-sclerotic phenomena are present in the context of the myometrial arteries. The above-mentioned phenomena are less evident in the base and tubo-uterine angles, where it is possible to find, even many years after the menopause, an endometrium which, if not proliferative, is only slightly hypotrophic. Hundreds of post-menopausal endometria have been studied to enable us[2] to reach this conclusion.

From these remarks one will realize the clinical advantage to be gained by being able to know the zone of the endometrium from which the biopsy test sample has been obtained.

Certainly, for most women (80%), the menopause involves such processes of endometrial atrophy: McBride cites 74% of cases, Novak and Richardson 77% and Foix 86%[3].

Another estrogen-sensitive tissue, the vagina, is also involved in the processes of atrophy. The vagina loses its soft and elastic qualities, the fornixes decrease in width, the mucosa becomes increasingly pallid and dry, smoothed out by loss of folds; the epithelium decreases progressively in thickness and at the same time glycogen disappears progressively, with consequent loss in the processes of auto-depuration and defence, and so the vagina becomes an easy prey to common germs. The degree of atrophy/dystrophy, with or without superimposed inflammation, may make the woman's sex life problematical, with possible dyspareunia.

In the light of these basic remarks on the relationships between the ovary, endometrium and vagina, it follows that by determining the estrogens in the blood or evaluating effects on the receptors (by biopsy and cytological testing) we may form *a precise picture of the estrogen level and can decide as to the wisdom of starting or continuing replacement therapy according to the case.* Not all women in post-menopause ought to be so treated; of course, not all of them can be, either, at the same rate.

The symptomatological pattern (genital and extragenital), however polymorphous, that accompanies the postmenopause applies to some 50% of the women; the intensity of the phenomenology depends on many different factors, such as how exactly the neuro-endocrine modifications have come about, date of onset and background personality.

If we also take into account the fact, which everyone is bound to have noticed, that the aspect of the ovaries, both microscopic and macroscopic, after the menopause varies, also the degrees of utero-vaginal atrophy (not infrequent also are cases where atrophic and/or dystrophic processes are absent in women many years after the menopause), we become more and more convinced that the key relationship at this juncture lies between the ovary, endometrium and vagina.

Hormonal dosage levels (for estrogens in particular, also for androgens), a *simple progesterone test* (to evaluate the residual estrogenic level, basic, and endometrial responsive capacity), *endometrial biopsy* in the event and the *index of estrogenicity* (colpocytological evaluation of the estrogen stimulus) represent the main routines.

The index of estrogenicity is calculated on the basis of the following formula, that in every smear four types of cells are distinguished and each is given a value, thus:

(1) Basal and parabasal cells   . . . .   value 0
(2) Intermediate cells 0.5
(3) Basophile superficial cells 0.8
(4) Acidophile superficial cells   1

Count 100 cells (or convert to a percentage if the cell number is not sufficiently high) and multiply the cells observed by the appropriate value. Thus, an overall index figure is obtained, called the *index of estrogenicity*;

obviously, it will lie somewhere between zero (cells all of the basal and parabasal stratum) and 100 (cells all of the superficial and acidophile stratum). A zero rating will show estrogen activity absent; below 50, a weak or approaching average activity in proportion as the count approaches 50; an index figure of 70–80 may be regarded as good, in terms of estrogen activity.

Probing these three sectors (ovary, endometrium and vagina), two or even one of them, given their interdependence, will therefore help furnish the information for a sound decision on the course of treatment to be prescribed, whether preventive or curative, in order to remedy the genital and/or extra-genital damage recognized as connected with the perimenopausal climacteric.

Estrogens represent the irreplaceable means of achieving this purpose (see Table 11.1); they may be used alone or associated with progestins, according to the scope in view, depending on the age of the patient and presence or absence of the ovaries. Administration will be preferably by mouth, since in cases of prolonged treatment it is undoubtedly the most convenient and tolerable; local means will be reserved exclusively for local alterations, verified in the genitalia.

Table 11.1   Steroid and non-steroid estrogens

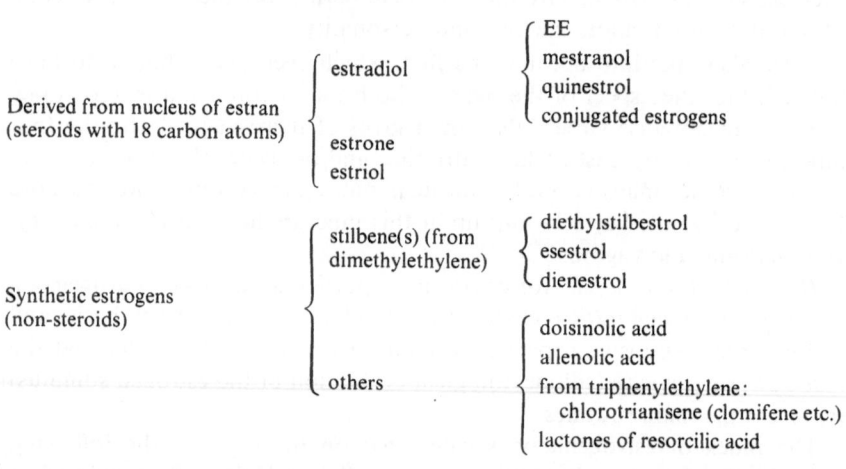

Derived from nucleus of estran (steroids with 18 carbon atoms)	estradiol	EE mestranol quinestrol conjugated estrogens
	estrone	
	estriol	
Synthetic estrogens (non-steroids)	stilbene(s) (from dimethylethylene)	diethylstilbestrol esestrol dienestrol
	others	doisinolic acid allenolic acid from triphenylethylene: chlorotrianisene (clomifene etc.) lactones of resorcilic acid

The question of restarting menses has to be considered, in particular if the woman patient so desires; this objective is possible up to an age limit which we set at about 55 – after 55 we administer estrogens only[4].

In precocious menopause, we strongly recommend the above type of therapy; in menopausal cases for surgery, with bilateral adnexectomy, we start estrogen–progestin treatment straight away, or estrogen; in cases with unilateral adnexectomy, treatment coincides with the onset of deficiency symptoms.

The choice of product is made according to the indications. and after careful thought as to any contraindications that may transpire in the event under general (clinical and laboratory) examination, be it gynecological, hormonal, cytological, endometrial or mammary; these examinations are to be repeated every 6 to 12 months during treatment. Estrogen–progestin treatment should be invariably periodic, whereas treatment with estrogens alone may be continuous or periodic (see later).

Per-therapeutic control is vital. As far back as 1974, we stated that the estrogen chosen ought to have *possibly analogous metabolism* to that which the organism enacts, with rapid and complete degradability so as to steer clear of any build-up phenomena; it must be suitable for prolonged treatments and without unpleasant side-effects, or as far as possible, such as water retention, mammary tension, abdominal tension, pelvic congestion, etc.[4].

EE and mestranol metabolize slowly and with difficulty: their strength is in part associated with this factor, also their toxicity.

The natural estrogens, then, are better (estriol, estrone and estradiol). These are, in fact, readily conjugated and eliminated; certainly, exogenous administration will never be superimposable on normal ovarian secretion.

The main thing is *not the derivation of the estrogen but rather its strength*; this is closely related to its receptor affinity, which in turn raises questions of absorption, bio-disposability of the free part (not SBP-bonded), basic endocrine situation, method of administration, etc. Receptor affinity will provide the relative strength[5], while absolute strength is measured relative to the dose employed. The time factor is another thing to remember, in *occupation of the receptors* on the part of the estrogenic substance[6,7]: it has been seen to vary considerably, according to the substance, and must undoubtedly tie in with the method of pharmacological administration to achieve the intended purpose. Studying some of the routines to determine estrogen activity (weight of uterus, DNA synthesis, mitotic index, cell distribution rating, number of cells, etc.) has shown that E_3, for example, induces the same response as E_2 at receptor level, but that the proliferative response of E_3 is inferior to that of E_2; to achieve in 24 hours the same effect of an E_2 dose, the same dose of E_3 must be administered every 5 h and five times over[7,8]. This shows that E_3 binds the nuclear receptor more weakly and so releases more rapidly.

We have used diverse estrogens and, from overall evaluation of their effects on the postmenopausal climacteric syndrome, our findings are that E_3, E_1 and the rals have given us the best results. This leads to the last thing to be decided concerning the method of treatment, in other words if it ought to be *continuous* or *periodic*.

We support discontinuous treatment: achieving determined indexes of cellullar trophism, with the guarantee of regular cell turnover, without predominance of growth factors and alternating with rest periods, of varied duration, to be established according to the instance; this enables us to avoid those protracted-stimulus situations where the high risks obviously lie.

Hormonal research on the ovary and study of the receptors, both endometrial and vaginal, given the relationships existing between these three sectors, will be invaluable to us in screening those women for whom postmenopausal estrogen replacement therapy may appropriately be started/ maintained over a varying period of time. The advantages for women, unthinkable before the days of estrogen–progestin or estrogen-only treatment, will be many; the effects on cenesthesis will be profound and favorable, with the happy result that a woman's standing is bound to rise in response to the improvement in her well-being.

SUMMARY

The relationships between ovary, endometrium and vagina can be shown by test routines which are easy to perform; note must be taken of these when postmenopausal estrogen therapy is going to be applied. Natural estrogens are preferable for this purpose, the choice depending on their strength; treatment procedures will be decided according to the individual case, personalized not only on the basis of the relationships between ovary, endometrium and vagina aforesaid but in the light of the individual's character and way of life.

References

1. Tseng, L. and Gurpide, E. (1972). Effect of estrone and progesterone on the nuclear uptake of oestradiol by slices of human endometrium. *Endocrinology*, **90**, 1041
2. Boemi, P., Pace, G., Cianci, A. and Di Stefano, F. (1978). Rapporti ovaro-endometriali nel climaterio. *59° Congresso Soc. Ital. Ostet. Ginecol.*, Parma 1978. (In press)
3. Netter, A. (1977). Menopause. *Encycl. Méd.-chir., Gynécologie*, 38, A-10, Paris 12
4. Boemi, P. (1974). Gli estrogeni nella terapia della sindrome climaterica. *Att. Ostet. Ginecol.*, **16–21**, 93
5. Bresciani, F. (1970). Ovarian steroid control of cell proliferation in the mammary gland and cancer. *Proc. Third International Seminar on Reproductive Physiology and Sexual Endocrinology*, Brussels, 1970
6. Bresciani, F., Nola, E., Sica, V. and Puca, A. G. (1973). Early stages in estrogen control of gene expression and its derangement in cancer. *Fed. Proc.*, **32**, 2126
7. Martin, L., Pollard, J. W. and Fagg, B. (1976). Oestriol, oestradiol-17β and the proliferation and death of uterine cells. *J. Endocrinol.*, **69**, 103
8. Haskins, A. L., Moszkowski, E. F. and Whistelock, V. P. (1968). The estrogenic potential of estriol. *Am. J. Obstet. Gynecol.*, **102**, 665

12
Prolactin in Post-menopausal Endometrial Hyperplasia and Adenocarcinoma

A. VOLPE, P. P. PELLEGRI, F. BOSELLI, V. MAZZA,
A. GRASSO, G. MACCARRONE, A. GOLES and
G. D. MONTANARI

In our previous study[1], concerning patients affected by endometrial adeno-carcinoma, we found prolactin levels statistically higher than in controls.

In a few cases treated with bromocriptine at high dosage we observed regressive modification in endometrial histopathology, but no variation on clinical follow-up. From these evaluations, we have continued our investigation, including also patients affected by endometrial hyperplasia.

MATERIAL AND METHODS

The present study refers to: 47 cases of endometrial adenocarcinoma, of which 35 were untreated and 12 previously operated on and treated with medroxyprogesterone; 17 cases affected by endometrial hyperplasia in various degrees; and nine controls without any endometrial pathology and without any steroidal treatment during the last 6 months (Table 12.1). The control group was matched for age, weight, blood pressure, years after menopause and carbohydrate metabolism (Table 12.2). As shown in Table 12.3, basal FSH, LH, E_1, E_2, T, PG, 17-OHPG, as well as hormonal response to GnRH, arginine, TRH and sulpiride were evaluated.

Table 12.1 Material

Untreated endometrial adenocarcinoma	35 cases
Treated endometrial adenocarcinoma (surgery and MAP*)	12 cases
Untreated endometrial hyperplasia	17 cases
Controls	9 cases

* 3 g/week for more than 2 months

Table 12.2 Comparison between patients with endometrial adenocarcinoma or hyperplasia and controls

Parameter	Endometrial adenocarcinoma (35 cases)	Endometrial hyperplasia (17 cases)	Controls (9 cases)
Years after the menopause	14.0 ± 7.4	15.0 ± 13.5	15.2 ± 7.0
Age	61.7 ± 7.9	56.7 ± 7.7	62.8 ± 6.9
Weight	73.7 ± 14.0	74.2 ± 14.0	68.1 ± 9.0
Mean blood pressure	111.9 ± 20.5	107.5 ± 11.2	112.2 ± 22.2
Positive glucose tolerance test	8 out of 13 cases	4 out of 5 cases	3 out of 5 cases

Table 12.3 Methods

FSH, LH, PRL[1]		
ESTRONE, ESTRADIOL[2]		
TESTOSTERONE, 17-OH-PROGESTERONE, PROGESTERONE[3]		
GnRH Test[1]	(100 µg i.v.)	FSH, LH at 0–15–30–45–60–90–120 min
Repeated GnRH Test[2]	(100 µg i.v. + 300 µg in saline solution during 180 min)	FSH, LH, E_1, at 0–15–30–45–60 min and every 30 min during 3 hours
TRH Test[4]	(200 µg i.v.)	PRL at 0–10–20–30–45–60–90–120 min
Arginine Test[5]	(25 g i.v. in 400 ml saline solution during 30 min)	GH at 0 min and every 30 min during 2 hours
Sulpiride Test[6]	(100 µg i.m.)	PRL at 0–30–60–90–120 min

[1] = All cases; [2] = 42 cases; [3] = 64 cases; [4] = 31 cases; [5] = 7 cases; [6] = 8 cases

All measurements were performed by radioimmunoassay (Kits Cea IRE, Sorin).

RESULTS AND DISCUSSION

During menopause, prolactin levels decrease as estrogen secretion by ovarian tissue is low (Figure 12.1). Hypophyseal reserve is also reduced, as demonstrated by the TRH test[2]. These findings would correlate with an actual reduction in the pituitary galactotrope-cell mass[3].

In menopausal women affected by endometrial adenocarcinoma, prolactin levels are significantly higher than in controls; moreover, in patients with endometrial hyperplasia, prolactin is also higher than in controls, but these

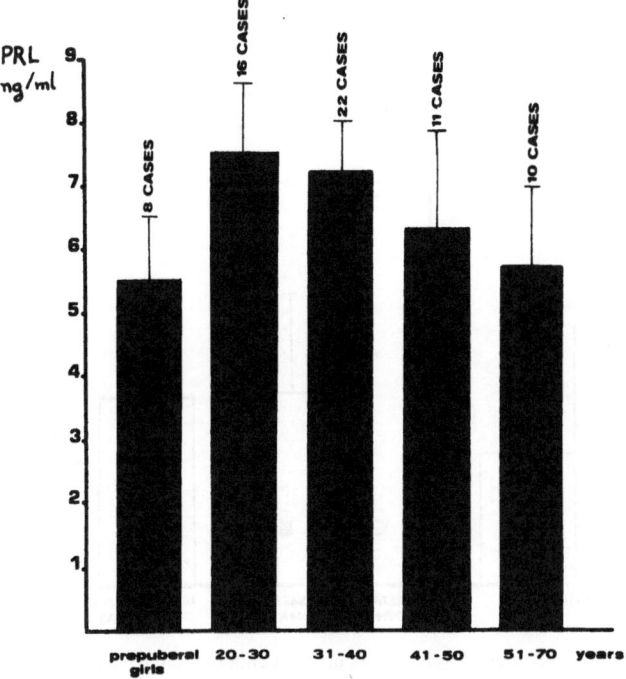

Figure 12.1 Prolactin levels according to different ages in woman

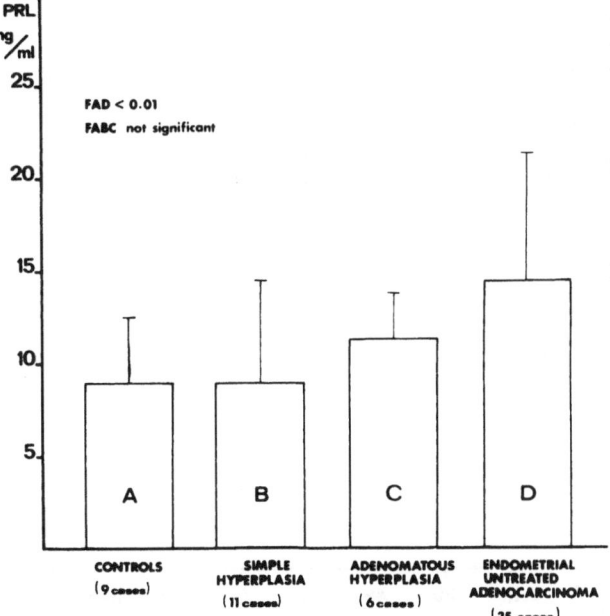

Figure 12.2 Prolactin levels in examined groups

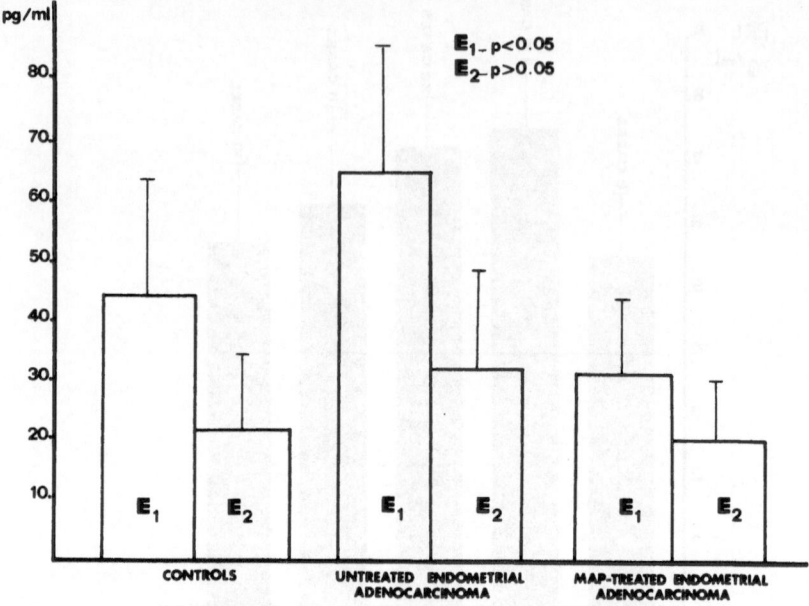

Figure 12.3   Estrone and estradiol levels in patients with endometrial adenocarcinoma and in controls

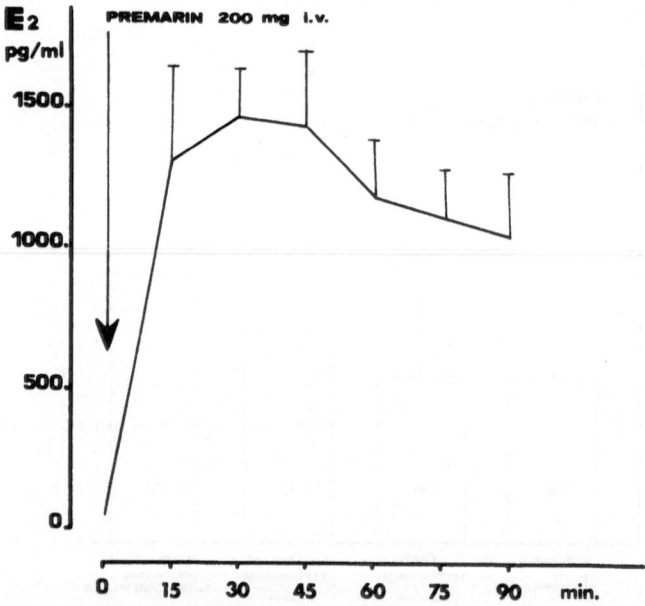

Figure 12.4   Estradiol levels after Premarin (estrone sulfate 48%) 200 mg i.v. (three cases)

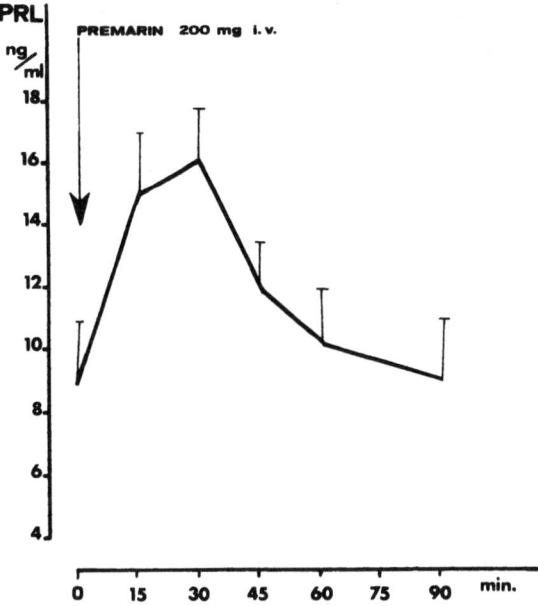

Figure 12.5 Prolactin levels after Premarin (estrone sulfate 48%) 200 mg i.v. (three cases)

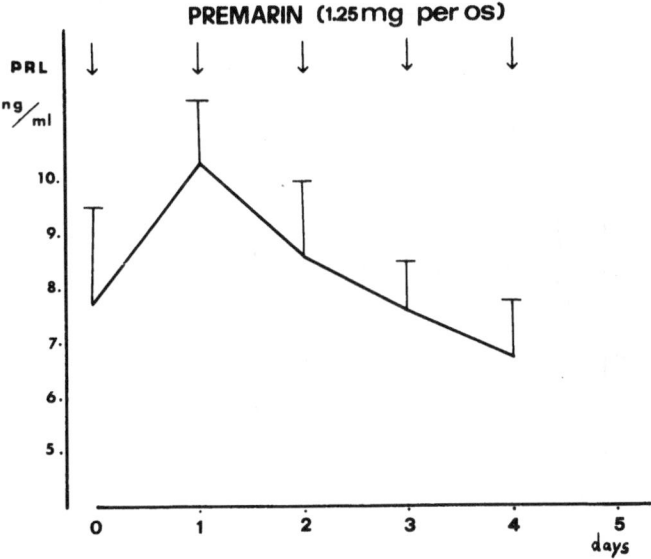

Figure 12.6 Prolactin levels after Premarin (1.25 mg per os) (five cases)

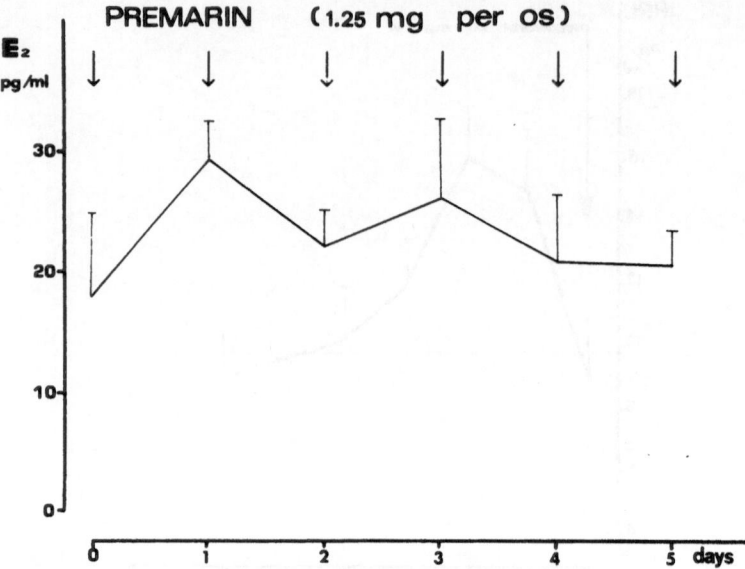

Figure 12.7   Estradiol levels after Premarin (estrone sulfate 48%) per os (five cases)

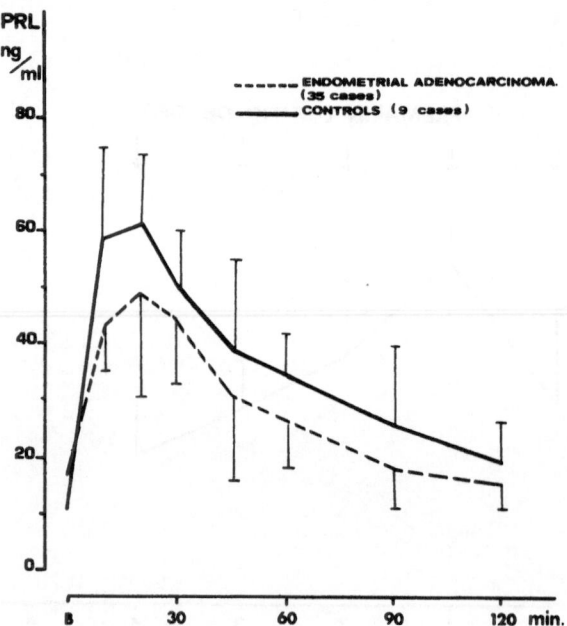

Figure 12.8   Prolactin response to TRH (200 μg i.v.) in patients with endometrial adenocarcinoma and in controls

data are not statistically significant (Figure 12.2). In all these cases, hyper-prolactinemia is probably related to hypothalamo-pituitary stimulus of estrogens. These increase prolactin secretion by acting on the hypophysis and perhaps on the hypothalamus, as is demonstrated by *in vitro* studies[4]. This action is mainly due to estradiol. However, in our patients estradiol is not significantly increased, while estrone is higher than in controls (Figure 12.3). This fact is probably due to metabolic conversion to estrone. 200 mg conjugated estrogens, with 48% of estrone sulfate, administered intravenously increase rapidly estradiol and prolactin levels (Figures 12.4 and 12.5). The same result, even if less remarkable, may be obtained with daily oral administration of 1.25 mg Premarin. It is interesting to note that, after 24 hours, although oral administration is continuing, prolactin and estradiol levels decrease (Figures 12.6 and 12.7). In patients affected by endometrial adenocarcinoma, we also observed low prolactin response to TRH (Figure 12.8) and sulpiride (Figure 12.9).

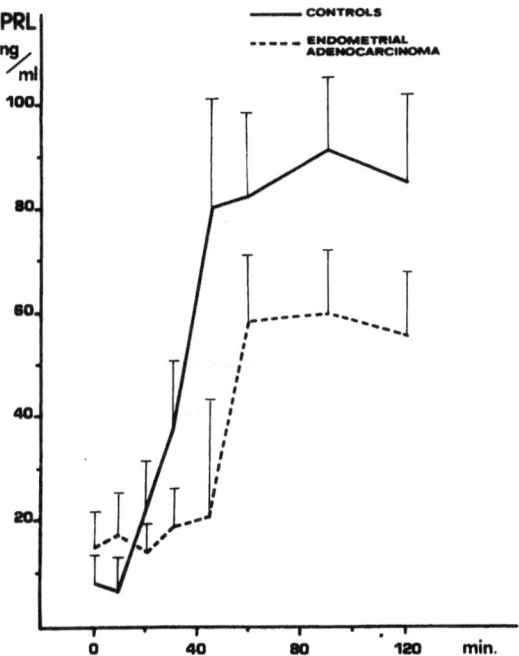

Figure 12.9   Prolactin response to sulpiride (100 mg i.m.) in patients with endometrial adenocarcinoma and in controls

Benjamin *et al.*[5,6] have reported the findings of hyperprolactinemia and other endocrine metabolic changes often manifest in these subjects as 'hypothalamo-pituitary dysfunction'. Dilman *et al.*[7,8] reported these findings as 'hypothalamic hyperactivity'. According to our experience, gonadotrophin levels were not significantly different in endometrial adenocarcinoma, hyperplasia and controls. A statistically significant decrease of these hormones was observed after high dose MAP treatment (Figure 12.10). In cases of adenocarcinoma, MAP inhibits endogenous secretion of LHRH from the hypothalamus. FSH, LH and estrone response to GnRH test is similar in the three examined groups (Figures 12.11, 12.12, 12.13 and 12.14). GH response to arginine is normal (Figure 12.15). Moreover, in cases treated with MAP at

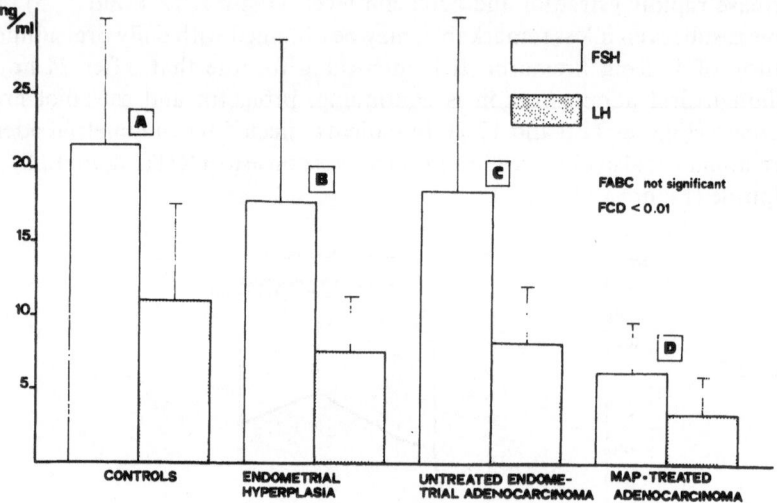

Figure 12.10   FSH and LH levels in the four examined groups

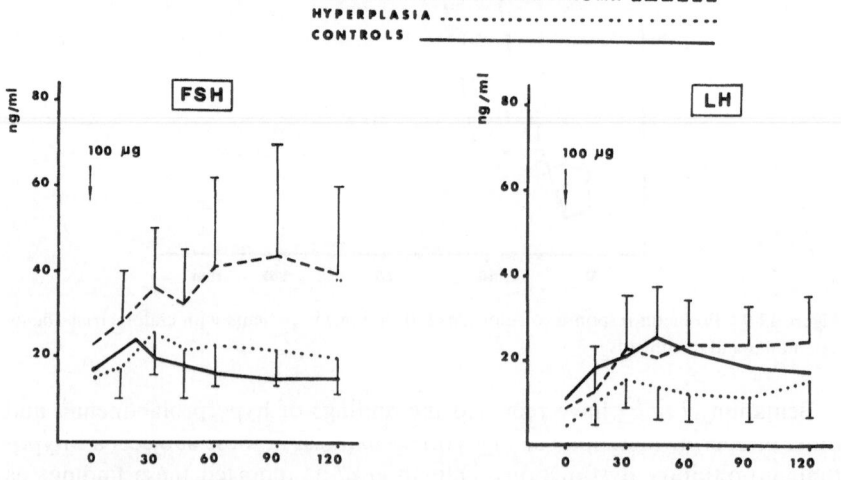

Figure 12.11   FSH and LH response to GnRH in the three examined groups

high doses, we have observed a decrease of gonadotrophin response to GnRH (Figure 12.16). Our results are in contrast with the findings of Franchimont et al.[9], but the difference is probably due to different doses of MAP used and to length of therapy. Testosterone, progesterone and 17-OH-progesterone plasma levels are similar among the examined groups (Figure 12.17).

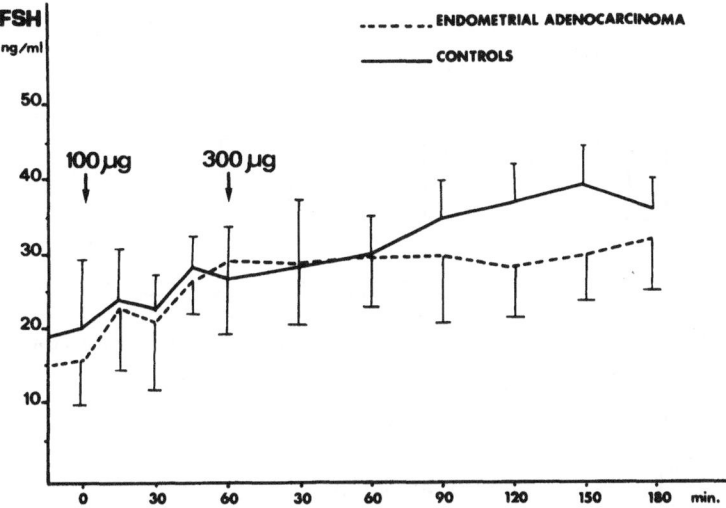

Figure 12.12 FSH response to GnRH in patients with endometrial adenocarcinoma and in controls

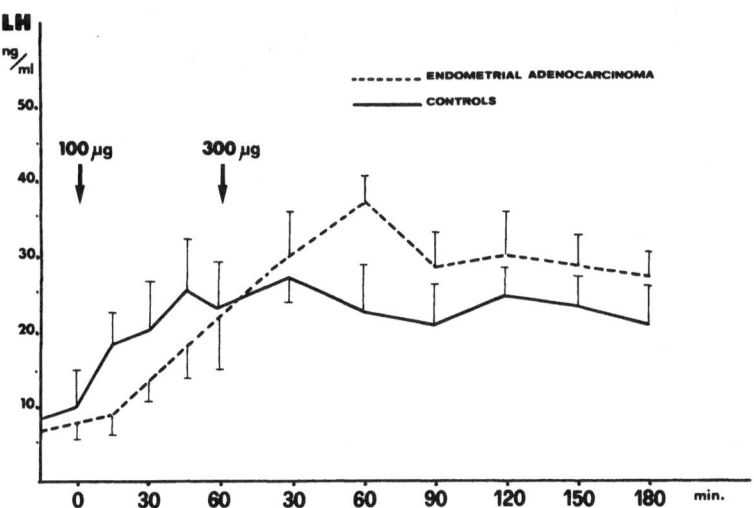

Figure 12.13 LH response to GnRH in endometrial adenocarcinoma and in controls

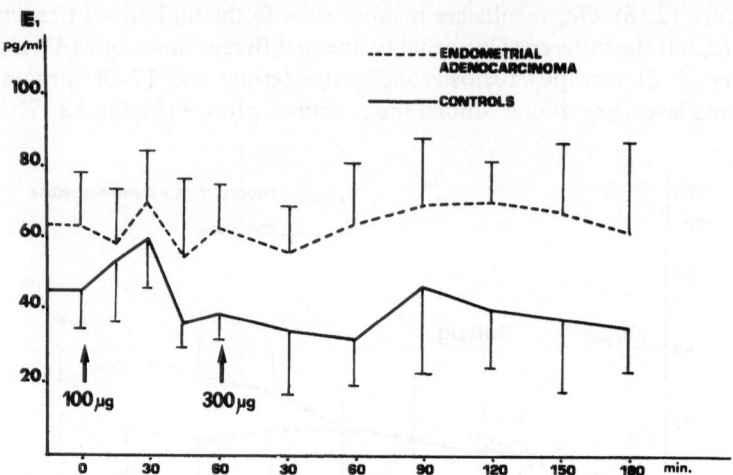

Figure 12.14 E₁ levels after GnRH in endometrial adenocarcinoma and controls

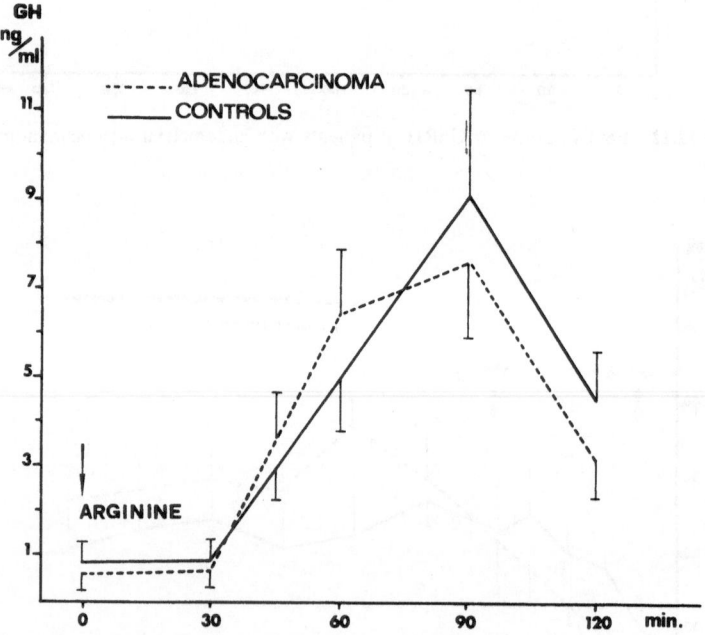

Figure 12.15 GH response to arginine in endometrial adenocarcinoma and in controls

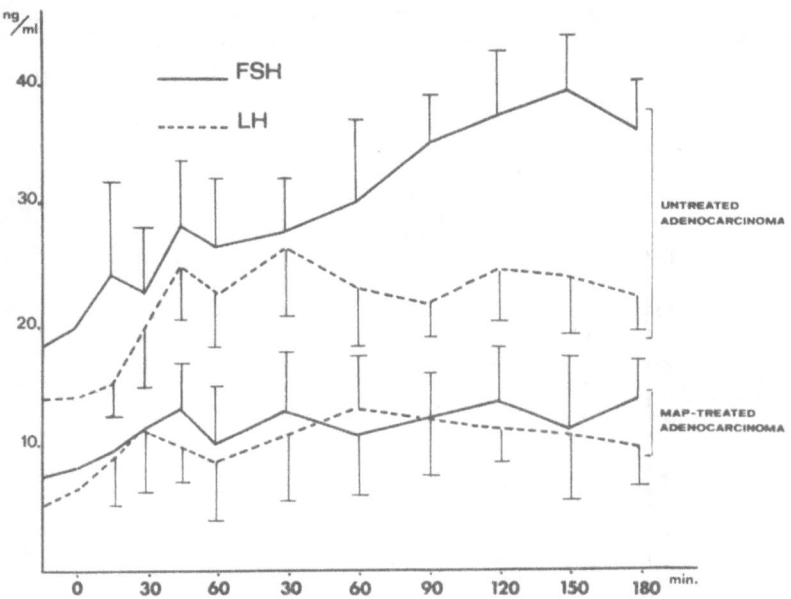

Figure 12.16 FSH and LH response to GnRH in untreated and MAP-treated endometrial adenocarcinoma

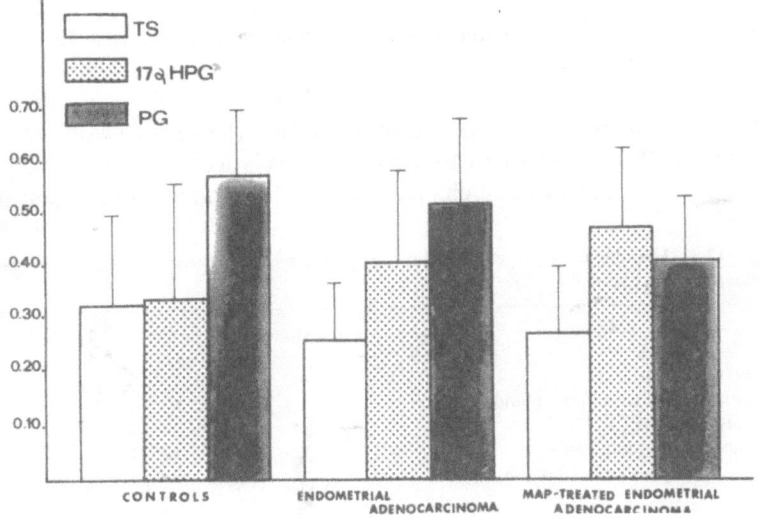

Figure 12.17 Testosterone, 17α-hydroxyprogesterone and progesterone in patients with adenocarcinoma and in controls

From these findings, we have tried experimentally to evaluate the effect of high dosage bromocryptine therapy in five cases of endometrial adeno-carcinoma. In three cases, therapy started during the pre-operative period, whereas two cases were in advanced phase of cancer. Daily maximal therapy

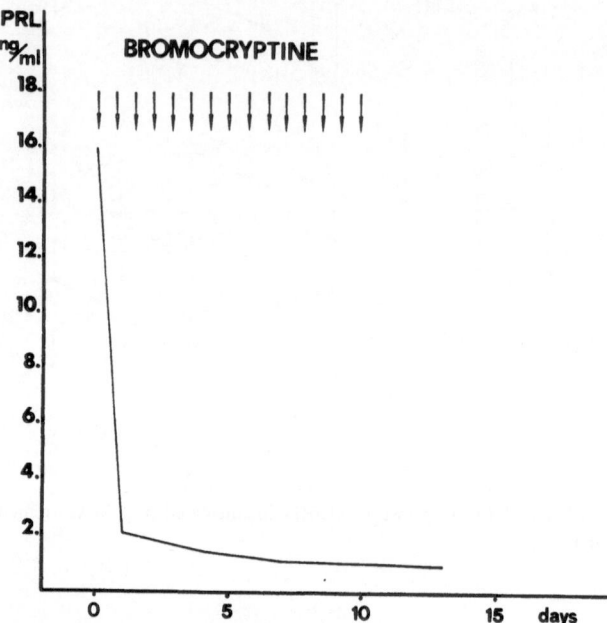

Figure 12.18   Prolactin levels during bromocryptine therapy (total dose from 250 to 700 mg; maximal daily dose 30 mg)

with 37.5 mg of bromocryptine was continued for a period of 3 weeks to a total amount of 700 mg. In all five cases, prolactin levels decreased to normal values (Figure 12.18). Histological changes were quite similar to those induced by

Table 12.4   Histological changes after bromocryptine in five patients affected by endometrial adenocarcinoma (Total dose 250–700 mg)

Response	Increased	Decreased	No change
Gland formation	4	0	1
Stratification of cells lining gland spaces	1	3	1
Mitosis (× 10 HPF)	1	4	0
Pyknosis of glandular cells	4	1	0
Vacuolation in cytoplasm of glandular cells	3	1	1
Necrosis	4	0	1
Secretory activity	3	1	1
Decidual change	1	0	4
Papillary formation	2	1	2

high dose progestagens, but these findings may be also observed in untreated adenocarcinoma. We want to point out the remarkable histologic regressive phenomena observed in two cases treated with more than 500 mg bromocryptine (Table 12.4). Bromocryptine therapy did not affect the long-term survival in these two cases.

It is impossible to state from our experiments whether or not the effect observed on the adenocarcinomatous cells is related to the drastic decrease of prolactin produced by bromocriptine or to a direct action of the ergot derivative on the neoplasm. In favour of the former hypothesis there is supportive evidence that prolactin can accelerate the appearance of the 3-methylcolantrene-induced uterus carcinoma[10].

References

1. Montanari, G. D., Volpe, A., Oliva, A., Baviera, G. and Mazza, V. (1979). *In:* G. D. Montanari and A. Volpe (eds.). *La Prolattina in Ginecologia.* (Padova: Piccin)
2. Jacobs, L. S., Synyder, P. J., Utiger, R. D. and Daughadey, W. H. (1973). *J. Clin. Endocrinol.,* **36,** 1069
3. Del Pozo, E., Hiba, J., Lancrainjan, I. and Kunzig, H. J. (1977). *In:* P. G. Crosignani and C. Robyn (eds.). *Prolactin and Human Reproduction.* (London: Academic Press)
4. MacLeod, R. and Lehmeyer (1974). *Cancer Res.,* **34,** 345
5. Benjamin, F., Casper, D., Serman, L. and Kolodny, H. (1969). *N. Engl. J. Med.,* **281,** 1448
6. Benjamin, F. and Deutsch, S. (1976). *Am. J. Obstet. Gynecol.,* **126,** 638
7. Dilman, V. M., Berstein, L. M., Bobrovy, F., Bohman, W., Kovalena, I. G. and Kylova, N. W. (1968). *Am. J. Obstet. Gynecol.,* **102,** 880
8. Dilman, W. M., Goluber, W. N. and Kylova, N. W. (1973). *Am. J. Obstet. Gynecol.,* **115,** 996
9. Franchimont, P., Gaspard, W., Van Cawenberge, R. and Depass, E. (1976). *In:* W. James,
   * M. Serio and G. Giusti (eds.). *The Endocrine Function of Human Ovary.* (London: Academic Press)
10. Forsberg, J. C. and Breistein, L. L. (1976). *Acta Pathol. Microbiol. Scand. A,* **84,** 384

13
The Prevention and Treatment of Endometrial Pathology in Post-menopausal Women receiving Exogenous Estrogens

J. W. W. STUDD, M. H. THOM, M. E. L. PATERSON
and T. WADE-EVANS

INTRODUCTION

Most gynecologists will now accept that approximately 25% of women of menopausal age would be sufficiently distressed by symptoms of estrogen deficiency to warrant specific estrogen therapy proven to be of benefit by many trials[1–3]. More recently, Hammond et al.[4] have demonstrated that replacement estrogen therapy has longterm metabolic benefits in significantly reducing the incidence of strokes, heart attacks, hypertension, osteoporosis and fractures. However, there is a widespread fear that this treatment will result in an increased incidence of endometrial carcinoma, although until 5 years ago it was generally believed that there was no such risk. There are now many case-controlled studies from the United States[5–9] showing between a five-fold and 15-fold increased risk of cancer of the uterus in these patients. This risk is both duration-dependent and dose-dependent.

These studies have been criticized in many ways, particularly by the selection of cases and controls, difficulty in interpretation of the endometrial histology and the unsupervised medication using unopposed estrogens long-term without any added progestogen[10]. Horwitz and Feinstein[11] have also suggested that bias exists in the methods of case control and have suggested alternative analytical methods for case-controlled studies where they found that unopposed estrogen administration carried a minimal risk far less than that alleged by Smith et al.[5], Zeil and Finkel[6], Mack et al.[7] and Jick et al.[9]. It is significant that Hammond et al.[12], while finding the undoubted benefits of longterm estrogen therapy, also reported an eight-fold increase in endometrial carcinoma in his patients taking unopposed estrogen.

PREVENTION OF HYPERPLASIA

Prolonged unopposed estrogen therapy induces endometrial hyperplasia[13] and, as a progression between cystic hyperplasia and adenomatous hyperplasia and adenocarcinoma is possible in susceptible patients[14-16], estrogen therapy in the postmenopausal woman must avoid any hyperplastic change in the endometrium. Even if unopposed estrogens are given cyclically with one week for endometrial shedding and uterine bleeding, it is clear that focal

Table 13.1   Current data ($n = 855$)

Regimen	n	Duration progestogen	Cystic hyperplasia
Syntex menophase	150	13	0%
Estradiol implant	40	13	0%
Estradiol implant	40	10	3%
Estradiol implant	145	5	9%
Estradiol implant	43	nil defaulted	56%
Cyclo-Progynova	58	10	2%
Cyclical Premarin low dose	76	nil	7%
high dose	233	nil	15%
high dose	70	7	3%

From reference 19

shedding of the superficial layer occurs and that most of the stimulated endometrium is left behind each month. This is in contrast with the patient having estrogen and supplementary progestogens in whom a 'pill-like', almost atrophic, picture of the endometrium is seen. This must be the objective of hormone replacement.

We have previously reported some results from our very large menopause clinic at Dulwich Hospital, London, and Birmingham Women's Hospital, and have revealed approximately a 15% incidence of hyperplasia with unopposed cyclical estrogens[17]. This is essentially in agreement with the studies of Campbell and Whitehead[18], except that our rates of hyperplasia for a given treatment regimen or bleeding pattern are slightly lower. Our current data, as shown in Table 13.1, is a simplified classification of 855 patients who have been under our supervision for up to 5 years, and have had an endometrial biopsy done by an outpatient Vabra curettage every year[19]. The data can be broken down in simple subpopulations which show that those women having low-dose cyclical Premarin (0.625 mg) have a 7% incidence of cystic hyperplasia. On the high-dose Premarin (1.25 mg) the incidence of cystic hyperplasia is 15%. If progestogen is added to this high dose regimen for 7 days each month, the incidence of hyperplasia falls to 3%. Cyclo-Progynova contains 10 days of a progestogen (+)-norgestrel and the hyperplasia incidence is only 2% with this preparation.

More than half our patients have subcutaneous implants of 50 mg estradiol and are instructed to take progestogen (norethisterone 5 mg) for 5–13 days each month. Sometimes the patients default, not taking the progestogen in a mistaken attempt to avoid bleeding, or to avoid some of the side-effects of progestogens such as breast discomfort, nausea, tiredness and dysmenorrhoea. These patients ultimately develop hyperplasia and heavy irregular vaginal bleeding. Fifty-six per cent of patients who do not take progestogens for 2 months or more develop hyperplasia. With 5 days of norethisterone the incidence is still high at 9%; with 10 days of norethisterone the rate is 3% and 13 days of norethisterone seems to prevent the occurrence of hyperplasia. It is of interest that Syntex Menophase, an oral preparation containing mestranol every day and 13 days of progestogen, also had a 0% incidence of cystic hyperplasia[17, 19]; thus it would appear that regardless of the type or the route of estrogens given, 13 days of progestogen is required to ensure that there is no endometrial hyperplasia.

Clinically our aim must be to use a combination of estrogen and progestogen which will produce the least possible incidence of hyperplasia and thus remove the risk of carcinoma and remove the need for an annual curettage. It is our belief that hyperplasia can be prevented by giving the lowest dose of estrogens required for removal of symptoms cyclically for 21 days out of 28, together with the addition of a progestogen for between 7 and 13 days each month.

TREATMENT OF HYPERPLASIA

The treatment of estrogen-induced endometrial hyperplasia has been reported[20]. In this study endometrial biopsies were taken from 850 patients who had been receiving various regimens of estrogen, sometimes without a progestogen, for climacteric symptoms for up to 30 years. These specimens were also obtained from outpatient Vabra suction curettage during the routine clinic visit, but a dilatation and curettage under general anesthesia was performed on patients in whom this proved impossible either due to distortion of the cervix by previous surgery or because of pain. The regimens often varied during the course of treatment as modifications were made in individual patients according to symptomatic response and their willingness to accept withdrawal bleeding or not. At any time approximately half of the patients had a subcutaneous implant of estradiol and all of these patients who have a uterus were informed of the need to take a monthly course of 5 or 7 days of progestogen. The others received oral therapy either cyclically for three weeks out of four, with or without a 7-day progestogen course, or continuously with a monthly course of 13 days of a progestogen in the form of Syntex Menophase. Some patients with endometrial pathology have been referred by other practitioners because of their irregular bleeding, so therefore this study is not able to ascertain the incidence of endometrial pathology on the various regimens at our two clinics, but was concerned entirely with the causation and treatment of these changes. When a patient was found to have cystic, adenomatous or atypical hyperplasia, oral estrogens were withheld and two 21-day courses of 5 mg norethisterone daily were prescribed separated by an interval of 1 week, when a withdrawal bleed occurred. The endometrial biopsy was repeated at the end of the second course, and if the endometrium remained abnormal, progestogens were prescribed separated by an interval of 1 week, when a withdrawal bleed occurred. The endometrial biopsy was repeated at the end of the second course, and if the endometrium remained abnormal, progestogens were prescribed daily until a hysterectomy was performed. All specimens were reported by a single observer (T.W.-E.) by light microscopy and selected specimens were prepared and examined by scanning electron microscopy.

Table 13.2   Cystic hyperplasia ($n = 60$)

Regimens	Duration progestogen	n pre-treatment	n post-treatment
Pretreatment	nil	3	0
Cyclical Premarin 0.625 mg	nil	2	0
Continuous Premarin 0.625 mg × 4 years	nil	1	0
Cyclical Premarin 1.25 mg	nil	13	0
Continuous Premarin 1.25 mg	nil	4	0
Cyclical Harmogen 3 mg	nil	1	0
Continuous Harmogen 3 mg	nil	1	0
Cyclical Progynova 2 mg	nil	2	0
Cyclo-Progynova	(+)-norgestrel × 10 days	1	0
Continuous stilbestrol × 10 years	nil	1	0
Continuous ethinyl estradiol × 10 years	nil	1	0
Implant estradiol 50 mg	norethisterone 5–7 days	9	0
Implant estradiol 50 mg	nil for at least 2 months	21	0

Cystic hyperplasia

There were 60 patients with cystic hyperplasia shown in Table 13.2; three of these occurred before treatment and they were all reversed to normal with one of the standard preparations, Cyclo-Progynova or Syntex Menophase, which contain 10 or 13 days of progestogen. The rest were given norethisterone in the way described. Hyperplasia was found in 17 women taking cyclical un- opposed estrogens and three patients taking continuous unopposed estrogens. Thirty patients had received an estradiol implant, but 21 of these had not taken the norethisterone as prescribed for 5 or 7 days each month. All of the 60 patients with hyperplasia had normal secretory or 'pill-like' endometrium after their correcting course of progestogen.

Adenomatous hyperplasia

There were eight cases of adenomatous hyperplasia shown in Table 13.3, six of these having a premenopausal history of menorrhagia. The patients had a greater association with abnormal menstrual history than the failure to take progestogen. Four of the eight patients did take progestogens and the other four did not. Six of the eight patients had their adenomatous hyperplasia reversed to normal with two 21-day courses of progestogens. The seventh case had returned to normal after five 21-day courses of progestogen.

Table 13.3   Adenomatous hyperplasia ($n = 8$)

Regimen	Duration progestogen	n pre- treatment	n post- treatment
Pretreatment	nil	2	0
Cyclical Premarin 1.25 mg	nil	2	0
Implant estradiol 50 mg	norethisterone 5–7 days	4	1

DO ESTROGENS CAUSE CANCER?

There is evidence that continuous estrogens, particularly in high doses, may, in women who are susceptible, cause cancer of the endometrium, but great care must be taken when attempting to extrapolate data related to theca cell tumors to the clinical problem of estrogen treatment for the menopause. The current reports which show the increased incidence of endometrial carcinoma describe very accurately American practice in the 1960s, that is, continuous therapy, often high-dose, occasionally cyclical; the use of stilbestrol and no addition of progestogen. The recent papers from Antunes et al.[8] and Hammond et al.[12] are particularly important because for the first time they describe details of estrogen therapy. In the 65 patients with carcinoma reported by Antunes *et al.*, none had taken progestogen. Half these patients were taking continuous therapy and nine were taking stilbestrol. Similarly, Hammond *et al.* reported 11 patients with cancer and only one – a patient with gonadal dysgenesis – had taken progestogen 'rarely' during the 24 years of cyclical therapy of Premarin 2.5 mg daily.

Recently, Jick *et al.*[9] have predicted a risk of cancer of the uterus of 20 per year per 1000 estrogen users. We are pleased to report that our experience does not reproduce this gloomy prediction. We have perhaps the largest menopause clinic in Europe, and, when the results of Dulwich Hospital and Birmingham Women's Hospital are combined, we can report that we have had no cancers in patients whose treatment we have initiated and supervised in more than 1000 patients over 5 years.

There have been, however, four patients with cancer of the uterus referred from elsewhere.

(1) A 65-year-old patient had a 10-year history or oral continuous therapy. She developed Stage I, Grade I carcinoma of the uterus and, after 4 weeks norethisterone, hysterectomy showed few small focal areas of well-differentiated carcinoma with no invasion into the myometrium. We regard this therapy as being grossly inappropriate.

(2) A 60-year-old patient had been taking ethinyl estradiol 0.05 mg daily continuously for 16 years. She was given an estradiol implant with 7 days progestogen orally without a preliminary curettage. Endometrial biopsy 6 months later showed an early carcinoma, which did not reverse with progestogen. This case demonstrates inappropriate continuous therapy for 16 years and the error of continuing estrogen therapy without a preliminary endometrial biopsy in these patients.

(3) A 54-year-old patient who took 9 months of cyclical Premarin and then had a 50 mg estradiol implant with 5 days of norethisterone for 18 months. Atypical hyperplasia was found but not treated, and 18 months later a second biopsy was considered to show well-differentiated adenocarcinoma. She was then referred to our clinic, pathology was confirmed by further curettage and hysterectomy following 1 month of 15 mg norethisterone showed atypical hyperplasia with no evidence of carcinoma.

The initial diagnosis was probably wrong in this case, and the administration of progestogen reversed the 'pseudomalignant hyperplasia'[21] into a less sinister pathology.

(4) A 68-year-old American patient had been taking between 5 and 12.5 mg Premarin every day for 30 years. She complained of four years of continual vaginal bleeding and a curettage showed a moderately differentiated adenocarcinoma. She refused surgery, but stopped Premarin and took 10 mg norethisterone daily for 6 weeks, and repeat curettage

confirmed the diagnosis. After a second opinion also suggested treatment in the form of surgery, she defaulted and was not seen again.

Four cases of adenocarcinoma referred to our clinic have been presented. Three are clearly the victims of inappropriate, poorly supervised therapy and the other was a pseudomalignant endometrium that showed a hyperplastic pattern following two courses of progestogen.

SCANNING ELECTRON MICROSCOPY

We are now studying in greater detail the surface ultrastructure of endometrial cells in order to assess the possibility of distinguishing between severe hyperplasia and early carcinoma. Initially we are attempting to characterize the cell surface characteristics of normal atrophic cells, proliferative cells, secretory cells and hyperplastic and malignant cells from patients with and without exogenous estrogens.

Endometrial biopsy specimens that were examined under the scanning electron microscope required careful preparation. They were first washed with saline to remove blood and mucus and then fixed for at least 2 hours in a mixture of sucrose, sodium cacodylate and glutaraldehyde solution. Cacodylate wash was then used to wash them for 1 hour, when they were dehydrated in graded ethanol–water solutions, and then treated with graded amyl acetate–ethanol solutions prior to critical point drying for about 2 hours. Finally they were mounted on SEM stubs and coated with colloidal gold.

The surface ultrastructure of normal proliferative endometrium similar to that described by Ferenczy and Richart[22] is shown in Figure 13.1. The specimen was taken from a patient who had been on an estrogen–progestogen preparation (Prempak 1.25 mg) for 2 years and was taken during the second week of the treatment cycle. The cells can be seen to be of uniform size and approximately one-third are covered with long cilia of uniform length. Numerous microvilli are seen on the remaining cells.

Figures 13.2 and 13.3 are from the same patient who had omitted the prescribed monthly courses of progestogen after an implant of estradiol. Figure 13.2 shows the surface ultrastructure of the specimen obtained when she returned to the clinic complaining of the inevitable heavy bleeding. The histology was reported as showing cystic hyperplasia. The cells are still of uniform size, but there has been a proliferation of cilia of more variable length. Figure 13.3 is the surface of part of the endometrium obtained after the usual two 21-day courses of norethisterone 5 mg daily, separated by an interval of a week. The obvious change after progestogen is that the number of cilia is greatly reduced. Some of the microvilli are fused and some cells appear wrinkled, and all are more pleomorphic. These changes are indicative of withdrawal of the estrogen stimulation and progestogen therapy.

Figure 13.4 is a detail of the specimen from the patient with carcinoma of the endometrium described in case 4. The cells can be seen to have marked surface changes, as described by Ferenczy and Richart[23]. There is considerable variation in cell size and appearance and no ciliated cells are visible. The surface of the enlarged cells show a loss of surface architecture and some of

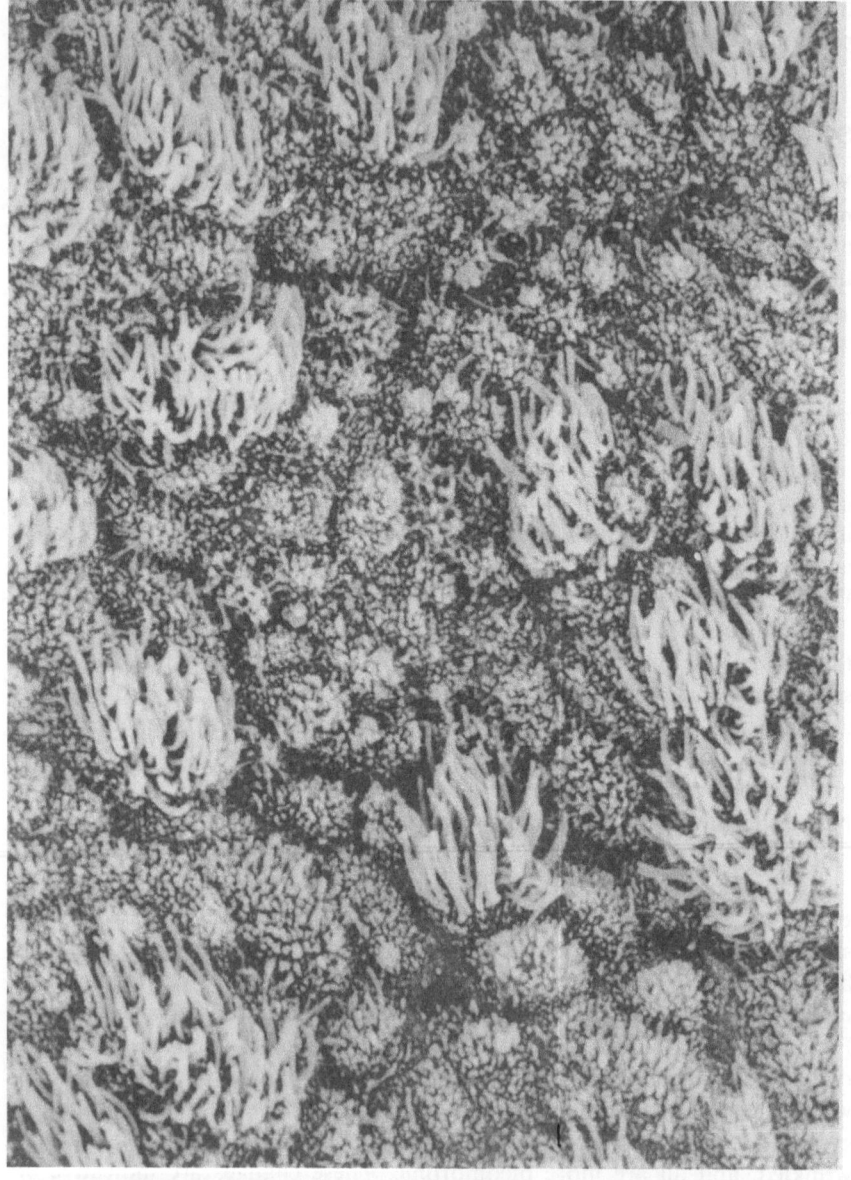

Figure 13.1   SEM view of the surface of normal proliferative endometrium

them measure up to 20μm in diameter. Microvilli are seen, but appear variable, abnormal and fused in places. The membrane of a cell in the top right-hand corner is folded and could represent a greater surface area for increased metabolic function of the tumor cells. These wrinkles seen with the

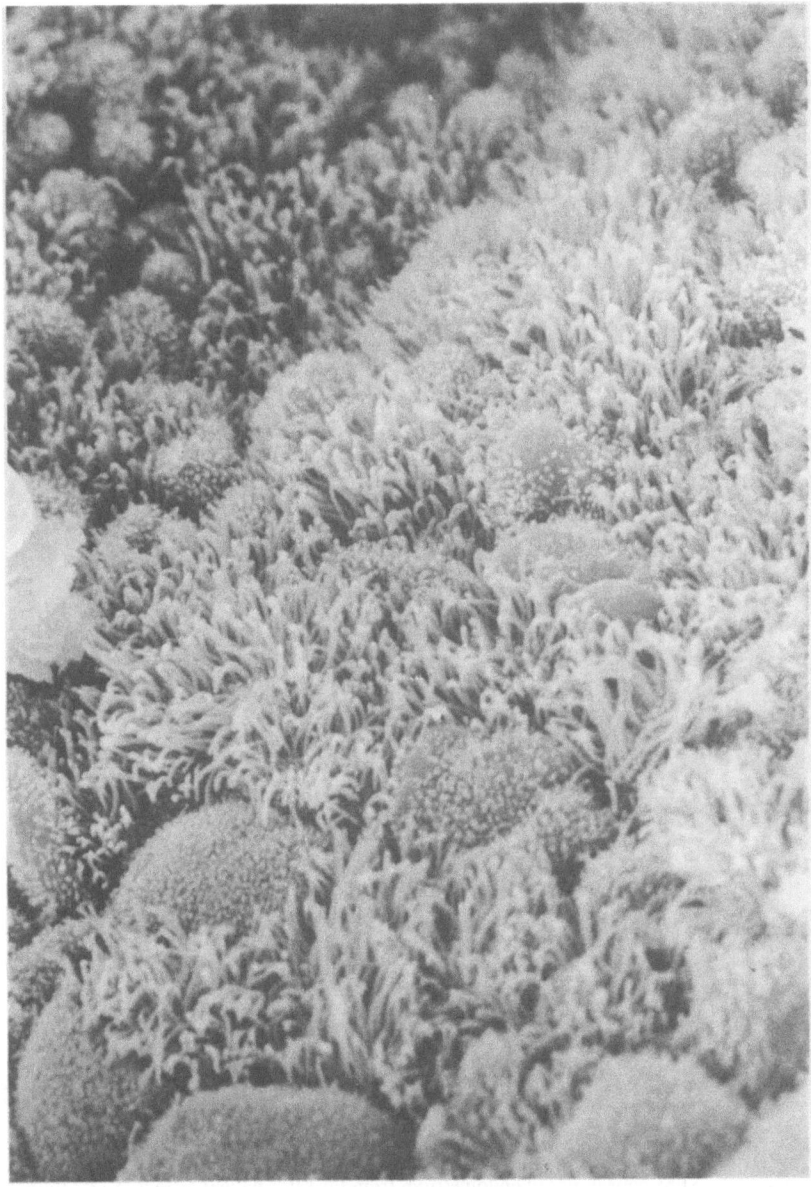

Figure 13.2   SEM appearance of cystic hyperplasia of the endometrium

scanning electron microscope may correspond to the variations and irregularities of the cell surface in adenocarcinoma cells studied with the transmission electron microscopy and noted by Nilsson *et al.*[24]. With loss of differentiation of the carcinoma viable histologically, the surface changes are even more dramatic.

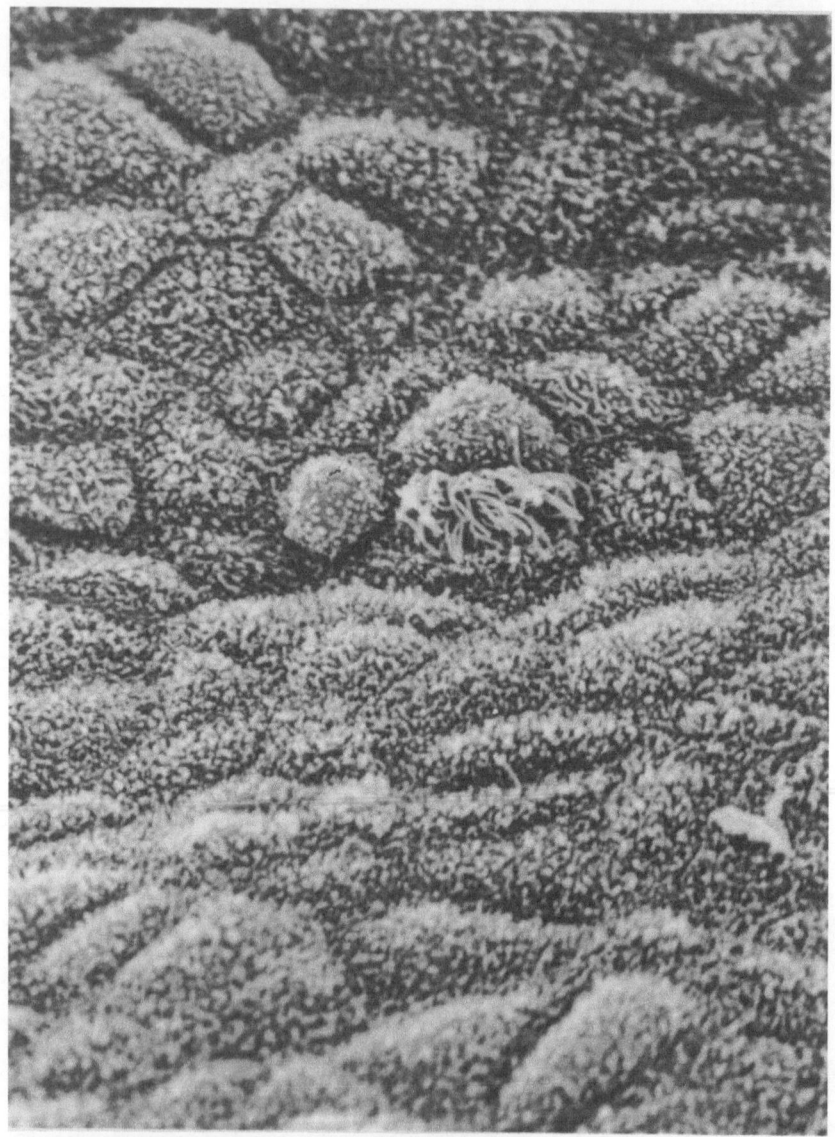

Figure 13.3   SEM appearance of endometrium from the same patient as Figure 13.2 following treatment with two 21-day courses of norethisterone

There remains considerable controversy concerning the risk of endometrial carcinoma with estrogen therapy. Our findings are that much of the anxiety produced by the case-controlled studies is the result of the type of therapy and supervision given to these women over the last 20 years. For the most part excessive doses were used, and there is much self-medication without adequate diagnostic surveillance of the endometrium or the use of a diagnostic test of progestogen when an apparently malignant hyperplasia was found. Above all, most patients had unopposed estrogens either continuously or cyclically and the addition of progestogens was, and still is, a rarity. There are exceptions in that Greenblatt[25] and Gambrell[26] have recommended the use of progestogens for 10 years or more, and have not found this increased incidence of endometrial carcinoma.

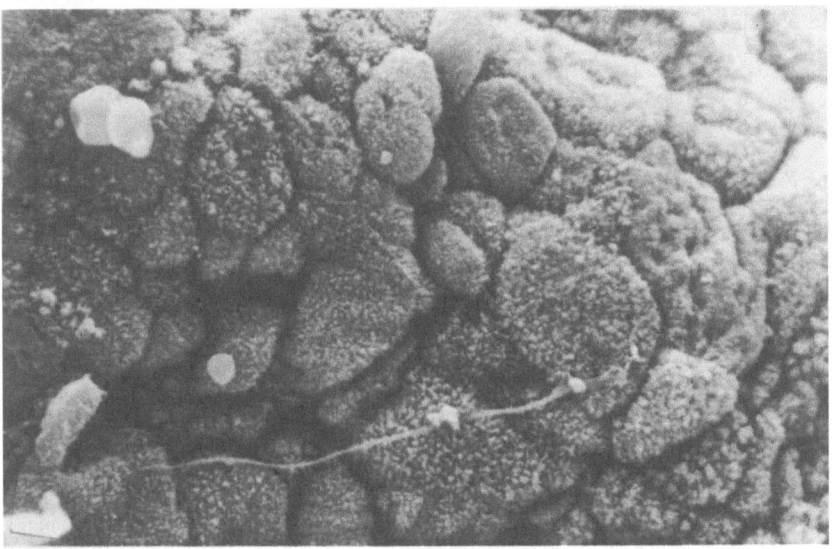

Figure 13.4   SEM appearance of adenocarcinoma of the endometrium from a patient taking unopposed estrogens for over 30 years

In conclusion, we believe that the danger of endometrial carcinoma can be eliminated by the addition of between 7 and 13 days of progestogen, and that, to our knowledge, there is no evidence in the medical literature that low-dose cyclical estrogen with 7 to 13 days progestogen is in any way associated with an increased risk of cancer of the endometrium.

Acknowledgment

We would like to thank Mr R. Senkus and Mr K. Davies for their invaluable help with the scanning electron microscopy.

References

1. Utian, W. H. (1972). The true features of the post-menopause and oophorectomy and their response to oestrogen therapy. *S. Afr. Med. J.*, **46**, 732

2. Campbell, S. and Whitehead, M. I. (1977). In R. B. Greenblatt and J. W. W. Studd (eds), *Clinics in Obstetrics and Gynaecology*, **4**, 31–47. (London: Saunders)

3. Studd, J., Chakravarti, S. and Oram, D. (1977). In R. B. Greenblatt and J. W. W. Studd (eds), *Clinics in Obstetrics and Gynaecology*, **4**, 3–29. (London: Saunders)

4. Hammond, C. B., Jelovsek, F. R., Lee, K. L., Creasman, W. T. and Parker, R. T. (1977). Effects of long-term estrogen replacement therapy. *Am. J. Obstet. Gynecol.*, **133**, 525

5. Smith, D. G., Prentice, R. and Thompson, D. J. (1975). Association of exogenous estrogens and endometrial carcinoma. *N. Engl. J. Med.*, **293**, 1164

6. Zeil, H. K. and Finkle, W. D. (1975). Increased risk of endometrial carcinoma among users of conjugated estrogens. *N. Engl. J. Med.*, **293**, 1167

7. Mack, T. M., Pike, M. C., Henderson, B. E., Pfeffer, R. I., Gerkins, V. R., Arthur, M. and Brown, S. E. (1976). Estrogens and endometrial cancer in a retirement community. *N. Engl. J. Med.*, **294**, 1262

8. Antunes, C. M. F., Stolley, P. D., Rosenheim, N. B., Davies, J. L., Tonascia, J. A., Brown, C., Burnett, L., Rutledge, A., Pokempner, M. and Garcia, R. (1979). Endometrial cancer and estrogen use. *N. Engl. J. Med.*, **300**, 1

9. Jick, H., Watkins, R. N., Hunter, J. R., Dinen, B. J., Madsen, S., Rothmark, J. and Waiter, A. M. (1979). Replacement estrogens and endometrial carcinoma. *N. Engl. J. Med.*, **300**, 218

10. Studd, J. W. W. and Thom, M. H. (1979). Estrogen use and endometrial cancer. *N. Engl. J. Med.*, **300**, 922

11. Horwitz, R. I. and Feinstein, A. R. (1978). Alternative analytic methods for case control studies of estrogens and endometrial cancer. *N. Engl. J. Med.*, **299**, 1089

12. Hammond, C. B., Jelovsek, F. R., Lee, K. L., Creasman, W. T. and Parker, R. T. (1979). The effects of long-term estrogen replacement therapy. II. Neoplasia. *Am. J. Obstet. Gynecol.*, **133**, 537

13. Gusberg, S. B. (1947). Precursors of corpus carcinoma. Estrogen and adenomatous hyperplasia. *Am. J. Obstet. Gynecol.*, **54**, 904

14. Welch, W. R. and Scully, R. E. (1977). Pre-cancerous lesions of the endometrium. *Hum. Pathol.*, **8** (5), 503

15. Gusberg, S. B. and Kaplan, A. L. (1963). Precursors of corpus cancer. IV. Adenomatous hyperplasia as Stage 0 carcinoma of the endometrium. *Am. J. Obstet. Gynecol.*, **87**, 662

16. Hertig, A. T., Sommers, S. C. and Bengloft, H. (1949). Genesis of endometrial carcinoma. III. Carcinoma *in situ*. *Cancer*, **2**, 964

17. Sturdee, D. W., Wade-Evans, T., Paterson, M. E. L., Thom, M. H. and Studd, J. W. W. (1978). Relations between bleeding pattern, endometrial histology and oestrogen treatment in menopausal women. *Br. Med. J.*, **1**, 1575

18. Campbell, S., McQueen, J., Minardi, J. and Whitehead, M. I. (1978). The modifying effect of progestogen on the response of the post-menopausal endometrium to exogenous oestrogens. *Postgrad. Med. J.*, **54** (Suppl. 2), 59

19. Patterson, M. E. L., Sturdee, D. W., Wade-Evans, T., Thom, M. H. and Studd, J. W. W. (1979). (In preparation)

20. Thom, M. H., White, P. J., Williams, R. M., Paterson, M. E. L., Wade-Evans, T. and Studd, J. W. W. (1979). The prevention and treatment of endometrial lesions in women on oestrogen therapy for climacteric symptoms. *Lancet*, **2**, 455

21. Oestergaard, E. (1974). Malignant and pseudomalignant hyperplasia adenomatosa of the endometrium in post-menopausal women treated with oestrogen. *Acta Obstet. Gynecol. Scand.*, **53**, 97

22. Ferenczy, A. and Richart, T. M. (1973). Scanning and transmission electron microscopy of the human endometrial surface epithelium. *J. Clin. Endocrinol. Metab.*, **36**, 999

23. Ferenczy, A. and Richart, R. M. (1973). Scanning electron microscopy of hyperplastic and neoplastic endometria. In O. Johan (ed.), *Scanning Electron Microscopy 1973, Part III.* Proceedings of the Workshop on SEM in Pathology, pp. 613–20. (Chicago: IIT Research Institute)

24. Nilsson, O., Kottmeir, H. L. and Tillinger, K. G. (1963). Some differences in the ultra-structure of normal and cancerous human uterine endometrium. *Acta Obstet. Gynecol. Scand.*, **45**, 73

25. Greenblatt, R. B. (1965). Estrogen therapy for postmenopausal females. *N. Engl. J. Med.*, **272**, 305

26. Gambrell, R. D. Jr. (1974). Perimenopausal and postmenopausal bleeding: mechanisms, pathology, management with progestational agents. In R. B. Greenblatt, V. B. Mahesh and P. G. McDonough), *The Menopausal Syndrome*, pp. 147–56. (New York: Medcam Press)

14
Treatment of Patients at Risk. Cross-over Study between Natural Estrogens

N. PASETTO, E. PICCIONE, F. PASETTO, L. BASCHIERI
and R. MATURI

The concept that estrogen therapy, in the menopausal and postmenopausal woman, may constitute a potential risk tending to determined morbid situations is generally accepted at the present day. It is based on data of two kinds:

(1) from case histories of oral contraceptive hormonal treatment in which the estrogen employed derives from synthetic C-17-alkylate formulations administered at a dosage level distinctly superior (about three to four times) that adopted in menopausal replacement therapy;

(2) from retrospective epidemiological studies on the presumed increased incidence of malignant neoplasia cases (uterine and mammary) in menopausal subjects who have used estrogens; plus objective information about estrogen–cancer relationships, namely:

(a) that endometrial carcinoma can be induced in animals through parenteral treatment with stilbestrol;

(b) that obesity presents a high risk of endometrial adenocarcinoma (because of higher circulating estrogens levels); and lastly

(c) that there is a direct relationship between estrogen treatment in quantity and duration and cystic glandular hyperplasia arising in the endometrium.

In so far as menopausal estrogen replacement therapy does not make use of synthetic C-17-alkylate estrogens, and in so far as findings to date concerning the cancer–estrogen association fall short of documented proof as to the existence of a cause–effect relationship, a potential-risk hypothesis may be considered tenable until such time as documentary evidence shows differently.

Estrogen therapy, like every other form of treatment based on highly active drugs, also involves side-effects which may be highly detrimental in the case of some patients. It is not always possible to tell in advance who are, or may be, the patients most at risk in regard to any such complications.

What has emerged clearly is that the occurrence of side-effects or complications is always 'dose-dependent', even 'type of estrogen-dependent'.

RISK FACTORS

Type of estrogen

All observations on estrogen complications refer to synthetic C-17-alkylate formulations. This has led to unjustified generalization about the estrogen risk[1]. Natural and synthetic estrogens present different metabolic characteristics and also different metabolic effects.

Metabolization

Administration of ethinylestradiol (EE) by oral means produces an immediate, massive and prolonged concentration of estrogen at hepatic level (compared with natural preparations).

In fact, since EE does not bind the vector plasma-specific proteins (as does most of the estradiol), and since it is solely the non-binding, that is to say free, form, the one active at cellular level, it follows that its administration leads to acute hematic peaking of active hormone.

Further, at endometrial level EE does not comprise a substratum for the action of the enzyme 17-β-estradiol-dehydrogenase, which has the function of breaking down the natural estradiol to estrone (thus to a less active compound) it develops at such a level a much more intense estrogen activity.

Its halflife, moreover, is much longer (7 hours) compared to natural estradiol (90 minutes); given that oral administration (the conventional method for synthetics) brings about an estrogen concentration in the portal system four to five times greater than in the peripheral venous network, at the intrahepatic level it sets up an exceptional condition of hyperestrogenism.

In the liver, the estrogens bind to specific cytoplasmic and intranuclear receptors[2], thus stimulating directly the various biosynthetic reactions which underlie these metabolic disturbances responsible for the various risk factors. This select action on the part of estrogen at the hepatobiliary level also entails greater cholestatic effect, and the administration of synthetic (C-17-alkylate) estrogens causes the phenomenon of build-up, increase and persistence of the estrogen effect. It is this particular concentration and retention of estrogen at the intrahepatic level, outside the physiological margins of fluctuation, which holds the key to interpreting the diverse metabolic effects between natural and synthetic formulations.

Clotting

Apart from the fact that it is at present impossible to ascertain the real significance of variations in some clotting factors, objectively there has been found to exist a substantial difference between natural and synthetic estrogen formulations with regard to clotting factors.

At conventional dosage levels in replacement therapy, the natural ones cause no variation or minimal variation in the intrinsic and extrinsic blood coagulation systems and platelet behavior[3]; alterations have been found with synthetic estrogens and may last for up to 9 months from end of treatment[4].

Vascular wall

Besides the clotting process, the contrast in effects between synthetic and natural estrogens is apparent also at the level of the vascular wall. Whereas a vascular protective role has been attributed to the natural ones[5], synthetic formulations by contrast would be responsible for deleterious alterations to the vascular wall, such as endothelial proliferation and fibrous conditions with subendothelial thickening. In some tissues particularly vulnerable to the exaggerated concentration and retention of synthetic estrogens, such as the liver and endometrium, an intense vascular neoformation has been noted, with parietal thickening. Responsibility for this deleterious effect has been thought to belong in part, aside from the dose-dependent factor, to the presence of the ethylin radical in C-17, given that the same alterations have been observed using androgen-derived formulations with the ethylin radical in C-17.

With regard to the vascular protective effect in natural compounds, recent work[6] on the presence of specific receptors for estradiol in the endothelial cells propounds a physiological role for natural estrogen on secreting properties of the endothelium in the sense that prostaglandins, the fibrinolytic system and HDL convey degradable excess cholesterol to the liver.

Impossibility of reproducing in menopause and postmenopause the normal hormone profiles of premenopausal ovarian endogenous secretion

By oral administration, rapid and intermittent stepping-up of blood flow rates can be obtained, but endogenous secretion has its own rhythm, allowing for daily variations. Secondly, oral administation produces a different blood picture from that of the premenopause; whatever the amount of estradiol or estrone that may be administered, estrone is always prevalent in the blood relative to estradiol.

At the intranuclear level, independently of the blood flow rates for estradiol and estrone, the prevalent estrogen is estradiol. The problem of more or less risk in administering estradiol or estrone by oral means thus disappears.

The relationship between estradiol and estrone in the blood is conditioned by the method of administration (oral/intestinal mucosa). Further, even with natural compounds, oral administration leads to estrogen levels in the portal system from four to five times higher than those present in the peripheral venous system.

With reference to gonadotropin behavior (FSH and LH) during estrogen therapy, evidence shows that the estrogen dose permitting the blood level to attain premenopausal levels is not sufficient to restore the premenopausal gonadotropin level. To resume this level, a high estrogen dosage would be required so as to bring about a hyperestrogen state[7].

Dose-dependent factor

That the side-effects are dose-dependent has been amply demonstrated in the laboratory and clinical practice, both for natural and synthetic formulations, and in respect of general metabolic effects, e.g. upon the genitalia.

Recent work on the blood levels of estrogens during treatment shows that, from the quantitative angle, estrogen therapy is not really at replacement level, since conventional dosage, based on empirical observations or because of the therapeutic end-effect, is frequently higher than that required to restore the premenopausal blood rate levels.

On the other hand, it is maintained by various authors that for replacement purposes the blood levels of estrogen required ought to be lower than those present in the organism during the fertile years. This may be valid from a physiological standpoint but, from the therapeutic point of view, the use of dosages above physiological levels is often required.

CROSS-OVER STUDY BETWEEN NATURAL FORMULATIONS

Within the scope of the estrogen effect, a distinction emerges in quality and quantity with regard to various natural formulations. This distinction is evident, in relation to estriol dosage levels, on the vagina and endometrium, and especially where catecholic compounds are concerned[8], which are inactive at endometrial level and particularly active at cerebral level.

A distinction in quality of effect appears also to be shown between natural and synthetic formulations in the context of effect on the nervous system; it seems to be absent or very slight in stilbene compounds and derivatives[9].

Since menopausal symptoms vary and are deemed to connect directly only in part with the state of estrogen deficiency, special interest attaches to study of the existence of a relationship between dose–effectiveness and type of symptoms in natural formulations (conjugated estrogens and estriol).

An outpatient study has been carried out during the last 2 years on a cross-over basis, using conjugated estrogens at a dosage level of 1.25 mg per day and estriol at a dosage level of 2 mg per day. Treatment continued for both natural formulaticns over 3 weeks in a given month and for a 2-month period.

The two groups each comprised 20 patients, in the age ranges from 46 to 55, 1 to 3 years into the menopause and presenting approximately analogous symptoms. The patients knew they were under hormone treatment and that the change of medication after a 2-month period was designed to help investigate which was the more effective, tolerable product. Effectiveness was assessed in the context of the various menopausal symptoms and response in psychosomatic terms was measured on the Campbell scale[14].

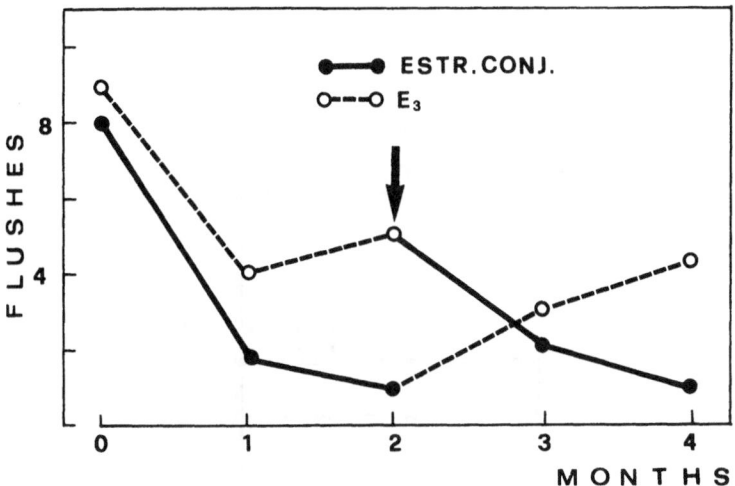

Figure 14.1   Cross-over study between conjugated estrogens and estriol on hot flushes

At vaginal level (maturation rating, vaginal dryness) and vesical level (cystalgia and micturition frequency), the two preparations showed more or less equal effectiveness.

The effect on psychosomatic and vasomotor symptoms was diverse in intensity, higher marks going to the conjugated estrogens at the dosage level adopted (Figures 14.1 and 14.2).

A different effect was found concerning symptoms under the heading of 'mental effect'. It is possible that this diverse effect, as to intensity, may be dose-dependent for estriol, since it alone at dosage levels decidedly higher (6 to 8 mg/day) than those advised (1 to 2 mg/day) seems able to show therapeutic

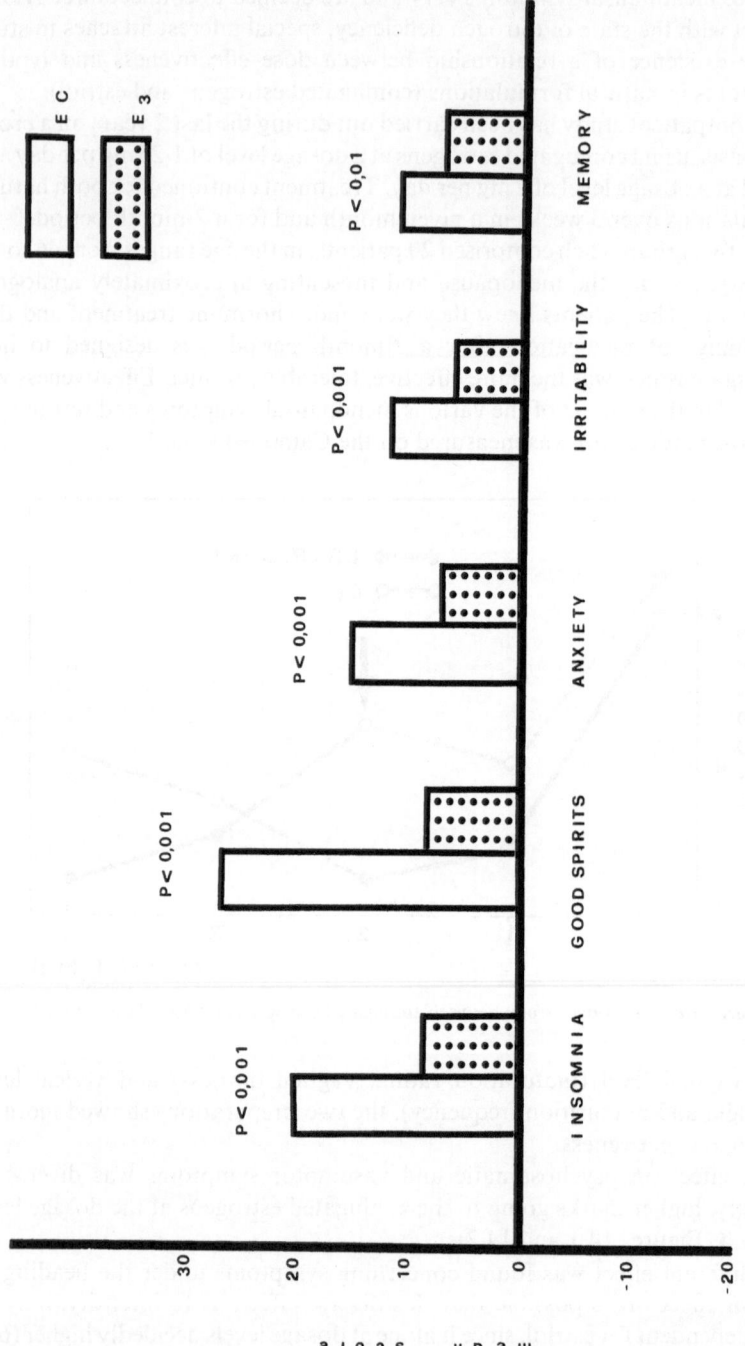

Figure 14.2 Differences in graphic rating scores for conjugated estrogens and estriol therapy

effect[15]. Given the brief treatment period, it is not possible to evaluate any placebo effect.

PATIENTS AT RISK

To speak of patients at risk concerning estrogen therapy means, apart from singling out contra-indications, also choosing treatment methods that carry the minimum risk of complications. Treatment options, at the present time, depend on adjusting the treatment to the individual subject, in equating a choice of estrogen type with the type of symptom prevailing, in using progestin or estrogen associated with androgens and in determining the length of treatment.

The treatment, it goes without saying, is not for all patients, only those who warrant it. For patients requiring short-term treatment, the problem does not arise. The difficulty comes with the need for long-term treatment, since no special guidelines are available for selecting which patients to treat, except on the basis of persisting symptoms; there is no known routine for recognizing which patients at risk can have long-term treatment.

Picking out the patients at risk, if at times extremely easy on anamnestic data alone, at other times is impossible.

Hypertension

High blood pressure increasing by reason of age is not modified by estrogen treatment at low dosage levels and if carried out with natural formulations. In cases where the response is hypertensive, this is due to patient characteristics or dosage levels which have been high in the first instance.

The pathogenetic background covers many factors, that is certain; a general view is taken that estrogen works through a two-fold mechanism, namely by action on the renicardiac–aldosterone system and direct action on sodium retention. On the basis of recent work showing the presence also in cerebral tissue of a renin-like enzyme and a renin substrate, action on the nervous system has also been put forward.

Contra-indications for the treatment must comprise persistent hypertension, renal and cardiovascular disturbances. If hypertension arises during treatment, it means reducing the dosage or suspending it; if treatment must continue, then recourse may be had to spironolactone in small doses. The alternative in the event, using progestins, does not lessen the hypertensive risk given the mineral–corticoid effect of the progestins.

Lower glucose tolerance

Lower glucose tolerance, relatively frequent with synthetic formulations, may appear also with natural preparations if used at high dosage levels; but in the small doses which are conventional it is widely held that no significant modifications are observed. Various hypotheses have been advanced in explanation, such as increase of transcortin, cortisol, somatotropic hormone or interference with glucagon secretion and alteration of the insulin–glucagon ratio in the portal blood.

Particular importance attaches to the method of administration, in so far as alterations are more clearly manifest with treatment by oral means. Simply reducing the dose may put matters right and the metabolism returns to normal within weeks.

Patients at risk comprise diabetics, subjects with an obstetric history suggestive of a prediabetic condition and obese subjects. Diabetes, if not associated with serious vascular changes, does not present an absolute contra-indication.

As an alternative treatment, estrogen may usefully be associated with an androgen administered by parenteral means, or a progestin. But it has to be remembered that progestin also involves the question of possible effects on the carbohydrate metabolism.

Cholestasis–cholelithiasis

This is a complication with all steroids and so may occur in using natural ones also, though apparently much more frequent with EE and especially mestranol. Estrogens depress or inhibit the biliary excretive function, this action being dose-dependent and reversible. They produce, in addition, a more saturated bile, consequently predisposing to lithiasis. Particularly at risk are those patients who had cholestasis and pruritus in pregnancy. Progestins on the whole present the same risk too, especially norethisterone and derivatives.

Thromboses and thromboembolism

Epidemiological tests and biochemical data on clotting have underlined how serious this complication is. It has been shown that an increase takes place in factors VII, VIII, IX, X and fibrinogen level and platelet aggregation and a reduction in antithrombin III in correlation with plasminogen and fibrinolysis of the vascular wall. All these observations concern use of synthetic estrogens in very high dosages and over a considerable period.

Also the method of administration is important, since oral means influence the coagulation system more than the parenteral. None of these alterations has been found with natural formulations at low dosage levels as, for example, 2 mg estradiol valerate, 1.25 mg conjugated estrogens and up to 6 mg estriol. Recently the use has been envisaged for screening of study of antithrombin III.

In line with the above, our findings drawn from case histories of patients under estrogen therapy over periods ranging from 1 to 5 years have not shown any variation in this regard, either with estradiol valerate or conjugated estrogens or estriol. Although at the present time no test is available to establish who may encounter thromboembolic complications, accurate evaluation means taking into account all known risk factors, such as smoking, or surgery or prolonged immobilization. The presence of varicose veins in the lower limbs is a risk factor for thromboses. The risk can be reduced by limiting treatment to only 2 or 3 days per week, or else by prophylactic use of salicylates or sulphinpyrazone. The use of progestin may offer an alternative.

Hyperlipidemia–pancreatitis

That the fertile woman has a lower incidence of coronary diseases than the opposite sex is a matter of general agreement. Why this happens is not absolutely clear.

The menopause itself brings about a rise, over the premenopausal phase, in the cholesterol triglyceride rate. Synthetic estrogens lead to an increase in triglycerides (by increased synthesis and liberation), associated with a small increase in cholesterol. The natural ones, at lower dosage levels, have no significant activity; the conjugated ones stimulate production and removal of VLD-triglycerides. A decrease has been observed with estradiol and estriol[10].

When there is a family background of lipidic disturbances or hyperlipidemia occurs, then a thorough assessment of the lipidic state is needed both prior to and during treatment. If hyperlipidemia type IV occurs, treatment can bring a strong increase in triglycerides and may possibly occasion pancreatitis. The proportions of the hypertriglyceridemia rise represent the critical factor in the onset of pancreatitis. But this complication, fortunately, is very rare. It is advisable to avoid treatment in cases of hyperlipidemia type IV and, when necessary, to verify lipidemic conditions frequently and carefully.

As a treatment option, it is worth remembering that progestins of nortestosterone derivation also, though to a lesser extent, act on lipidemia, whereas gonanic compounds display a protective effect, neutralizing the estrogen effect.

Endometrial and mammary cancer

This comprises the gravest risk in long-term treatment, but opinions vary widely on the real dimensions of this risk. The carcinogenesis is very complex, calling many factors into account: according to Lauritzen[10], the estrogens are endowed with an optional co-carcinogenetic role and it appears arguable whether estrogen alone can occasion neoplasia without other predisposing factors and really carcinogenetic factors. All the same, it is the general view that estrogens administered alone and over prolonged periods can increase the risk of endometrial cancer.

At the present time, there is no test available capable of predicting accurately which patients are going to encounter neoplastic degenerative difficulties. It follows that if various risk factors are at work, the decision to treat requires a particularly cautious approach.

For the endometrium, the researches of Campbell, Studd and (in the biochemical field) of King clearly demonstrate the protective role of progesterone and the need to observe low dosage margins both for estradiol valerate and the conjugated estrogens; dosage levels considered medium to low in relation to clinical effectiveness can turn out to be excessive at endometrial level. From this there follows the need for treatment to be adapted to the individual, according to the symptoms presented, and for cyclical treatment to be adopted in association with progestin.

For progestin, it is advisable to distinguish type, dose, treatment cycle, which should be from about 8–10 to 13 days. In the choice of progestin, preference may be given to those formulations which, conserving the anabolic androgen effect, can be helpful in regard to osteoporosis.

Annual tests of the endometrium need to be conducted by aspiration/cytological examination or complete histological examination. For the breast, at present it is not known if what has been verified in biochemical terms at endometrial level, as between estrogen and progesterone, applies also to mammary tissue. In high-risk cases, it is worth considering the advisability of treatment by progestin alone or else estroprogestin or estro-androgen. Progestin appears indicated for breast and endometrium, also because of the fact that increasing the clearance rate of androgens helps the liver to reduce the 5-α and so slow androgen–estrogen conversion.

Epidemiological studies[11, 12] have indicated that estriol is constructive in preventing mammary neoplastic transformation. Opinions differ about this protective role of estriol; also under discussion at the present time is its description as a weak or 'impeded' estrogen in the light of the latest research on relations between estrogen action and intranuclear permanence of the receptor complex[13]. With continuous exposure to estriol action, as treatment verifies and as happens in nature anyway, its effect would be estradiol-like. At endometrial level, it does not constitute a substrate for 17β-dehydrogenase.

There is less than general agreement also on the use of progestin in estrogen therapy of the menopause, because of the risk of superficial thromboses and because of cerebrovascular disturbances and for its psychosomatic effect, completely opposite from that of estrogen.

References

1. Lauritzen, C. (1978). Management of the patient at risk. *Front. Hormone Res.*, **5**, 230. (Basel: Karger)
2. Eisenfeld, A. J. *et al.* (1978). Oral contraceptives. Possible mediation of side effects via an estrogen receptor in liver. *Biochem. Pharmacol.*, **27**, 2571

3. Studd, J. *et al.* (1978). The effect of hormone replacement therapy on glucose tolerance, clotting factors, fibrinolysis and platelet behaviour in post-menopausal women. In: I. D. Cooke (ed.). *The Role of Estrogen/Progestogen in the Management of the Menopause.* (Lancaster: MTP Press)

4. Aylward, M., Maddock, J., Lewis, P. A. and Rees, P. L. (1977). Oestrogen replacement therapy and blood clotting. *Curr. Med. Res. Opin.*, **4**, Suppl. 3, 83

5. Wolinsky, H. (1972). Effects of estrogen and progestagen treatment and the response of the male rat aorta to hypertension/morphological and chemical studies. *Circ. Res.*, **30**, 341

6. Colburn, P. and Buonassisi, V. (1978). *Science*, **201**, 817

7. Utian, W. H. *et al.* (1978). Effect of premenopausal castration and incremental dosages of conjugated equine estrogens on plasma follicle-stimulating hormone, luteinizing hormone and estradiol. *Am. J. Obstet. Gynecol.*, **132**, 297

8. Martucci C. and Fishman, J. (1977). Direction of estradiol metabolism as control of its hormonal action. Uterotrophic activity of estradiol metabolites. *Endocrinology*, **101**, 1709

9. Kopera, H. (1973). In: *Front. Hormone Res.*, p. 120. (Basel: Karger)

10. Lauritzen, C. (1976). Oestrogen and endometrial cancer. *Clin. Obstet. Gynecol.*, **4**. (London: Saunders)

11. MacMahon, B. *et al.* (1973). Etiology of human breast cancer: a review. *J. Natl. Cancer Inst.*, **50**, 21

12. Lemon, H. M. (1975). Estriol prevention of mammary carcinoma induced by 7,12-dimethyl-benz(a)anthracene and procarbazine. *Cancer Res.*, **35**, 1341

13. Clark, J. H. *et al.* (1978). Estrogen receptor binding and growth of the reproductive tract. *Pediatrics*, Suppl. 62, 1121

14. Campbell, S. (1976). In: S. Campbell (ed.). *The Management of the Menopause and Post-menopausal Years*, p. 149. (Lancaster: MTP Press)

15. Tzinbounis, V. A. *et al.* (1978). Estriol in the management of the menopause. *J. Am. Med. Assoc.*, **239**, 1638

15
Estrogen Therapy preparatory to Vaginal Surgery in Advanced Menopause

G. B. CANDIANI and S. G. CARINELLI

The lamina propria of the vagina and oeso-cervix is rich in elastic tissue, disposed in typical architectural arrangement. Thin elastic fibres lie in the lamina propria, forming a relatively thick tissue becoming slightly denser around the vessels. Coarser fibres, thickly packed, gather in the lee of the basal membrane of the lining epithelium, however, to form a characteristic sub-epithelial stratum; on this, fibres stand out perpendicular to the main axis of the vagina, anchoring onto the elastic network of the lamina propria. The subepithelial elastic stratum is the structure most sensitive to modifications of the lamina propria, induced by physiological and pathological factors[1-3].

Modifications of the elastic tissue of the vagina and cervix have been studied before; recently, we have checked previously published findings against our own, made from surgical biopsy material, with the aim of evaluating in particular the subepithelial stratum modifications (Table 15.1). From our records, it emerges that marked atypias of the elastic tissue were present in

Table 15.1 Elastic tissue of vagina relative to hormonal state

	Vaginas examined	Atypias of elastic tissue
Women of fertile age	33	11 (33%)
Women in postmenopause	12	8 (67%)
Total	45	19 (42%)

67% of women patients in postmenopause and in those over 48 years of age, while in women of fertile age, atypias of the elastic tissue were present in only 33% of cases and in women under 48 years of age in 21% of cases. Modifications of the vaginal and cervical mucosa induced by age and the subject's hormonal state are indeed correlative, therefore, with alterations in the elastic tissue.

Recently, we have undertaken a study of the elastic tissue of the lamina propria of the vaginal–cervical tract after estrogen therapy, preparatory to vaginal surgery corresponding to advanced menopause. Over the 5-year period from 1973 to 1977, a total number of 1861 celiotomy operations and 346 non-celiotomy operations were performed; laparo-hysterectomy operations numbered 665 and colpo-hysterectomy operations 401. These preliminary figures make it plain that vaginal surgery figures largely in the work-load of this clinic, partly because of a lead given here some 50 years ago (Table 15.2).

Table 15.2   Five-year period 1973–77

Celiotomy operations	1861
Non-celiotomy operations	346
Laparo-hysterectomies	665
Colpo-hysterectomies	401

As to the celiotomies by vaginal path, within the same 5-year period from 1973 to 1977, it is of interest to note how in the distribution by age-group the vaginal operation peaks among the 'forties and 'fifties, the clinical indications referring for the most part to metrorrhagic symptoms resistant to medical therapy; a fairly high rate still obtains after the age of 65, when the indications for the operation will depend on alterations in the pelvic statics (Table 15.3).

Table 15.3   Celiotomy operations *per vagina*: distribution by age group in the 5-year period 1973–77 ($n = 401$)

<30	31–40	41–45	45–50	51–55	56–60	61–65	>65
0	34	74	110	64	27	38	54

Precise indications for surgery are set out in detail in Table 15.4. Of 401 operations, it will be seen that 224 cases, equivalent to 55.87%, are referable to the pathology of ptosis of the pelvic organs.

In the final table (Table 15.5), the type of vaginal surgery is given as a percentage figure, in the course of which colpo-hysterectomy was in all cases carried out. This serves to show how important to the vaginal gynecologist the preparation of vaginal tissues can be; their collection from vesica, uterus and rectum is anatomically basic in considering the various structures concerned in the pathology of pelvic statics.

Now, estrogens are known to hypertrophize in a similar manner the vaginal epithelium; they do not induce eutrophic modifications to connective and muscular structures of the apparatus for suspension of the uterus. These data are of fundamental interest insofar as if the amputated uterine ligaments can offer adequate support to tamp the peritoneal hiatus after removal of the uterus, it is nevertheless indispensable for the vagina, residual from colpectomy, to be restored in trophic terms in order to constitute a sound anchor to the above-mentioned ligamental structures.

Table 15.4 Indication for vaginal celiotomy operations, 5-year period 1973–77

Alteration in pelvic statics	224	55.87%
Hypertrophic sclero-utero-fibromas	126	31.42%
Carcinoma *in situ* and dysplasia	32	7.98%
K endometrium	11	2.74%
Other indications	8	1.99%

Table 15.5 Colpo-hysterectomy operations for pathology of pelvic statics, 5-year period 1973–77

With anterior and posterior colpoplasty	215	73.00%
With anterior colpoplasty only	46	16.00%
With posterior colpoplasty only	28	9.50%
With Marshall–Marchetti burch	4	1.50%

Wherefore, if a marked architectonic atypia of the elastic component is observed (67% of cases) in the postmenopause and after traumatic damage from child-bearing, it has been observed that after treatment with estriol at a dosage level of at least 2 mg per day for a period of from 30 to 60 days, there obtains a renewal of the epithelial layers characterized by a high karyopyknotic index and intense PAS-positivity.

This 'pharmacological re-training' of the vaginal receptor accompanies regularization of the elastic network and so has two advantages to contribute on the clinical plane, namely:

(a) it obviates iatrogenic pathology of the structures bordering the uterus, through realization of optimum planes of cleavage which minimize the denervation of the vesica, leaving the Halban band adherent, and so traumatize the ureter which can readily be slipped in an upwards direction;

(b) it improves the short- and long-term effects of surgery which demolishes yet at the same time aims to be mainly restorative.

In conclusion, even if the present study of the elastic network results are incomplete both from the number of findings so far covered and, probably, from the methodology used, it seems that the encouraging results obtained by use of estriol do support the continuation of this experimental clinical study. We are heartened, in this regard, by the lack of postoperative complications associated with techniques used and the good results obtained also given a low percentage frequency of urinary incontinence after surgery.

Insofar as the definitive choice of estrogen is concerned, preparatory to vaginal surgery, further documentation will be required in order to establish the type of formulation most appropriate, since we have till now been relying on estriol and have no experience of using natural conjugated estrogens.

References

1. El-Kholi, G. Y. and Mina, S. N. (1975). Elastic tissue of the vagina in genital prolapse. A morphological study. *J. Egypt. Med. Assoc.*, **58**, 196
2. Carinelli, S. G., Senzani, F. and Remotti, G. (1979). Le fibre elastiche superficiali nell'esocervice uterina e nella vagina, in condizioni normali e dopo terapia radiante. *Ann. Ostet. Ginecol. Med. Perin.*, **100**, 27
3. Carinelli, S. G., Cefis, F., Bruni, M., Senzani, F., Candiani, G. B. and Remotti, G. (1979). Il tessuto elastico della lamina propria in alcune malformazioni della vagina e della cervice. In corso di stampa su: *Ann. Ostet. Ginecol. Med. Perin.*
4. Anderson, H. E. (1958). Clinical use of estrogen in uterine prolapse. *J. Am. Med. Assoc.*, **168**, 173
5. Raz, S., Zeigler, M. and Caine, M. (1973). The role of female hormones in stress incontinence. *XVI Congrès de la Soc. Internat. d'Urologie*, Amsterdam
6. Kistner, R. W. (1969). Atrophic vaginitis and other atrophic changes in the postmenopausal patient in the female climacteric. *Ayerst Lab.*, **1** (2)

16
The Correction by Estrogens of Calcium Disorders Induced by Estrogen-deficient States

H. P. KLOTZ

The role of estrogens in maintaining bone calcium stores is quite certain. It is clearly demonstrated by bone decalcification in untreated gonadal agenesis (Turner's syndrome) and in the early and severe osteoporosis seen in women following oophorectomy in the absence of estrogen substitutes.

The physiological antagonism between parathormone (PTR) and estrogen was reported in 1941 by Klotz et al.[1,2]. The hypercalcemic action of PTH is opposed by the hypocalcemic action of estrogen. Since that time, numerous studies have emphasized this antagonism both in vivo and in vitro[3], and have attributed postmenopausal osteoporosis to an increase in bone receptors to PTH, by virtue of the disappearance of the antagonistic hormone[4,5]. According to Van Oassen et al., estrogens also act by antagonizing the action on the bone of GH, hence the frequent finding of hypophosphatemia in estrogen-deficient states.

Finally, it is possible that estrogens also act by a third mechanism: the stimulation by estrogens of the secretion of calcitonin. The authors have demonstrated this effect of estrogens on plasma thyrocalcitonin levels in the oophorectomized animals[6].

The therapeutic influence of estrogens in postmenopausal osteoporosis was first stressed by Albright et al. in 1941[7], but this form of treatment was very controversial. The first overall study was that of Wallach and Henneman[8], the conclusions of which were very favourable. Gallagher and Nordin[9,10] have noted in recent years that after the menopause estrogens suppress the slight increase in blood calcium levels and the more marked increase in urinary calcium usually present in such subjects, which they attribute to increased bone resorption. They have codified a convenient method for the measurement of this bone resorption by calculation in the morning urine (from 8 to 10 a.m.), in an individual fasting since the previous evening, the ratio Ca:creatinine, which should be <0.10, and the ratio hydroxyproline:creatine, which must be <0.20. An increase in these ratios calculated at this time of the day is indicative of bone resorption. Dequeker et al.[11] have confirmed the influence of estrogens on bone by radiometry of the second metacarpal, and by photon absorptiometry of the distal end of the radius.

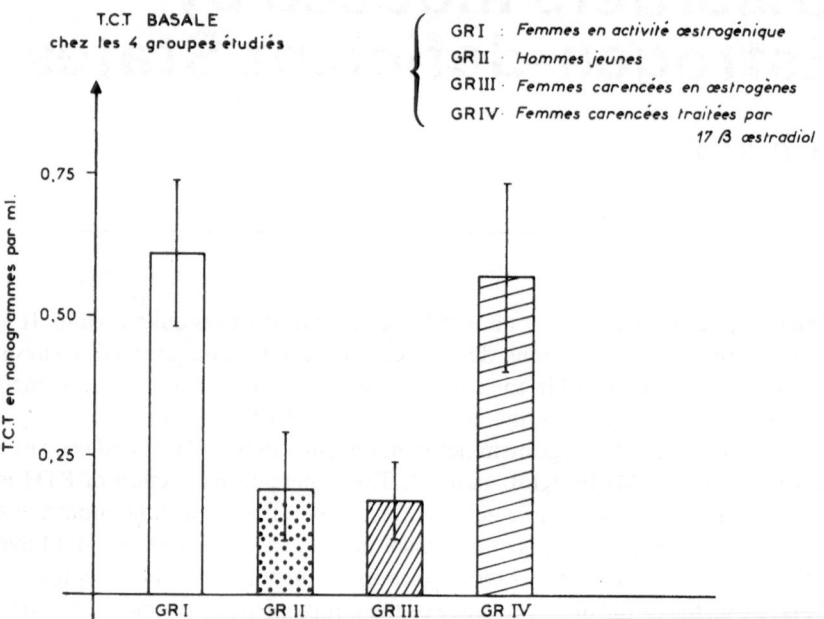

Figure 16.1 Effect of estrogen on basal calcitonin in human bone in the four groups studied. GR I: Women with estrogenic activity; GR II: Young men; GR III: Women deficient in estrogen; GR IV: Deficient women treated with 17β-estradiol

The authors have themselves observed two types of finding (Figure 16.1, Tables 16.1 and 16.2). On the one hand, severe decalcifying osteosis, sometimes even associated with quasispontaneous fractures, in women who are still young (around 40), oophorectomized many years before and left without hormone treatment. In such patients, we have succeeded in stopping progression of the process and suppressing the risk of fractures by long-term estrogen therapy. The first cases of this type were reported in the thesis of our pupil Pierre Detroy, Paris (1959).

Secondly, early and latent osteoporosis after the natural menopause in which the morning bone resorption coefficient (Ca:creatinine) is highly pathological and returns to normal as a result of estrogen treatment only, whether β-estradiol gel, tablets of ethinyl estradiol or conjugated estrogens of equine origin. Estriol is also active on bone provided high doses are used, in excess of 6 mg/day.

Table 16.1 Influence of progressively increasing doses of estrone on the levels of plasma calcitonin in female castrated rats

Batch no. (6 per batch)	Dose of estrone (µg/day)	Calcitonin level (milli-UMRC/ml)
1	0	
2	0.5	0.160
3	1	0.560
4	1	0.500
5	1	0.550
8	2	0.660
6	0	

Table 16.2 Influence of total estrone dose on plasma calcitonin in female castrated rats

Batch no. (6 per batch)	Total estrone dose (µg)	Calcitonin level (milli-UMRC/ml)
1	0	
2	6.5	0.160
3	13.5	0.560
4	14	0.500
5	34	0.550
8	8	0.660
6	0	

We have also seen untreated menopausal women with a normal morning bone resorption coefficient. In terms of the understanding of postmenopausal osteoporosis we therefore attach great importance to seeking one or more associated factors: inadequate diet or intestinal absorption of calcium or of vitamin D, inadequate physical activity, spontaneous or iatrogenic excess of thyroxin, or a spontaneous or drug excess of cortisol. When present, all these associated factors should be corrected simultaneously.

In practice, our programme of management is as follows:

(1) In the case of early oophorectomy before the age of 45, substitute estrogen therapy is felt to be necessary to protect the skeleton (all contraindications and precautions being respected). Aitken[12] emphasizes the need to begin such treatment during the 3 years following the oophorectomy.

(2) In the case of natural menopause, apparently uncomplicated if the morning bone resorption coefficient is pathological (greater than 10) treatment is given. If not, the patient is merely kept under observation unless there is another indication for hormone therapy (general trophic, etc.).

(3) In the case of postmenopausal osteoporosis, detectable on the basis of radiological or laboratory findings, estrogens are always prescribed, which in association with calcium and anabolic agents often leads to the relief of pain and functional incapacity in immobolized patients with severe pain.

Contraindications to treatment are, of course:

A past history of carcinoma of the breast.

A definite past history of phlebitis or embolism.

A past history of fibroid in a patient who has not undergone hysterectomy.

Too advanced an age at the time of the diagnosis of osteoporosis. It is difficult to define such an age, though it may be said that there is generally agreed hesitation to start estrogen therapy after the age of 68.

A carcinoma, even latent 'incipiens' of the endometrium or of the breast. Thus before starting estrogen therapy, it is essential to confirm that routine vaginal cytology and mammography are normal. These examinations should be repeated periodically throughout the period of treatment.

References

1. Klotz, H. P., Barbier, P., Miranda, R. and Cantorovich, B. (1949). Action des oestrogènes sur la calcémie du chien normal et parathyréoprive. *Ann. Endocrinol.*, **10**, 445
2. Justin-Bésançon, L., Klotz, H. P. and Barbier, P. (1949). Etude clinique de l'action du benzoate d'oestradiol sur la calcémie. *Bul. Mém. Soc. Méd. Hôp. Paris*, **11** and **12**, 451
3. Atkins, D., Zanelli, J. M., Peacock, M. and Nordin, B. E. C. (1972). The effect of oestrogens on the response of bone to parathyroid hormone *in vitro*. *J. Endocrinol.*, **54**, 107
4. Heaney, R. P. (1965). A unified concept of osteoporosis. *Am. J. Med.*, **39**, 877
5. Nordin, B. E. C., Young, M. M., Bulusu, L. and Horsman, A. (1970). Osteoporosis re-examined. In R. Barzel (ed.). *Osteoporosis*, pp. 47–67. (New York: Grune and Stratton)
6. Klotz, H. P., Delorme, M. L., Ochoa, F. and Aussemera, C. (1975). Hormones sexuelles et sécrétion de calcitonine. *Sem. Hôp. Paris*, **51**, 1333
7. Albright, F., Smith, P. H. and Richardson, A. M. (1941). Postmenopausal osteoporosis: its clinical features. *J. Am. Med. Assoc.*, **116**, 2465
8. Wallach, S. and Henneman, Ph. (1959). Prolonged oestrogentherapy in postmenopausal women. *J. Am. Med. Assoc.*, **71**, 1637
9. Gallagher, J. C. and Nordin, B. E. C. (1973). Oestrogens and calcium metabolism. In Van Keem and Lauritzen (eds.). *Ageing and Estrogens. Front. Hormone Res.*, Vol. 2, pp. 98–117. (Basel: Karger)
10. Gallagher, J. C., Young, M. M. and Nordin, B. E. C. (1972). Effects of artificial menopause on plasma and urine calcium and phosphate. *Clin. Endocrinol.*, **1**, 57

11. Dequeker, J., Roh, Y. S., Dessel, D. van, Gautama, K. and Burssens, A. (1973). Bone mineral estimation *in vivo* by photon absorptiometry. Influence of skeletal size and its value for detecting osteoporosis. *J. Belge Méd. Phys. Rhum.*, **28**, 293

12. Aitken, J. M., Hart, D. M. and Lindsay, R. (1973b). Oestrogen replacement therapy for prevention of osteoporosis after oophorectomy. *Br. Med. J.*, **2**, 515

17
Calcium Metabolism in the Postmenopause and Sex Steroid Therapy: Post-menopausal Osteoporosis and Sex Steroids

R. LINDSAY

INTRODUCTION

Considerable controversy still surrounds the etiology of osteoporosis in ageing women. Albright, Smith and Richardson in 1941[1] originally drew attention to its relationship to the menopause, and in a simple hypothesis proposed an etiological association between loss of ovarian function and the subsequent development of osteoporosis. Metabolic balance studies indicated that both estrogen and androgen should be effective in the treatment of osteoporosis[2]. However, treatment with androgens fell into disrepute when it became obvious that they were ineffective unless given in virilizing doses[3] and, using the relatively insensitive techniques then available, cross-sectional studies suggested that, at best, estrogen would only prevent skeletal loss[4], and that such an effect might only be temporary. Further, Donaldson and Nassim[5] were unable to find any significant association between osteoporosis and oophorectomy.

There was, however, still a substantial amount of circumstantial evidence that ovarian function in some way was related to skeletal mass. Osteoporosis is predominantly a disease of women[6]. Bone mass reaches a maximum value in the female population at about the age of 35 years[7], at the time when ovarian weight[8] and estrogen output[9] are both maximal. Utilizing newer quantitative techniques such as photon absorptiometry[10], we have endeavoured to examine the relationship between ovarian function and skeletal homeostasis and the role of the sex steroids in prevention of postmenopausal bone loss.

The osteoporotic woman

Clinicians in different specialties are aware of the problems of osteoporosis. There is a gradual loss of height as dorso-lumbar vertebrae wedge and finally collapse. Such catastrophes may occur after what would be regarded in the young as quite trivial trauma (stooping, stepping down from a high vehicle, or a stumble without fall). The resulting pain, incapacity and general morbidity are out of all proportion to these insignificant incidents immediately preceding vertebral collapse. It is important to realize that the invisible asymptomatic loss of bone from the skeleton, by this time, has been steadily progressive from the middle years and that once bone is lost to this extent the situation is irreversible, although further reduction in bone mineral can be inhibited.

Other fractures are observed in the ageing woman more commonly than in the male. Notorious are fracture of the lower end of the radius (Colles fracture) and fracture of the femoral neck. This latter, occurring generally among the older population group, results in significant mortality as well as making an important contribution to morbidity among the elderly.

BONE LOSS AND CALCIUM STATUS IN OOPHORECTOMIZED WOMEN

To allow us to study more closely the mechanisms involved in bone loss, we elected to follow a population of women likely to be more at risk than the average. Therefore it seemed in many ways a more logical approach to observe a cohort of younger women, utilizing the technique of the controlled clinical

Table 17.1 Biochemical changes in postmenopausal women

	Premenopausal	Postmenopausal	Postmenopausal (estrogen treated)
Serum calcium (mg/100 ml)	9.56 ± 0.08	9.84 ± 0.08	9.52 ± 0.04
Serum phosphate (mg/100 ml)	2.82 ± 0.09	3.32 ± 0.06	2.94 ± 0.06
Alkaline phosphatase (K.A. units)	7.06 ± 0.39	7.96 ± 0.42	7.00 ± 0.31
Urine Ca/Cr (mg/mg)	0.091 ± 0.007	0.114 ± 0.01	0.071 ± 0.006
Urine OHp/Cr (mg/mg)	0.015 ± 0.002	0.026 ± 0.003	0.011 ± 0.002
$\dfrac{TmPO_4}{GFR}$ (mg/100 ml)	2.90 ± 0.1	3.39 ± 0.09	2.87 ± 0.11

Ca/Cr = Ratio of calcium to creatinine in urine after overnight fast
OHp/Cr = Ratio of total hydroxyproline to creatinine in urine after overnight fast
$\dfrac{TmPO_4}{GFR}$ = Tubular maximum for phosphate reabsorption per unit glomerular filtration rate

trial to investigate not only the phenomenon of bone loss itself, but also the possibility that therapy, in this instance with estrogen, might effectively *prevent* reduction of mineral content and the consequent catastrophes. To that end our initial studies entailed observing several cohorts of women who had come to hysterectomy, with or without oophorectomy, while regular menstruation was still present (up to the time of operation). Much of the early data from these studies has now been published[11-13], but it is relevant to review the important findings, particularly from the oophorectomized groups. The sudden production of an artificial menopause is associated with an increased serum and urinary calcium, an increase in the amount of hydroxyproline-containing peptide in urine, and a change in phosphate excretion resulting in increased retention of phosphate (Table 17.1).

These biochemical changes persist[13] and are accompanied by increased loss of bone mineral content estimated at the midpoint of the third right metacarpal (Figure 17.1) or mid or distal radius (Figure 17.2), and, although

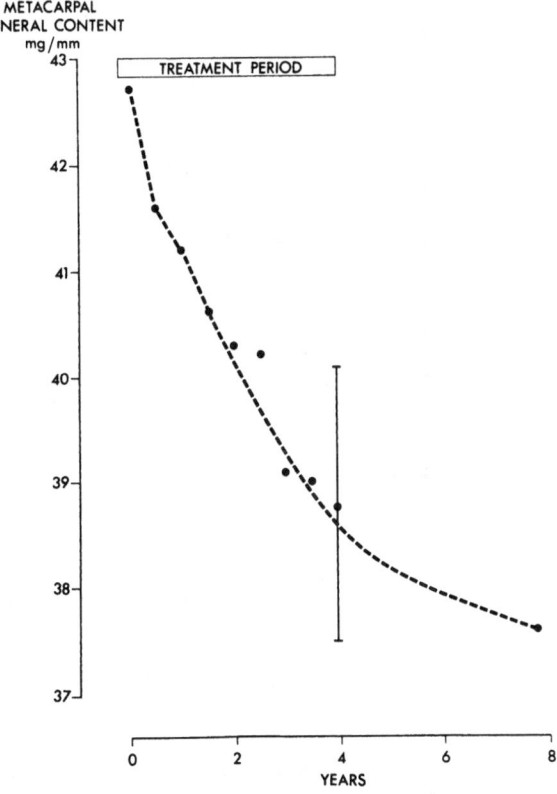

Figure 17.1 Metacarpal mineral content estimated by photon absorptiometry in patients' oophorectomized premenopausally and followed for the subsequent 8 years (from ref. 31 by kind permission of the Editor, *Lancet*). Means ± maximum SEM

osteoporosis is primarily a disease affecting the spine[14], some autopsy studies have suggested that these peripheral bone measurements may be reasonable estimates of spinal mineral content, particularly in women[15]. As measurements of the spine (*in vivo*) are difficult to make, and notoriously inaccurate, we feel that our estimates of bone loss at these peripheral sites, even though these are predominantly sites consisting of cortical, are relevant to the disease 'spinal osteoporosis'. (Even the distal radius site 2 cm from the peripheral end of the radius consists of at least 60% cortical bone).

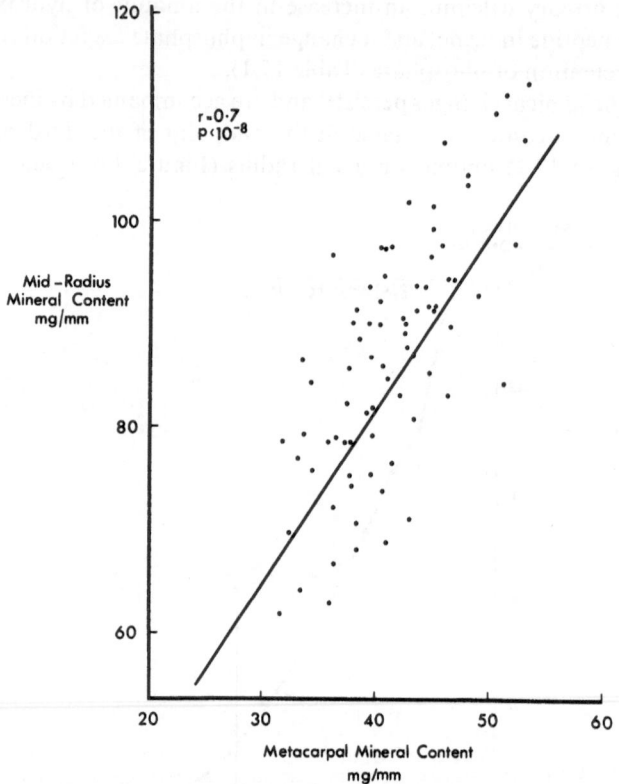

Figure 17.2 Relationship of the mineral content at the mid-point of the third right metacarpal to the mineral content at the mid-point of the right radius in the same patients. A similar relationship can be shown between either measurement and mineral content at a distal radius site (2 cm from distal end). All measurements by photon absorptiometry (from ref. 45 by kind permission of the publisher)

In these original studies assessment of bone loss after oophorectomy was carried out in three separate groups of women followed for 2 months, 3 years and 6 years after oophorectomy. We found that oophorectomy, when carried out premenopausally, was followed by a period of increased rate of bone loss lasting 3–6 years (Figure 17.1), when the average rate of loss of mineral at the metacarpal site was nearly 2% per annum[16]. This early phase of bone loss was followed by a period of continual reduction in bone mineral which appeared to last indefinitely, at an average rate of 0.7% per annum. To date we have followed some women for 12 years, and although individual rates and patterns of bone loss vary enormously, once started the process appears inexorable. Not all oophorectomized women lose bone, however, and we have examined our groups of women in detail to attempt to unravel some of those factors which might be important in determining rate of loss of bone mineral.

Determinants of bone loss in untreated women

Bone loss in untreated oophorectomized women can be related to several factors. Daniel[17] pointed out that the majority of women who present with symptoms of osteoporosis are slim and smoke cigarettes. The latter we have not examined, but body build is undoubtedly important in determining rate of bone loss.

Firstly, height is only very loosely related to rate of bone loss at the metacarpal site (Figure 17.3), but there is a more significant association between weight and bone loss (Lindsay et al. – unpublished observations), and calculation of body fat from the relationship of height to weight confirmed the

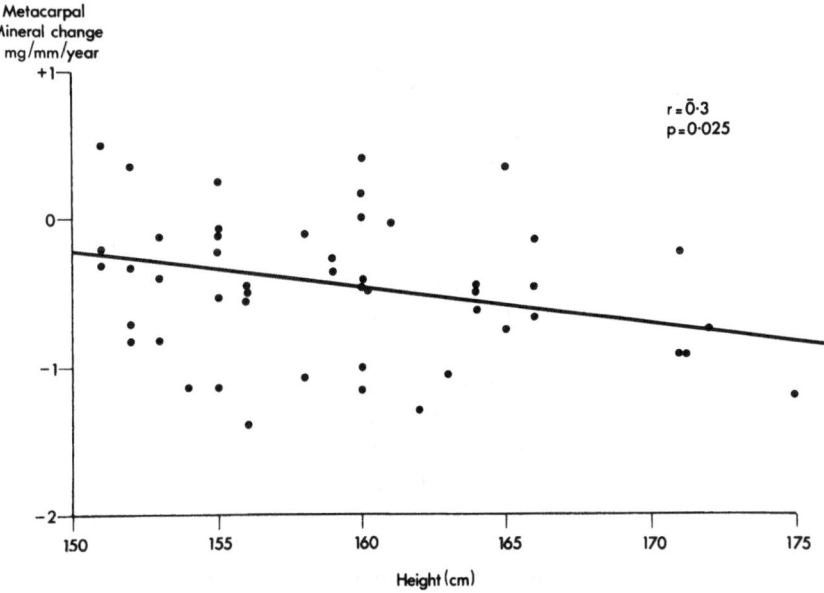

Figure 17.3 Relationship of height (in centimeters at the initial visit) to the subsequent rate of change of bone mineral content at the mid-point of the third right metacarpal. All patients were oophorectomized untreated women followed for 3–5 years from operation

importance of obesity in determining rate of mineral loss. From the data of Grodin *et al.*[18] we already knew of the suggestion that the majority of the circulating estrogen in postmenopausal or oophorectomized women was produced by peripheral conversion of adrenal androgen and that this conversion probably took place mainly in adipose tissue. We have confirmed a significant relationship between circulating endogenous estrogen and the degree of obesity[19] and a somewhat similar, but altogether looser, relationship between circulating estrogen and metacarpal bone loss[20]. However, the situation may be more complex than this. Figure 17.4 illustrates the relationship

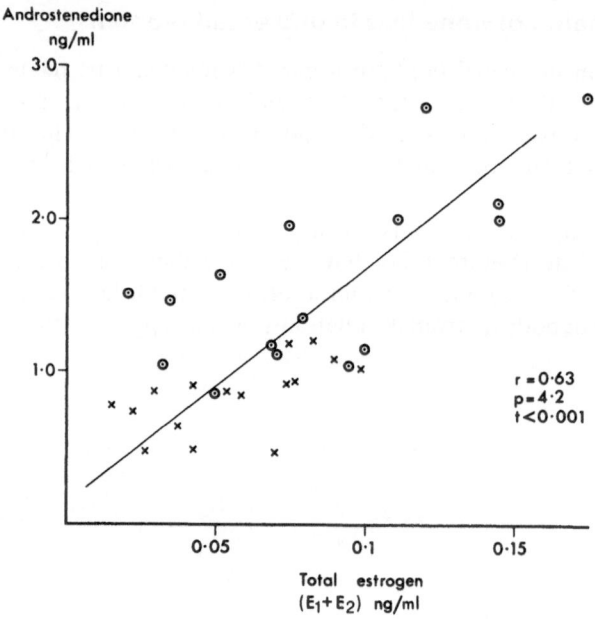

Figure 17.4 Androstenedione and 'total' estrogen (estradiol + estrone) plasma levels in oophorectomized, untreated women. Symbols (×) indicate women with higher than average rates of bone loss; (⊙) women with low rates of bone loss

between bone loss and some of the relevant sex hormones produced. Those women losing bone most quickly have lower levels of circulating androstenedione and 'total' estrogen (estrone plus estradiol), and there is a significant association between androstenedione and total estrogen, but not (in our studies) between circulating androstenedione and either estrogen individually.

As stated, the majority of endogenous estrogen in the postmenopausal or oophorectomized women apparently comes from peripheral conversion of adrenal androgens. Variations between women in mean circulating estrogen levels could result, therefore, either from differences in adrenal steroid production or alteration in the rate of peripheral conversion of androgens to estrogens. Alternatively, changes in binding protein levels could account for the observed variations. The latter is unlikely and no evidence of altered conversion rate has been found[21]. Therefore we examined the role of the adrenal gland in two experiments. Serial measurements of urinary free cortisol were made at 3-monthly intervals on 24-hour urine specimens collected by 74 women participating in a controlled trial of estrogen therapy[13]. Prior to, during and following the period of monitoring cortisol production, metacarpal mineral was estimated by photon absorptiometry at 6-monthly intervals. Analysis of the results revealed that those women with highest mean urinary free cortisol had greatest rate of bone loss[22].

In an acute study of adrenal function, we performed ACTH stimulation tests following dexamethasone suppression in two groups of women whose rate of change of metacarpal mineral we had documented. The women were divided naturally into separate groups, one of which was losing significant amounts of bone and the other a group whose mean rate of bone loss, measured by our technique, was minimal ($<0.5\%$ per annum). The groups were matched for age, weight, time from menopause, etc. In both groups the results of acute adrenal stimulation were virtually identical, there being no significant difference in cortisol production following maximal stimulation. The increment was in fact *smaller* (although not significantly so) in the group losing bone, which perhaps suggests some impairment of adrenal reserve[23], although this is purely speculative.

The changes in calcium homeostasis implied by our findings and those of other workers have been studied in detail by Heaney and co-workers[24, 25]. They have shown consistent changes in calcium homeostasis and bone remodeling occurring across the menopause. In a careful study in which they examined bone remodeling in 151 normal perimenopausal women, they demonstrated a change in computed skeletal balance from -0.021 g/day (calcium) to -0.038 g/day occurring across the menopause[25]. Such a figure is equivalent to a net annual loss of bone of about 1.5%, agreeing fairly closely with the expected average figure and that recorded in our studies. We have not been able to document any differences in plasma levels of PTH, calcitonin or 25-hydroxyvitamin D in women losing bone when compared to age-matched women whose bone mineral status was stable when estimated by serial photon absorptiometry or radiogrammetry.

ESTROGEN THERAPY AFTER OOPHORECTOMY

Three groups working independently, and using different techniques, have now shown that estrogen therapy prevents bone loss in both postmenopausal and oophorectomized women[12, 13, 26, 27].

In our original studies[12] we used mestranol in an *average* daily dose of about 25 µg. Recent data have confirmed that prevention of bone loss is a feature of all estrogens, with the possible exception of estriol (Figure 17.5) *in normally prescribed doses*[28]. It is possible, although we have yet to confirm the data, that as little as 0.3 mg conjugated equine estrogen per day will be sufficient to prevent bone loss, although higher doses may be required in the short term for control of menopausal symptoms.

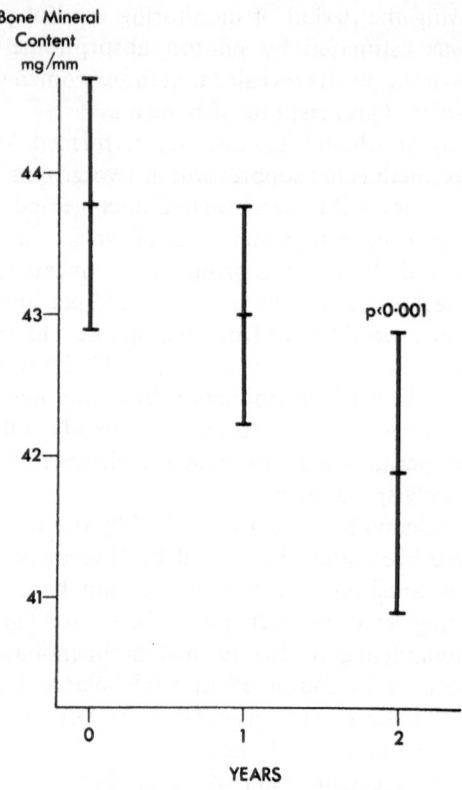

Figure 17.5 Bone loss during therapy with estriol treatment. Estriol was provided in an average daily dose of 10 mg estriol hemisuccinate to 46 postmenopausal patients (of whom 14 had had oophorectomy performed). Mean rate of bone loss is about 1.9% per annum (from ref. 28 by kind permission of the Editor, *Maturitas*)

In one of our groups of oophorectomized women in whom onset of treatment was delayed for 3 years from oophorectomy, there was a significant increase in peripheral bone mineral mass[13] (Figure 17.6), estimated by photon absorptiometry and confirmed using a radiographic densitometric technique[29] (Figure 17.7). We have seen some evidence (as yet unpublished) of similar changes in groups in whom onset of treatment is delayed for several years beyond a normal menopause. It is evident (from Figure 17.7) that the loss of bone to be expected from a cross-sectional study of normal women[7] is

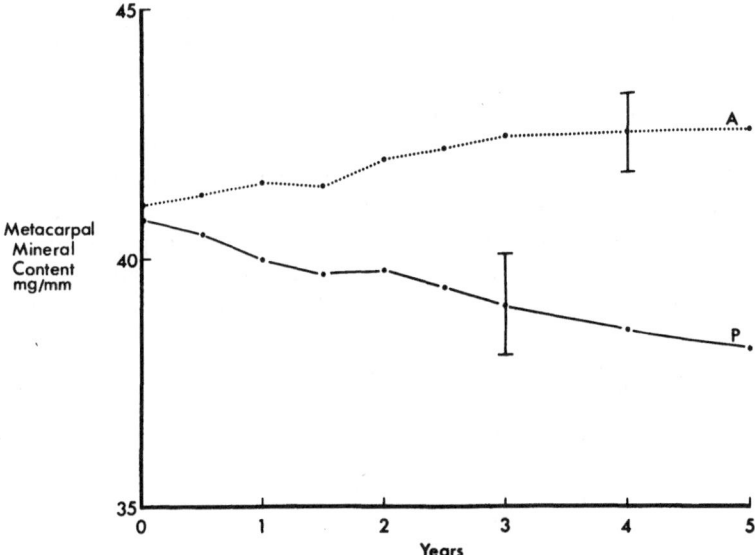

Figure 17.6   Metacarpal mineral content during a 5-year follow-up period of 120 patients who had been oophorectomized 3 years prior to time zero. The women were randomly divided into two groups and prescribed either mestranol (A) or an identical placebo (P). Measurements were by photon absorptiometry. A total of 63 women received an average daily dose of 24.8 µg mestranol (from ref. 13 by kind permission of the Editor, *Lancet*)

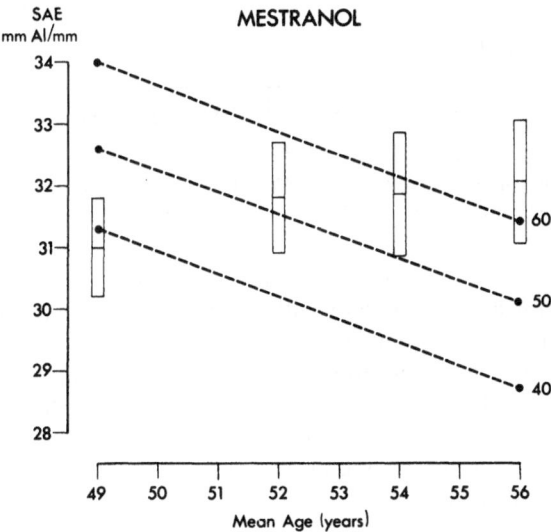

Figure 17.7   Changes in metacarpal mineral (radiodensitometry: SAE – Standardized Aluminium Equivalent in mm aluminium per mm bone – for a description of the method see ref. 28). Estrogen-treated group is identical to Figure 17.6 and indicated by mean ± SEM (boxes). Dotted lines indicate the expected behaviour of a normal Glasgow population of similar age group (numbers 40, 50, 60 indicate percentile values – from ref. 7)

not seen in the longitudinal follow-up of women treated with estrogen. The control group (placebo treated), however, shows a rate of bone loss which is comparable to that expected from the cross-sectional study (Figure 17.8).

The biochemical effects of estrogen therapy on calcium metabolism are well known (Table 17.1). There is a reduction in serum calcium and a fall in the urinary excretion of calcium, both of which persist even if estrogen treatment is continued for some years[13]. Associated with estrogen therapy there is also an increased phosphate excretion, reduction in serum phosphate and a dramatic fall in urinary hydroxyproline. Unfortunately, within individuals none of these changes correlate closely with the effect of estrogen or mineral loss[30].

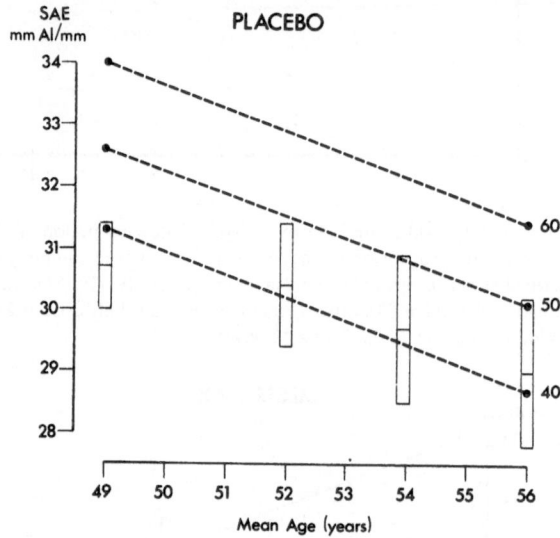

Figure 17.8 For comparison with Figure 17.7. Changes in metacarpal mineral by radio-densitometry in 57 patients in Figure 17.6 treated with placebo

Recently, we have demonstrated that prevention of bone loss may not be unique to estrogens, since therapy with a pure progestogen appears also to be effective[31]. With the requirement in several countries to prescribe estrogen in cyclical fashion with the addition of a progestogen to prevent endometrial hyperplasia, this observation may be important. As yet there is little information about the efficacy of combination or sequential therapy in postmenopausal women, but we see no reason to suspect that it will prove less effective than estrogen alone.

Duration of estrogen treatment

No study at present has determined the duration of estrogen treatment required for prevention of fracture. We recently had the opportunity to study a group of 14 patients who had completed 4 years' therapy in our trial of mestranol therapy[32]. All had been taking the active preparation and all discontinued therapy after 4 years. At a follow-up review 4 years later, the mean mineral content of that group was similar to that of an age-matched group of women who had been taking placebo therapy for 8 years (Figure 17.9). Removal of estrogen therapy appeared to have resulted in an increased loss of bone, analogous to that occurring across the menopause[24, 25], albeit slightly more exaggerated. It suggests that to be effective estrogen therapy may have to be continued indefinitely.

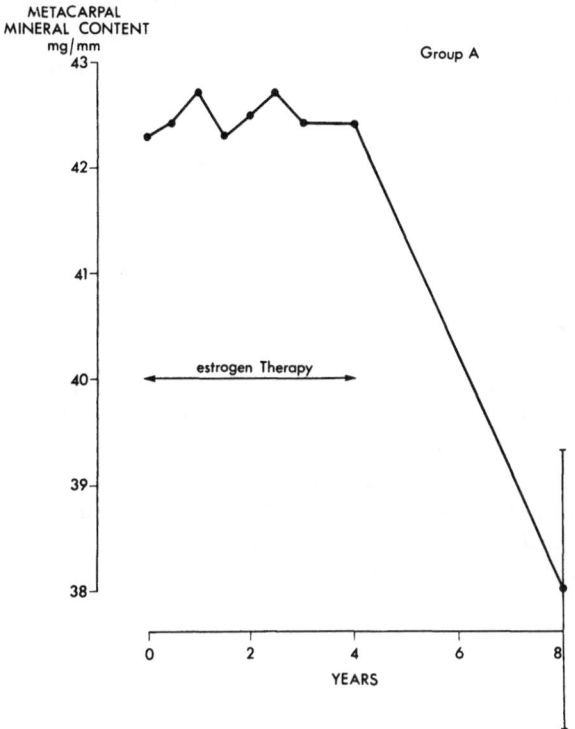

Figure 17.9 The effect of removal of estrogen therapy on metacarpal mineral content in oophorectomized women. A group of 14 women were treated with mestranol (average daily dose 27.6 μg) for 4 years. Treatment was discontinued and the group reviewed after a further 4 years (from ref. 32 by kind permission of the Editor, *Lancet*)

This observation raises important questions, social, ethical and financial, which we have discussed in detail elsewhere[32]. However, it is clear from this study that no definite evidence exists to allow us to decide on the appropriate treatment period for complete prevention of osteoporosis and protection against fracture.

THE POSTMENOPAUSAL WOMAN

Although the majority of our data has been collected using oophorectomized women, as far as we can see there is no qualitative difference between oophorectomized women and women who have undergone a spontaneous menopause. In one study completed[31] thus far, a mixed group of post-menopausal and oophorectomized women responded equally successfully to estrogen treatment, with no evidence of deterioration in bone mass. The two other prospective studies published[26, 27] have confirmed this. In a detailed study of the behavior of both postmenopausal and oophorectomized women, in terms of mineral metabolism, we found that there was some evidence that estrogen (estrone and estradiol) and androstenedione levels were lower in oophorectomized than in postmenopausal women[22], although this is not a universal finding[33]. We felt that since there were significant correlations between circulating total estrogen and androstenedione, the major portion at least of the available estrogen in the postmenopausal woman must be obtained from adrenal androgen precursors, and this must be true in both oophorectomized and postmenopausal women[33].

DISCUSSION

Our studies confirm and extend the observation that osteoporosis is a disorder occurring after oophorectomy or a natural menopause. It is a preventable condition using small doses of estrogens. As far as we can determine, estrogen therapy is effective for as long as it is given ($\sim$ 10 years to date) and the result of estrogen withdrawal is catastrophic. As our population of women ages, it is likely that a further age- (and not sex-) related bone loss will be superimposed upon the observed postmenopausal change. This 'senile osteoporosis' is probably related to reduced physical activity[34], reduction in calcium absorption from the gut[35], and perhaps also in some populations 'sub-clinical' vitamin D deficiency[36]. This condition is, we feel, a separate disorder from postmenopausal osteoporosis, so effectively prevented with estrogen treatment.

The mechanism by which estrogen prevents bone loss is still uncertain, and is discussed in detail in the accompanying chapters[37, 38]. It is important to mention that supplementation of the diet with calcium (to about 1.5 g elemental calcium per day) prevents to some extent bone loss in a post-menopausal population[26, 27]. In neither study, however, was calcium as effective as estrogen.

It is estimated that 50% of women over the age of 60 years may suffer from osteoporosis[39], and it is not surprising that in view of the considerable morbidity many therapies have been tried with varying success. Fluoride has enjoyed a considerable vogue, but some studies have suggested an increased incidence of microfractures[40] and macrofractures[41]. No studies of any sort are available demonstrating antifracture efficacy of fluoride[39]. Other therapies also have little place in the management of the menopausally related shift in calcium balance so elegantly demonstrated in the work from Heaney's laboratory[24, 25].

Although our studies indicate the efficacy of estrogen in prevention of loss of bone mineral, they do not demonstrate antifracture efficacy. To date no prospective controlled study has demonstrated fracture prevention. Suggestive evidence is available[6], and one case-control study recently published[42] has suggested that the risk of fracture was reduced by a factor of 7 when estrogen exposure began with 5 years of the menopause. Assessment of lateral spinal radiographs of patients who have been in our trial for 7–10 years suggests that wedge formation is inhibited by estrogen therapy[43]. Nevertheless, the risk/ benefit ratio must be assessed by each physician for each individual patient prior to deciding to provide what is likely to be almost life-long therapy in order to ensure adequate protection from osteoporosis. Previously[16] we have stated that such therapy should be undertaken only in specialized clinics, where experienced clinicians can ensure regular patient monitoring. In the present climate[44], and until alternative therapy is available, we see no reason to change this advice. Since prevention is likely to be more successful than cure, future research must be directed at defining those women at risk and providing for them adequate preventive therapy prior to skeletal collapse.

References

1. Albright, F., Smith, P. H. and Richardson, A. M. (1941). Postmenopausal osteoporosis: its clinical features. *J. Am. Med. Assoc.*, **116**, 2465
2. Albright, F. (1947). Osteoporosis. *Ann. Intern. Med.*, **27**, 861
3. Gordan, G. S., Picchi, J. and Roof, B. S. (1973). Antifracture efficacy of long-term estrogens for osteoporosis. *Trans. Assoc. Am. Phys.*, **86**, 326
4. Davis, M. E., Strandjord, N. M. and Lanzl, L. H. (1966). *Estrogens and the Aging Process:* The detection, prevention and retardation of osteoporosis. *J. Am. Med. Assoc.*, **96**, 129
5. Donaldson, A. and Nassim, J. R. (1954). The artificial menopause with particular relevance to the occurrence of spinal porosis. *Br. Med. J.*, **1**, 1228
6. Gordan, G. S. and Vaughan, C. (1976). *Clinical Management of the Osteoporoses.* (Acton, Mass.: Publishing Sciences Group Inc.)
7. Smith, D. A., Anderson, J. B., Shimmins, J., Speirs, C. F. and Barnett, E. (1969). Changes in metacarpal mineral content and density in normal male and female subjects with age. *Clin. Radiol.*, **20**, 23
8. Lauritzen, C. (1972). Endocrinology of the menopause and postmenopausal period. In P. E. Lebech, K. Ulrich and A. Helles (eds.). *Klimakteriet*, p. 17. (Kabenhaven Frederiksberg: Bogtrykkeri)
9. Pincus, G., Ramanoff, L. P. and Carlo, J. (1954). The excretion of urinary steroids by men and women of different ages. *J. Gerontol.*, **9**, 113
10. Cameron, J. R. and Sorenson, J. (1963). Measurement of bone mineral *in vivo*: an improved method. *Science*, **142**, 230
11. Aitken, J. M., Hart, D. M., Anderson, J. B., Lindsay, R., Smith, D. A. and Speirs, C. F.

(1973). Osteoporosis after oophorectomy for non-malignant disease in premenopausal women. *Br. Med. J.*, 1, 325

12. Aitken, J. M., Hart, D. M. and Lindsay, R. (1973). Oestrogen replacement therapy for prevention of osteoporosis after oophorectomy. *Br. Med. J.*, 2, 515

13. Lindsay, R., Hart, D. M., Aitken, J. M., MacDonald, E. B., Anderson, J. B. and Clark, A. C. (1976). Long-term prevention of postmenopausal osteoporosis by oestrogen. *Lancet*, i, 1038

14. Callagher, J. C., Aaron, J., Horsman, A., Marshall, D. H., Wilkinson, R. and Nordin, B. E. C. (1973). The crush fracture syndrome in postmenopausal women. *J. Clin. Endocr. Metab.*, 2, 293

15. Aitken, J. M., Smith, C. B., Horton, P. W., Clark, D. L., Boyd, J. F. and Smith, D. A. (1974). The interrelationships between bone mineral at different skeletal sites in male and female cadavera. *J. Bone Jt. Surg.*, 56B, 370

16. Lindsay, R. and Hart, D. M. (1978). Oestrogens and postmenopausal bone loss. *Scott. Med. J.*, 23, 13

17. Daniel, H. W. (1976). Osteoporosis of the slender smoker. *Arch. Intern. Med.*, 136, 298

18. Grodin, J. M., Siiteri, P. K. and McDonald, P. C. (1973). Source of oestrogen production in postmenopausal women. *J. Clin. Endocrinol. Metab.*, 36, 207

19. Lindsay, R., Coutts, J. R. T. and Hart, D. M. (1977). The effect of endogenous oestrogen on plasma and urinary calcium and phosphate in oophorectomised women. *Clin. Endocrinol.*, 6, 87

20. Lindsay, R., Coutts, J. R. T., Sweeney, A. and Hart, D. M. (1976). Endogenous oestrogen and bone loss following oophorectomy. *Calcified Tissues Res.*, 22 Suppl., 213

21. Marshall, D. H., Crilly, R. G. and Nordin, B. E. C. (1977). Plasma androstenedione and oestrone levels in normal and osteoporotic postmenopausal women. *Br. Med. J.*, 2, 1177

22. Lindsay, R., Hart, D. M., Manolagas, S., Anderson, D. C., Coutts, J. R. T. and Maclean, A. (1979). Sex steroids in pathogenesis and prevention of postmenopausal osteoporosis. In U. Barzel (ed.). *Osteoporosis II*, pp. 135–146. (New York: Grune and Stratton)

23. Manolagas, S. C., Anderson, D. C. and Lindsay, R. (1979). Adrenal steroids and the development of osteoporosis in oophorectomised women. *Lancet*. (In press)

24. Heaney, R. P., Recker, R. R. and Saville, P. D. (1978). Menopausal changes in calcium balance performance. *J. Lab. Clin. Med.*, 92, 953

25. Heaney, R. P., Recker, R. R. and Saville, P. D. (1978). Menopausal changes in bone remodelling. *J. Lab. Clin. Med.*, 92, 964

26. Recker, R. R., Saville, P. D. and Heaney, R. P. (1977). Effect of estrogens and calcium carbonate on bone loss in postmenopausal women. *Ann. Intern. Med.*, 87, 649

27. Horsman, A., Gallagher, J. C., Simpson, M. and Nordin, B. E. C. (1977). Prospective trial of oestrogen and calcium in postmenopausal women. *Br. Med. J.*, 2, 789

28. Lindsay, R., Hart, D. M., Maclean, A., Garwood, J., Clark, A. C. and Kraszewski, A. (1979). Bone loss during oestriol therapy in postmenopausal women. *Maturitas*. (In press)

29. Lindsay, R. and Anderson, J. B. (1978). Radiographic determination of bone density. *Radiography*, 517, 21

30. Aitken, J. M., Hart, D. M., Lindsay, R., Smith, D. A. and Wilson, G. M. (1974). Prevention of bone loss following oophorectomy in premenopausal women. *Isr. J. Med. Sci.*, 12, 608

31. Lindsay, R., Hart, D. M., Purdie, D., Ferguson, M. M., Clark, A. C. and Kraszewski, A. (1978). Comparative effects of oestrogen and a progestogen on bone loss in postmenopausal women. *Clin. Sci. Mol. Med.*, 54, 193

32. Lindsay, R., Hart, D. M., Maclean, A., Clark, A. C., Kraszewski, A. and Garwood, J. (1978). Bone response to termination of oestrogen treatment. *Lancet*, i, 1325

33. Peters, H. (1979). The ageing ovary. In P. A. Van Keep, D. M. Serr and R. B. Greenblatt (eds.). *Female and Male Climacteric: Current Opinion 1978*. (Lancaster: MTP Press)

34. Chalmers, J. and Ho, K. (1970). Geographical variations in senile osteoporosis. *J. Bone Jt. Surg.*, 52, 667

35. Gallagher, J. C., Aaron, J., Horsman, A., Marshall, D. H., Wilkinson, R. and Nordin, B. E. C. (1973). The crush fracture syndrome in postmenopausal women. *Clin. Endocrinol. Metab.*, **2**, 293

36. Baker, M. R., McDonnell, H., Peacock, M. and Nordin, B. E. C. (1979). Plasma 25-hydroxy-vitamin D concentrations in patients with fractures of the femoral neck. *Br. Med. J.*, **1**, 589

37. Klotz, P. (1979). Estrogen therapy of calcium metabolism disorders due to estrogen deficiency. Chapter 16, this volume

38. Gordan, G. S. (1979). Prevention and treatment of postmenopausal osteoporosis. Chapter 18, this volume

39. Marx, S. J. (1978). Restraint in use of high-dose fluorides to treat skeletal disorders. *J. Am. Med. Assoc.*, **240**, 1630

40. Baylink, D. J. and Bernstein, D. S. (1967). The effects of fluoride therapy on metabolic bone disease. *Clin. Orthop.*, **55**, 51

41. Inkovaara, J., Heikinheimo, R. and Jarvinen, K. (1975). Prophylactic fluoride treatment and aged bones. *Br. Med. J.*, **3**, 73

42. Hutchinson, T., Polansky, S. M. and Fernstein, A. R. (1978). A new application of case-control research demonstrating that postmenopausal estrogens protect against hip and radial fractures. *Clin. Res.*, **26**, 486A

43. Lindsay, R. and Hart, D. McK. (1979). Prevention of axial bone loss by long-term oestrogen therapy. *Endocrinology '79.* (Demonstration)

44. Editorial (1979). Oestrogen therapy and endometrial cancer. *Lancet*, **1**, 1121

45. Lindsay, R., Hart, D. M., Maclean, A., Garwood, Jane, Aitken, J. M., Clark, A. C. and Coutts, J. R. T. (1978). In I. D. Cooke (ed.). *The Role of Estrogen/Progestogen in the Management of the Menopause.* (Lancaster: MTP Press)

18
Prevention and Treatment of Postmenopausal Osteoporosis

G. S. GORDAN and C. VAUGHAN

In the last 4 years a body of information has been accumulating to confirm Professor Klotz's original concept that estrogens exert their beneficial effect on bone by way of calcitonin[1]. Confirmatory studies from the laboratories of Milhaud[2] in Paris and MacIntyre[3] in London give strong support to Professor Klotz's theory.

Doctor Lindsay in Chapter 17 describes his very important work, which demonstrates beyond doubt that estrogen deficiency leads directly to bone loss in ethnically predisposed women; that surprisingly small doses of estrogen prevent this loss; and that a long-acting progestogen has similar protective value. Androgenic–anabolic steroids have proved disappointing in the treatment of postmenopausal osteoporosis[4], but these agents may have some value in the quite different osteoporoses of immobilization or hypercorticism (Cushing's syndrome).

Osteoporosis is defined as insufficient but normally calcified bone mass. The osteoporoses are the most common of the metabolic bone diseases and result from a number of different processes, the three most common being: first, estrogen deficiency due to menopause or bilateral oophorectomy; second, immobilization; and third, hypercorticism. There are other less frequent osteoporoses, each quite different from the other, so that one cannot extrapolate the diagnostic features or effects of treatment from one type to another with quite dissimilar pathogenetic features. Postmenopausal osteoporosis is the most common variety, yet it is still not known precisely how many millions of women are affected. Perhaps this is because of its widespread distribution affecting all races except the black, and its insidious, asymptomatic onset. Whatever the reason, the outcome is that wherever you go, all over the world, you see elderly women shrunken and bent over, walking slowly with great difficulty, obviously in pain. In such women, a routine X-ray film shows that the loss of height, cervical kyphosis (dowager's hump) and the compensatory lumbar lordosis are the inevitable consequences of vertebral fractures.

We have ample historical evidence that fragility of the skeleton and increased incidence of fractures of vertebrae, wrists and hips in elderly women has long been a well-known phenomenon. Sir Astley Cooper noted in 1824 that in old age bones become 'thin in their shell and spongy in their texture', but he could not explain why. Bruns, in 1881, was puzzled to find that elderly women sustained more fractures of the wrist and femur than men over 50, despite less occupational hazard, and postulated that they must have tripped over their long skirts! Yet the relation of skeletal fragility to loss of ovarian function was not made until 1940, when the brilliant American endocrinologist, Fuller Albright, put this all together and coined the term post-

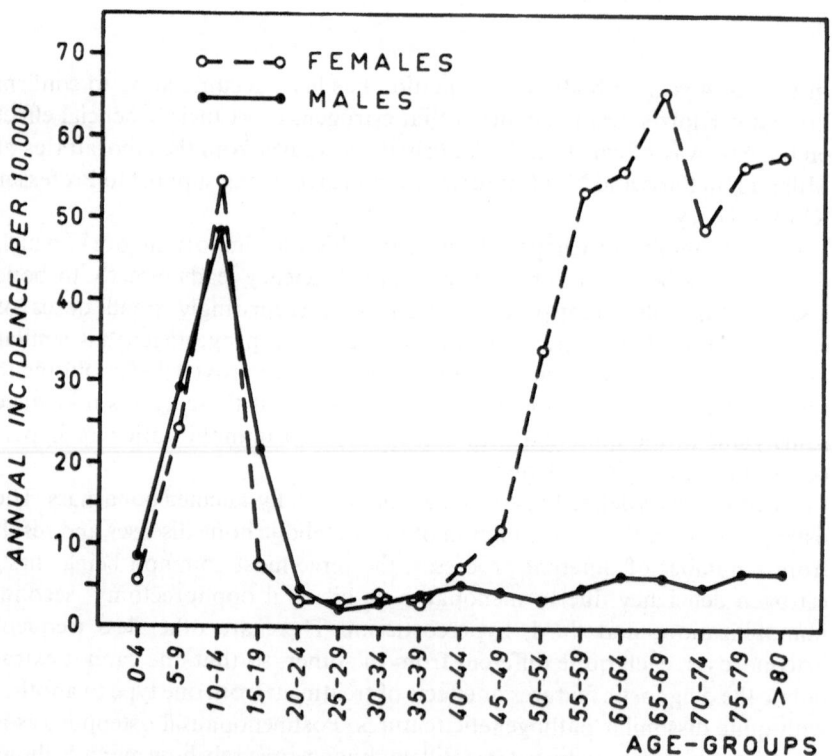

Figure 18.1 Annual incidence of fractures of the distal end of the radius or ulna, or both, in Malmö, Sweden. Note the increased rate after age 45 in women but not in men. (From ref. 6 with kind permission of the authors and the Editor of *J. Bone Jt. Surg.*)

menopausal osteoporosis[5]. Despite a number of learned challenges to Albright's theory, excellent epidemiologic data and, most recently, objective measurements of bone mass by a number of different techniques, have solidly confirmed Albright's prescient theory of the central role of estrogen deficiency in the pathogenesis of osteoporosis in women. The cogent epidemiologic data of Alffram and Bauer in 1962 showed that the incidence of wrist fractures in women over age 45 is up to 12 times higher than in age-matched men[6]. The preponderance of such fractures in women is surprising when one considers that many more men are exposed to accidents related to heavy manual labor. Clearly the long-skirt hypothesis of Professor Bruns is no longer tenable, but the high incidence of fracture in elderly women persists (Figure 18.1). The much greater frequency of hip fracture in Scandinavian women than men was also clearly demonstrated by Alhava and Puittinen[7] in 1973 (Figure 18.2).

Regrettably, we do not have similar data in the United States because we have a highly mobile population which creates many difficulties when one attempts to obtain meaningful epidemiologic data. Also in the United States, the Bureau of Vital Statistics does not record how many women die of hip fractures. We know the numbers are very great, but we can only extrapolate estimates from other sources, since our Vital Statistics Bureau lists deaths according to the secondary causes, e.g. thromboembolism, pneumonia, atelectasis, etc., and not to the primary cause – the hip fracture which led to anesthesia, major surgery and at least partial immobilization. We do have

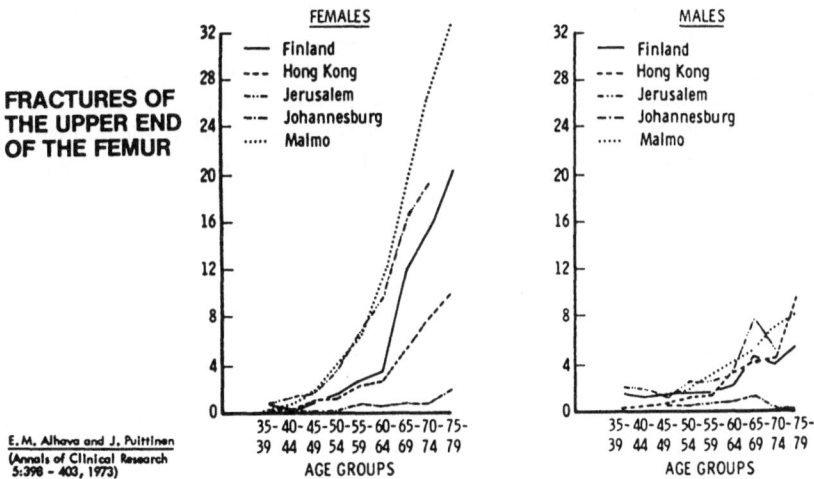

FRACTURES OF THE UPPER END OF THE FEMUR

E. M. Alhava and J. Puittinen
(Annals of Clinical Research
5:398 – 403, 1973)

Figure 18.2   Annual incidence of hip fractures in five cities showing lower and later incidence in white men. Note, however, the Johannesburg data, from the Bantu, show no significant increase of hip fracture with age in either sex despite poor diet, frequent pregnancies, prolonged periods of lactation and a high incidence of lactase deficiency which interferes with the absorption of milk products, the principal source of calcium. (With kind permission of the authors and the Editor of *Ann. Clin. Res.*)

data from the Professional Activity Surveillance Hospitals in the United States for 1974–75 which showed 11 299 hip facture *deaths* in a population accounting for 29% of all patients hospitalized in non-government, short-stay hospitals[8]. Their data ranked hip fracture as the 14th cause of death, accounting for 653 of every 10 000 female deaths. If this number applies to the 862 761 female deaths in the United States in 1974–75, an extrapolated female hip fracture death rate would be 56 289 in that one year. PSRO statistics for the United States show 211 000 hip fractures per year with a similar high mortality.

At present the Scandinavian epidemiologic data are still the most reliable and convincing because the population in Malmö is relatively homogeneous and stable and all the records have been channelled into one central hospital for many years. These data show that the frequency of hip fracture doubles *every 5 years* in Scandinavian women over age 65, attaining the astonishingly high figure of 40% after age 80. In all, 20% of Swedish women can expect to suffer one or more hip fractures sometime in their lives[6].

In a large co-operative study in the United Kingdom, Barnes found the vast majority of hip fractures occurred in women over the age of 65 and 34% of these died within 6 months after sustaining their fracture[9]. While osteoporotic vertebral fractures are painful and debilitating, often leading to invalidism and deformity, and osteoporotic wrist fractures are painful and create difficulties in performing daily activities, both of these can be treated on an out-patient basis. Hip fracture, however, is the ultimate complication of postmenopausal bone loss and is an entirely different matter. These are pathologic fractures which follow little or no trauma in elderly women, and because of the severity of the osteoporosis in the femoral neck they almost always must be treated surgically, either by nailing or total hip replacement. The complications of such major procedures are well known. In addition, the majority of these women are henceforth unable to take care of themselves and end up incarcerated in nursing homes. The costs to the individual and to society are tremendous: female hip fractures in the United States constitute a billion dollar a year industry. If, as we believe, most of these are preventable, human and economic savings could be enormous.

Both sexes lose bone with aging. This phenomenon has been termed 'physiological bone loss' and occurs earlier and is more precipitous in women; however, it is not a function of aging alone but is directly related to menopausal status[10] (Figure 18.3). The younger woman who is oophorectomized well before her expected age of natural menopause, and is not given hormone replacement therapy, is at greatest risk to develop pathologic postmenopausal osteoporosis, while those women who have a late menopause have a longer period of natural protection. Men at all ages and in all ethnic groups have a greater bone mass, a more dense skeleton, than women and they show no significant loss of bone mass before age 70; subsequently this loss is gradual (Figure 18.4).

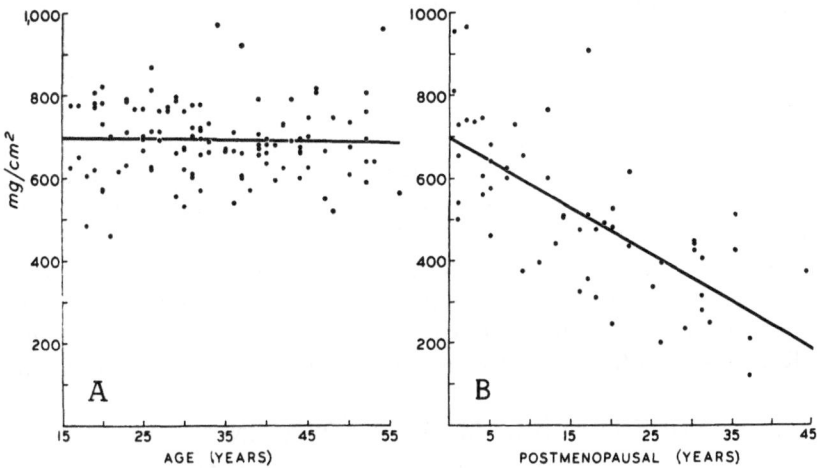

Figure 18.3 Bone mineral mass in normal premenopausal women according to age (A) and in normal postmenopausal women in relation to number of postmenopausal years (B). (Reprinted with permission from ref. 10)

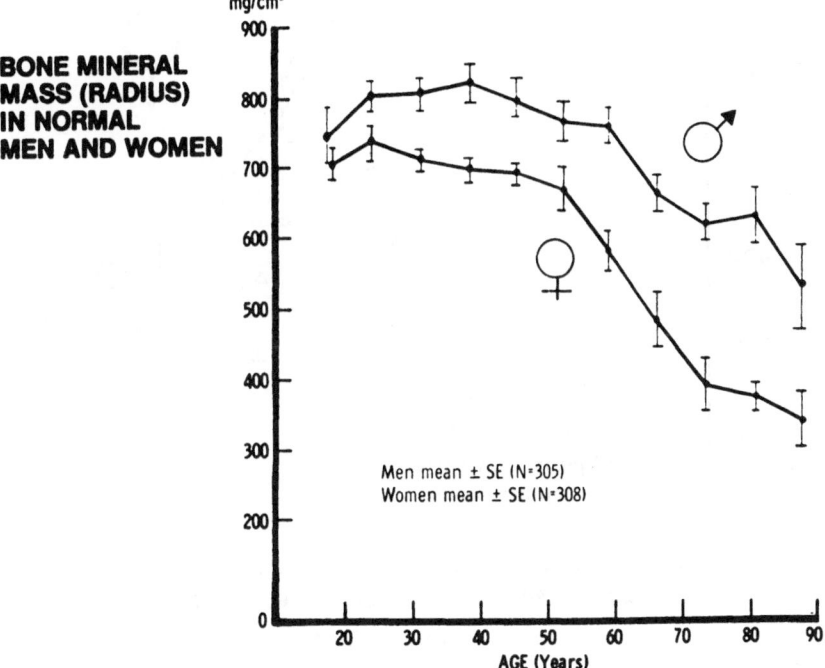

Figure 18.4 At all ages men have more bone than women. The greater severity and earlier onset of bone loss in women is more apt to lead to pathologic osteoporosis. (From ref. 10 with kind permission of the authors and the Editor of *Isr. J. Med. Sci.*)

Bone mass and the extent of physiological bone loss with aging varies with ethnic groups: the black races have the most dense skeletons and consequently the greatest protection against osteoporosis; the while races have the least. Data on the rate of bone loss in black, brown and yellow populations are sparse, but we know that Bantu women in South Africa do not show the marked increase in hip fracture after menopause that is seen in other races (*cf.* Figure 18.2). This finding is surprising because the Bantu are a poor people with generally a low-protein, high-carbohydrate diet, frequent pregnancies, prolonged periods of lactation and a high incidence of lactase deficiency which makes milk products, their best source of calcium, indigestible. In the United States the incidence of hip fracture in elderly black women is also very low[11].

Recent studies from various countries all show that women with osteo-

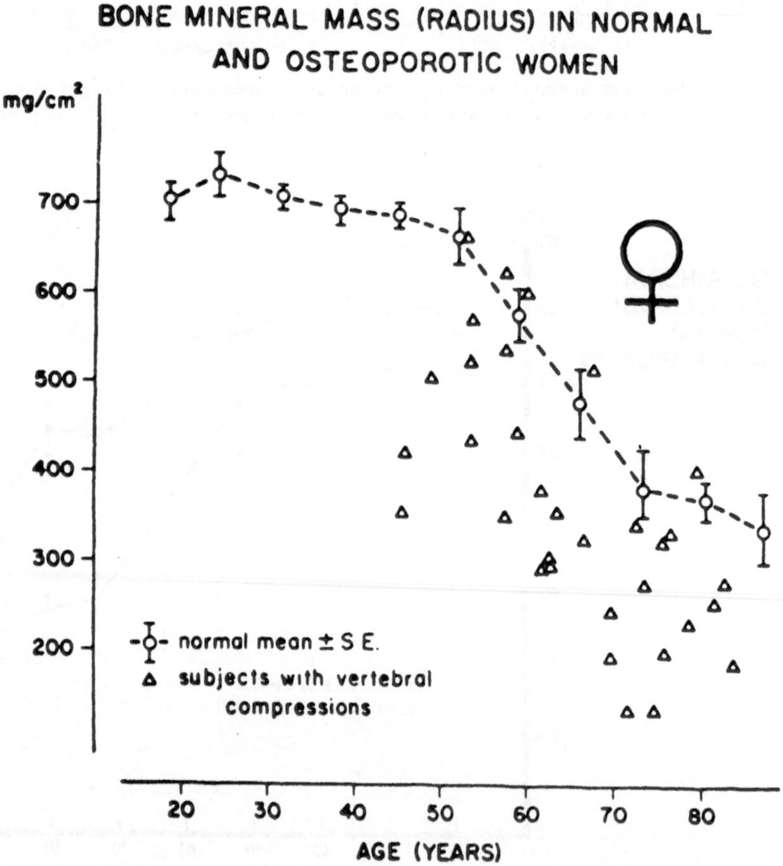

BONE MINERAL MASS (RADIUS) IN NORMAL AND OSTEOPOROTIC WOMEN

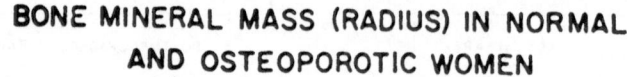

Figure 18.5 Note that most women with vertebral compression fractures have lost more bone than other women of the same age; however, bone loss is related to loss of ovarian function and not age *per se*. Some of these women have bone mass less than one-third of the premenopausal norm. (From ref. 10 with kind permission of the authors and the Editor of *Isr. J. Med. Sci.*)

porotic hip fractures have lost a significant amount of bone, sometimes as much as two-thirds of the premenopausal norm, and it is now obvious that osteoporotic fractures are complications of bone loss of such magnitude that the skeleton can no longer withstand normal or only slightly increased biochemical stress[10] (Figure 18.5). As many afflicted women say, 'I didn't fall and break my hip. My hip broke and I fell.'

The insidious and asymptomatic nature of early postmenopausal bone loss before fractures occur is comparable to the increased intra-ocular pressure in early glaucoma long before optic atrophy or blindness supervene. Perhaps an even better analogy is hypertension before the onset of stroke or coronary artery occlusion. Now that we can objectively measure loss of bone mass it is appropriate to institute proved methods of prophylaxis for osteoporosis before pathologic fragility and fractures occur in ethnically predisposed women. We now know that the loss of bone after loss of ovarian function averages 3% per year for the first 6 years, then 1–2% each year thereafter. We can predict that, by age 65, one half of all white women will have lost a significant amount of bone, that is two standard deviations below the premenopausal norm; whereas there is no significant loss of bone before menopause or oophorectomy (cf. Figure 18.3).

Bone is constantly being remodelled. Except during childhood growth and, in certain disease states, e.g. acromegaly, bone formation and bone resorption are coupled and homeostatically balanced. Albright pointed out that one can augment skeletal mass either by increasing bone formation or decreasing bone resorption. In 1963 we reported our bone tracer study showing that, in a very large number of osteoporotic women, estrogens, androgens and anabolic steroids caused a drop in the bone formation rate at the same time that the patients went into positive calcium balance[12]. Clearly, these findings show that in the human female skeleton these hormones are anticatabolic, not anabolic. Our findings were confirmed in 1969 by Riggs et al.[13] using the very different technique of microradiography, and it is now generally acknowledged that the sex hormones increase bone mass by reducing the rate of bone resorption to a greater degree than they reduce the rate of bone formation. Recently, Heaney et al. showed that at the menopause there is a sharp increase of about 20% in the bone resorption rate which can be prevented by as little as 18.8 μg ethynyl estradiol, or its equivalent, daily[14, 15].

It is vitally important to examine the total effect of estrogens on bone mass when interpreting these kinetic and microradiographic data. Total bone mass is preserved by the homeostatic coupling of bone formation and bone resorption. Although bone formation drops about 15% with sex hormone therapy the total bone mass is preserved or even increased because bone resorption falls more, usually about 20%. In fact, five recent studies[16–21] have all shown that estrogen prophylaxis or treatment in oophorectomized or postmenopausal, or even young, women is accompanied by an actual increase in bone mass as a consequence of a reduced level of bone remodelling.

We have followed more than 220 women with advanced, pathologic post-menopausal osteoporosis for upwards of 30 years. Unlike the very small doses of estrogen which have been shown to be effective in preventing post-menopausal bone loss, the effective, therapeutic dose for women who have already gone on to fractures must be full replacement, that is 1.25 mg conjugated estrogens, or the equivalent, for 20–25 consecutive days each month. This virtually prevents further fractures as long as the medication is continued and enables women incapacitated by the pain of osteoporotic fractures to resume normal, or near normal, physical activity. Even though there is no significant increase in bone formation, skeletal integrity has been achieved, and although these women now have a lower bone formation rate this is not deleterious to their total bone mass, or health, but is merely a normal homeostatic response to turning off bone resorption. However, since estrogens are not anabolic for the human skeleton the amount of lost bone that can be restored is very limited. Therefore, we strongly advocate that estrogen treatment be started before an excessive amount of bone tissue has been lost. Before estrogen treatment is started, however, the patient and her physician need to agree on a life-long commitment to this regimen, or an equally effective substitute therapy, to avoid further fractures. In our study, 9 of 24 women taken off estrogens for breakthrough bleeding soon suffered new vertebral fractures. This finding has been confirmed by Lindsay and Hart[21], who found that estrogen-treated women who stopped taking their pills lost back all the bone they had previously gained. Very recent data indicate that this complication occurs because the bone resorption rate immediately increases sharply on withdrawal of estrogen, whereas the subsequent increase in the bone formation rate takes considerably longer before a homeostatic balance is once again achieved at a higher level of bone remodelling. It is clear, therefore, that if one starts a program of estrogen prophylaxis, or treatment, for postmenopausal osteoporosis it must be continued indefinitely, and if it becomes necessary for medical, or other reasons, to discontinue estrogen therapy an appropriate substitute must immediately be provided, e.g. progestogen, calcium or calcitonin.

The diagnosis of osteoporosis always requires clinical, chemical and radiological examinations. Only rarely is bone biopsy required, and then usually to rule out another condition, notably metastatic cancer or myeloma. Since a number of diverse conditions mimic postmenopausal osteoporosis, including some of the other osteoporoses, the diagnosis can never be made on the basis of X-ray film alone. Early bone loss can only be detected by measurement of bone mass, e.g. cortical thickness, photon absorptiometry, radiographic densitometry, computed tomography, dual-beam spectrophotometry or neutron activation analysis. The earliest osteoporotic fractures occur in the weight-bearing vertebrae. Consequently, we were not surprised when our computed tomography data showed loss of vertebral spongiosa long before the more readily available methods of cortical thickness or photon absorptiometry could detect bone loss in the appendicular skeleton[22]. However, it must always be borne in mind that objective measurements of loss of bone mineral mass alone, or radiolucency on conventional X-ray films, are not enough to make the diagnosis of osteoporosis. Similar losses of bone mineral mass occur in many other conditions, including osteomalacia, osteitis fibrosa, osteogenesis imperfecta tarda or metastatic carcinoma. Clinical examination shows that both early postmenopausal bone loss and advanced pathologic postmenopausal osteoporosis are not associated with blue sclerae, Cushing's syndrome, goiter, generalized bone tenderness or history of a primary cancer. Laboratory data in postmenopausal osteoporosis show that the serum calcium, phosphate, alkaline phosphatase and electrophoretic protein pattern are all within normal limits.

Menopausal hypercalcemia can present a problem in differential diagnosis. We have now seen 15 postmenopausal women in whom a rise in serum calcium and phosphate levels slightly exceeded the usual upper limit or normal. Regrettably, these women had all been mistakenly diagnosed as cases of hyperparathyroidism and had all undergone negative operations for parathyroid adenomas, including sternum-slitting in two cases. Attention to the serum phosphate level, which is elevated rather than low as in hyperparathyroidism, and measurement of the tubular reabsorption of phosphate, which is normal rather than low, easily differentiates this menopausal hypercalcemia from true hyperparathyroidism. These cases appear to be exceptional and none simulated osteoporosis.

We are all familiar with the clinical picture of the elderly woman with advanced postmenopausal osteoporosis. She is shrunken, kyphotic, walks slowly and gingerly, with her feet spread apart for better balance. Her skin is paper-thin due to a loss of collagen, and mucous membranes, particularly the vaginal mucosa, are atrophied. Often she suffers chronic localized back pain with acute episodes after each new vertebral fracture, but bone tenderness does not become generalized as in osteomalacia or some cases of myeloma. At this stage it may be difficult to measure her height accurately because she is bent over, her ribs rest on her iliac crests and dorsal kyphosis is compensated by lumbar lordosis. Loss of height can be estimated by reduction in the (normally 1 : 1) height : arm-span ratio; each crush fracture results in about 1 centimeter of height loss and kyphosis further subtracts from the height and the ratio.

X-ray films show 'empty box' vertebrae. The spongiosa is almost entirely mobilized and the cortex is thin. Deformities of the vertebrae are common, including crush fractures, wedging with the apex anterior, and ballooning due to pressure from the tough intervertebral discs. Schmorl's nodules are sometimes seen but are not pathognomonic, while vertebral osteophytes are almost never seen in postmenopausal osteoporosis. The aorta is often heavily calcified; sometimes it may appear more opaque than the radiolucent spine.

The high morbidity and mortality associated with hip fracture makes it desirable to predict which osteoporotic women are at risk. Changes in the trabecular pattern of the femoral neck are seen in advanced osteoporosis[23], but these are not specific enough to provide a useful predictive index. Measurements of cortical thickness in the femoral neck have a greater predictive value in delineating sub-groups at greatest risk of developing a femoral fracture but, as yet, there is still too much overlap between groups to apply this technique to individuals[24].

In differential diagnosis, the two conditions most commonly confused with postmenopausal osteoporosis because of radiolucency are early metastatic cancer or myeloma. However, clinical and laboratory examination usually differentiates these serious diseases without great difficulty. Uncomplicated postmenopausal osteoporosis is not associated with a rise in the serum alkaline phosphatase or calcium, the electrophoretic protein pattern is not altered and there is no loss of weight or generalized bone tenderness. In difficult cases, especially when there is a history of a primary tumor, it may be necessary to do a bone biopsy, but the necessity for such a painful, invasive procedure is now rare. Osteomalacia very rarely mimics osteoporosis. Some groups, notably in Great Britain, have claimed an associated finding, possibly aggravated by lack of sunshine and vitamin D, but we have not. The clinical and radiological pictures of osteomalacia and osteoporosis are usually quite different. In osteomalacia there is abundant osteoid avid for calcium, the bones are soft and bowing is common, quite unlike the brittle, porous bones of osteoporosis. Generalized bone tenderness is common in osteomalacia and the patient often has a history of steatorrhea or malabsorption. The alkaline phosphatase level is high, while the serum calcium and/or serum phosphate are low. The pathognomonic X-ray signs of osteomalacia are pseudofractures or Looser zones (Milkman's syndrome). However, in rare cases of osteomalacia any or all of these may be absent and a bone biopsy will be required to make the correct diagnosis.

When postmenopausal osteoporosis has progressed to pathologic fractures the condition can no longer be cured, but it can be arrested and partially reversed. Pain is a poor criterion for effectiveness of therapy because it may be relieved by a number of agents. We found that an estrogen (methallenestril) and a psycho-active placebo (Dexamyl[R]) relieved pain in seven of 12 osteoporotic women in a short-term study using the double-blind technique, while the androgen (fluoxymesterone) did not. A lactose placebo gave relief in half the cases. It is likely that this placebo effect is a short-lived phenomenon which would be effective only until the patient sustained another fracture. Postmenopausal osteoporosis is noted for periods of clinical exacerbation and remission; therefore, the only useful criteria for effectiveness of treatment are whether the agent(s) stop further fractures or prevent further loss of bone mass. Over a period of 30 years we have shown that cyclic, full-replacement doses of estrogens – ethinyl estradiol $50\,\mu g$, or methallenestril 6 mg, or stilbestrol 1 mg, or conjugated estrogens 1.25 mg, daily for 20–25 consecutive days each month, with or without a progestin – will stop further fractures.

This anti-fracture efficacy of estrogens was sufficient even in women with very far advanced disease, some of whom had been bedridden for years. Naturally, these patients required a considerable amount of supportive rehabilitation and physical therapy, but all were ultimately restored to normal or near normal levels of physical activity. Lower doses of estrogens did not protect against further fractures, neither did androgens or anabolic steroids, although all of these were effective in restoring positive calcium balance. Recent studies indicate that calcitonin is also effective in arresting osteoporosis in some post-menopausal women, but at present these data are short term.

Table 18.1   Postmenopausal osteoporosis: long-term treatment (1948–1973)

Treatment	Observed fractures	Patient years	Rate Fractures/1000 patient years
1. Estrogens			
(a) Premarin ᴿ 1.25 mg	5*†	1507	3
(b) Premarin ᴿ 0.6 mg	4	157	25
(c) On stopping estrogen	5	—	—
2. Androgens and 'anabolics'	8	204	40

(1a) vs. (2): p < 0.01
* 1 in epileptic seizure
† 1 in auto accident

We began our long-term therapeutic study of far advanced, symptomatic postmenopausal osteoporosis in 1948 (Table 18.1). At that time the only radiologic parameter available to us was the conventional X-ray film which, of course, can only detect far advanced bone loss. We entered patients into our study randomly until 1955; their average age was 62 years. The original intent was to treat the disease with agents known to restore positive calcium balance: estrogens, androgens and 'anabolic' steroids (really all weak androgens). The primary objective endpoint was the number of fractures. All of the estrogens used in our study were effective as long as full replacement doses were used cyclically for 20 or more consecutive days each month. The patients were crossed over to the opposite hormone if they could not tolerate the medication or if another fracture occurred. We found that the cross-over went only one way because the androgens and the 'anabolics' were poorly tolerated because of acne, hirsutism, voice changes and often a markedly increased libido. Even more important to us was the fact that they did not protect the skeleton. We only accumulated 204 patient years with androgenic steroids and the fracture rate was essentially the same (40 per 1000 patient years) as in an untreated population of similar age and menstrual status.

Our patients were instructed to take one pill at bedtime every night, omitting the first 5–7 days each calendar month. We told them they could expect a period of withdrawal bleeding when they stopped their pills. Most of the women on full replacement doses of estrogen resumed monthly 'periods'. We very carefully explained the difference between withdrawal and breakthrough bleeding and emphasized that they must report *every* episode of breakthrough bleeding, however small, to us immediately. Every such episode was referred to the gynecologist for complete evaluation, including dilatation and curettage. Twenty-four of our patients had one or more episodes of breakthrough bleeding and had their estrogen dose reduced or stopped by the gynecologist. Nine of them promptly sustained another vertebral fracture. In consultation with the gynecologist, we were able to restore the full replacement dose in seven of these women and they were subsequently protected from further fractures. Two of the women could not be given further estrogen treatment because of congestive heart failure and they had additional osteoporotic fractures. We now think, on the basis of very recent data, that these two women might have benefited from a trial of calcitonin therapy. There are now three studies showing that calcitonin, either as large doses of the salmon preparation with oral calcium supplements[25, 26], or low doses of porcine calcitonin alone[27], had beneficial effects on bone mass as demonstrated by neutron activation analysis or on calcium kinetics.

We detected three cases of endometrial cancer in our study. All were early, non-invasive cancers found on dilatation and curettage for breakthrough bleeding and all have remained cured by hysterectomy. When we compared the number of patients in our study by age and length of treatment with an appropriate group in the same community we expected to see 20 cancers but, in fact, only eight occurred and none of these were of the breast, the most common cancer of women. We believe that our method of treatment of far-advanced postmenopausal osteoporosis, including our intensive patient instruction and close co-operation with the gynecologists, provides a safe and reasonable way to protect these elderly women from further fractures without exposing them to an increased risk of cancer or other life-threatening situation, certainly not an increased risk of cancer death.

Demographic data showing the rapidly growing population of elderly women who are ethnically predisposed to develop postmenopausal osteoporosis clearly signals the urgent need for a well-planned program of prophylaxis. We now have readily available techniques to objectively measure loss of bone mass. Black-skinned women appear to be protected, but all other races show an increased incidence of fracture with aging. Five prospective studies have now shown conclusively that oral estrogens, even in very low doses, protect the skeleton against postmenopausal bone loss. A long-acting injectable progestin has also shown similar protective value[28], as have high-dose oral calcium carbonate supplements[29] or frequent intramuscular injections of calcitonin[25-27]. In a study not yet published, Judd has shown that very small doses of conjugated estrogens (Premarin[R]) 0.3 mg daily, or ethynyl estradiol 10 µg daily, both of which are too small to alter the Maturation Index of the vaginal epithelium, are as effective as full replacement doses of estrogen in lowering the urinary calcium:creatinine ratio[30]. These data suggest that doses of estrogen lower than those found osteotrophic by Lindsay et al.[28] and Recker et al.[29] may suffice to prevent postmenopausal bone loss.

The most recent data demonstrating the protective effect of estrogens on bone was reported by Ross, from Mack's Cancer Surveillance Unit in Los Angeles, California. Using the same computer techniques which indicated increased diagnosis of endometrial cancer in estrogen users, these workers have now shown a greatly decreased incidence of hip fracture in women taking estrogen[31] (Table 18.2).

Table 18.2   Incidence of hip fractures in women taking estrogen

	Months of estrogen treatment			
	0	1–60	61–204	205
Castrates	1.00	0.49	0.19	0.13
All women	1.00	0.93	0.55	0.41

As might be expected, the effect was greatest and was seen earlier in castrates who had half the risk of hip fracture in the first 5 years of estrogen therapy, one-fifth the risk from 5–17 years and one-eighth the risk thereafter.

The recent report by Recker, Saville and Heaney[29] showed that calcium carbonate supplements of 2.6 g daily protected against postmenopausal bone loss. The dose used is high and it is also possible that calcium carbonate possesses some special properties since several studies using other calcium preparations have been disappointing. We can predictably expect some hypercalciuria and the possibility of stone formation if this dose of calcium is continued for a long period. Hypercalcemia could also, conceivably, be a dangerous complication of such therapy, though with careful instruction and monitoring of the patient this is not likely. Despite these limitations, Recker's report is very welcome because it provides us with another mode of treatment for those women who cannot, or will not, take hormones.

In conclusion, it has been clearly shown by all workers in this field that each type of prophylaxis or treatment has a risk:benefit ratio. The rationale for treatment must be understood by, and be acceptable to, each patient because commitment to therapy must be life-long. Subsequent evidence amply confirms the ruling of the advisory committees of the Food and Drug Administration that 'estrogens are effective in preventing postmenopausal bone loss and the benefits outweigh the risks.' It has long been recognized that the majority of those women who survive osteoporotic hip fractures remain severely disabled. Many are completely bedridden for the remainder of their lives and the quality of their life is greatly diminished. Prophylaxis is the only ethical solution to this major public health problem. It is particularly sad that at the very time we have developed methods to measure bone loss objectively, and have learned how to prevent it, many women are stopping their estrogen therapy or are afraid to start this treatment. They are unaware that estrogen deficiency kills and seriously injures tens of thousands of women, while properly supervised estrogen therapy is one of the safest and most gratifying of all treatments available. In our opinion, with presently available information, postmenopausal osteoporosis, with its serious morbidity and mortality, should go the way of smallpox and poliomyelitis. We hope that readers are convinced by the data shown here and will try to educate their patients, the lay public and regulatory agencies to stamp out this preventable, deforming and lethal disease.

References

A more complete bibliography can be found in reference 32.

1. Klotz, H-P., Delorme, M-L. *et al.* (1975). Hormones sexuelles et sécrétion de calcitonine. *Sem. Hop.*, **51**, 1333
2. Milhaud, G., Benezech-Lefevre, M. and Moukhtar, M. S. (1978). Deficiency of calcitonin in age-related osteoporoses. *Biomedicine*, **29**, 272
3. Hillyard, C. J., Stevenson, J. C. and MacIntyre, I. (1978). Relative deficiency of plasma-calcitonin in normal women. *Lancet*, **2**, 961
4. Gordan, G. S., Picchi, J. and Roof, B. S. (1973). Anti-fracture efficacy of long-term estrogens for osteoporosis. *Trans. Assoc. Am. Physicians*, **86**, 326
5. Albright, F., Bloomberg, E. and Smith, P. H. (1940). Postmenopausal osteoporosis. *Trans. Assoc. Am. Physicians*, **55**, 298
6. Alffram, P. A. and Bauer, G. C. H. (1962). Epidemiology of fractures of the forearm. *J. Bone Jt. Surg.*, **44-A**, 105
7. Alhava, E. M. and Puittinen, J. (1973). Fractures of the upper end of the femur as an index of senile osteoporosis in Finland. *Ann. Clin. Res.*, **5**, 398
8. Commission on Professional and Hospital Activities (1977). *Hospital Mortality, P.A.S. Hospitals, United States, 1974–1975.* (Ann Arbor: P.A.S. Press)
9. Barnes, R. and Brown, J. T. (1976). Subcapital fractures of the femur: prospective review. *J. Bone Jt. Surg.*, **58-B**, 2
10. Meema, S. and Meema, H. E. (1976). Menopausal bone loss and estrogen replacement. *Isr. J. Med. Sci.*, **12**, 601
11. Gyepes, M., Mellins, H. Z. and Katz, I. (1962). The low incidence of fracture of the hip in the Negro. *J. Am. Med. Assoc.*, **181**, 133
12. Gordan, G. S. and Eisenberg, E. (1963). The effect of oestrogens, androgens and corticoids on skeletal kinetics in man. *Proc. R. Soc. Med. (London)*, **56**, 1027
13. Riggs, B. L. and Jowsey, J. (1969). Effect of sex hormones on bone in primary osteoporosis. *J. Clin. Invest.*, **48**, 1065
14. Heaney, R. P., Recker, R. R. and Saville, P. D. (1978). Menopausal changes in calcium balance performance. *J. Lab. Clin. Med.*, **92**, 953
15. Ibid. (1978). Menopausal changes in bone remodelling. *J. Lab. Clin. Med.*, **92**, 964
16. Meema, S., Bunker, M. L. and Meema, H. E. (1975). Preventive effect of estrogen on postmenopausal bone loss. *Arch. Int. Med.*, **135**, 1436
17. Lindsay, R. and Aitken, J. M. (1976). Long-term prevention of postmenopausal osteoporosis by oestrogen. Evidence for an increased bone mass after delayed onset of oestrogen treatment. *Lancet*, **1**, 1038

18. Goldsmith, N. F. and Johnston, J. O. (1975). Bone mineral: effects of oral contraceptives, pregnancy and lactation. *J. Bone Jt. Surg.*, **57A**, 657
19. Dalén, N. P. and Furuhjelm, M. (1978). Changes in bone mineral content in women with natural menopause during treatment with female sex hormones. *Acta Obstet. Gynecol. Scand.*, **57**, 435
20. Nachtigall, L. E. and Nachtigall, R. H. (1979). Estrogen replacement therapy. I. Ten-year prospective study in relationship to osteoporosis. *Obstet. Gynecol.*, **53**, 277
21. Lindsay, R. and Hart, D. M. (1978). Bone response to termination of oestrogen treatment. *Lancet*, **2**, 1325
22. Ettinger, B., Genant, H. K., Gordan, G. S. and Cann, C. E. (1979). A prospective study of peripheral and vertebral bone loss in post-oophorectomy women. Presented at *Computed Tomography and Densitometry Workshop*, June 8, 1979, San Francisco. *J. Comput. Tomography*. (In press)
23. Singh, M. and Riggs, B. L. (1973). Femoral trabecular pattern index for evaluation of spinal osteoporosis. *Mayo Clin. Proc.*, **48**, 184
24. Hagberg, L. and Nilsson, B. E. (1977). Can fractures of the femoral neck be predicted? *Geriatrics*, **32**, 55
25. Wallach, S. and Cohn, S. H. (1977). Effect of salmon calcitonin on skeletal mass in osteoporosis. *Curr. Ther. Res.*, **22**, 556
26. Chestnut, C. H. and Baylinck, D. J. (1979). Calcitonin therapy in postmenopausal osteoporosis: preliminary results. *Clin. Res.*, **27**, 85
27. Milhaud, G., Talbot, J-N. and Coutris, G. (1975). Calcitonin treatment of postmenopausal osteoporosis. Evaluation of efficacy by principal components analysis. *Biomedicine*, **23**, 223
28. Lindsay, R. and Hart, D. M. (1978). Comparative effects of oestrogen and a progestogen on bone loss in postmenopausal women. *Clin. Sci.*, **54**, 193
29. Recker, R. R., Saville, P. D. and Heaney, R. P. (1977). Effect of estrogens and calcium carbonate on bone loss in postmenopausal women. *Ann. Int. Med.*, **87**, 649 (and Letter to Editor, *ibid*, **89**, 149)
30. Judd, H. L. (1979). Personal communication
31. Ross, R. K. (1979). Costs and benefits of postmenopausal estrogen therapy. Presented at the *24th Annual Postgraduate Obstetrics and Gynecology Symposium, Southern California Permanente Medical Group and Kaiser Foundation Hospitals of Los Angeles*, March 31, 1979, Los Angeles
32. Gordan, G. S. and Vaughan, C. (1976). *Clinical Management of the Osteoporoses*. (Acton, Mass.: Publishing Sciences Group)

19
The Clinical Epidemiology of Breast and Uterine Cancer

R. I. HORWITZ and A. R. FEINSTEIN

INTRODUCTION

The ideal way to determine whether estrogens cause endometrial or breast cancer would be to conduct an experiment. In a randomized clinical trial, postmenopausal women would be assigned to take or not take estrogen replacement therapy. Both groups of women would be followed thereafter with similar diagnostic methods to detect the occurrence of a neoplasm. For the study of endometrial cancer intra-endometrial examinations would be performed at regular intervals, while the study of breast cancer might require that treated and untreated patients have breast examinations with equal frequency and intensity. Although this type of clinical trial is scientifically desirable, most women would not accept or maintain such a randomized assignment to be treated or untreated.

In the absence of randomization, there are two general epidemiologic research strategies. The first is a longitudinal cohort study, in which postmenopausal women who have made their own decision to receive or not to receive estrogens would be followed for a suitably long period of time thereafter. To determine the rate at which cancer develops in the two groups, the members of each group would receive the same diagnostic examinations that might have been carried out in an experimental trial. The results of the cohort study would be expressed as a risk ratio, which is the rate of disease (breast or endometrial cancer) in those exposed to estrogens, divided by the rate in those not exposed.

Although a cohort study might be more acceptable to the women than a clinical trial, the performance of the cohort would probably be unacceptable to the investigator. Because the incidence of cancer is low – at the rate of perhaps one per thousand postmenopausal women – and because the 'incubation period' (for the development of cancer after estrogen exposure) may be many years, the attempt to achieve satisfactory statistical data would require the direct clinical observation of huge numbers of women for a protracted period of years. The logistics of such a study are so difficult it will probably never be conducted.

The second alternative research strategy is the retrospective case–control method. This type of research is relatively quick, inexpensive and easy to perform because it is conducted in a backward manner. The investigator begins with a group of *cases* who are women already proven to have the disease under study (e.g. breast or endometrial cancer). The investigator then arbitrarily chooses a group of *controls* who are women not shown to have the suspected disease. The two groups are then asked about their previous usage of estrogens. The results are expressed as an odds ratio, which is the exposure ratio in the cases (number of estrogen takers among women with the disease) divided by the exposure ratio in the controls (number of estrogen takers among women without the disease).

The case–control method has become epidemiologically popular despite the occurrence of well-known errors that have resulted from the use of this approach[1]. All of the evidence linking estrogens to cancer of the endometrium, and much of the data on estrogens and breast cancer, have come from this type of observational study. Because the results of case–control and cohort research are subject to serious distortion by various types of bias, investigators must adhere to strict methodologic standards to arrive at credible scientific evidence.

In this report we shall determine whether the epidemiologic evidence that links estrogens to cancer of the breast and endometrium has avoided several important sources of bias. For each of the alleged associations, we shall briefly present the available data and discuss how the sources of bias may account for the conflicting results in the studies of these topics.

ESTROGENS–ENDOMETRIAL CANCER

All of the data that have been used as the main support (or refutation) for the suspicion that estrogens cause endometrial cancer have come from retrospective case–control studies. The main source of the controversy rests on the willingness of investigators to accept the conventional tactics of case–control studies as a substitute for the scientific methods that might be employed in an experimental trial or suitably performed longitudinal cohort study. The main problem is the issue of community surveillance bias and the rates of diagnostic detection of the endometrial cancer.

Community surveillance refers to the medical examinations that occur before a person becomes a case or control in the hospital. A bias in surveillance can occur unless medical attention was sought and received before hospitalization in a way that allows the exposed (estrogen-taking) and the non-exposed people an equal chance to become detected as cases when endometrial cancer occurs.

The bias arises because the patients who are collected in the hospital as members of the case–control study start out in the community as exposed cases, non-exposed cases, exposed controls and non-exposed controls. Each of these four community groups then undergoes various rates of diagnostic surveillance before reaching the hospital to become the components of the case–control study. If the rates of surveillance are similar in each of the four community groups, the hospitalized cases and controls will properly represent their proportionate numbers in the community. If the rates are disparate, however, so that women who are both exposed and diseased receive an increased diagnostic surveillance in the community, the four case–control groups chosen in a conventional manner will misrepresent the true proportion of persons in the community who are both exposed and diseased. Since this bias, if present, has already occurred before the cases and controls are chosen for a case–control study, its distortions cannot be remedied by statistical adjustments of data collected in the conventional manner. Instead, the removal or reduction of the bias requires special procedures for the selection of patients and subsequent analysis of data.

To demonstrate the importance of community surveillance bias and the need for new methods of research in the relationship of estrogens and endometrial cancer, we performed two separate case–control studies[2]. The first used conventional methods to choose cases of endometrial cancer and a separate control group of women with other gynecologic cancer. The alternative diagnostic procedure method was developed to equalize the 'forces of diagnostic surveillance' by letting cases and controls emerge from a group of women referred to the hospital for the same diagnostic procedure. The results are then stratified according to the reasons for hospital referral. The results of the two comparative studies are presented in Table 19.1.

Table 19.1 Comparison of results using conventional and diagnostic-procedure methods of selecting patients for case–control study of estrogens and endometrial cancer

	Conventional method	Diagnostic procedure method
Number of women in study	238	298
Odds ratio (unstratified) with 95% confidence limits	11.98 (4.0–47.7)	2.30 (1.3–4.3)
Stratified odds ratio with 95% confidence limits		
A. Patients with uterine bleeding	10.76 (1.6–454.6)	1.71 (0.9–3.4)
B. Patients without uterine bleeding	6.00 (0.09–89.8)	1.83 (0.03–21.0)

In the conventional study the odds ratio for the unstratified data was 11.98. When the population was stratified according to the reason for hospital referral, the odds ratio was 10.76 for the groups presenting with uterine bleeding and 6.00 for the groups that presented with other, non-bleeding complaints. The results of this conventional study are consistent with the conclusions of the reports that linked estrogens and uterine cancer.

For the alternative study, with cases and controls selected by the diagnostic procedure method, the odds ratio for the unstratified data was 2.30. Although this ratio is strikingly smaller than that obtained by conventional sampling methods, the result continues to reflect the consequence of estrogen-influenced surveillance bias. When this bias was further reduced by stratifying the results according to the reason for hospitalization, the odds ratio was 1.71 for the group presenting with uterine bleeding and 1.83 for the non-bleeding group.

The results of the conventional method of sampling agree with the findings of other investigators who have used conventional tactics, whereas the results of the alternative diagnostic procedure method agree with those of the two older studies. As illustrated by Table 19.2, the odds ratio in conventional studies has ranged from 4.9 to 8.0. For diagnostic procedure studies, the values were 0.5 and 1.1 in studies that stratified for uterine bleeding, and 3.1 in the study that did not attempt stratification[3–10].

Table 19.2   Estrogens and endometrial cancer: sources of patients and results

	Principal investigator	Control group	Odds ratio
Conventional sampling	Smith[3]	other gyn. CA	7.5
	Ziel[4]	health plan	7.6
	Mack[5]	community	8.0
	McDonald[6]	community med.	4.9
	Antunes[7]	non-gyn. dis.	6.0
Diagnostic sampling	Gray[8]	not stratif.	3.1
	Dunn[9]	bleeders	1.1
	Pacheco[10]	bleeders	0.5

These disparities can be reconciled by the effects of community surveillance bias on the results of case–control studies. As seen in Figure 19.1, in a case–control study the investigator attempts to approximate accurately the results that would be obtained by a longitudinal cohort study. To achieve this, unbiased case–control groups must be assembled. In these groups, the ratio of diseased to non-diseased patients who are exposed (a/b) and non-exposed (c/d) is proportionately equal to the ratios in the community cohort. Thus, the resulting odds ratio from the case–control study is a valid approximation of the true ratio obtained in the cohort study.

Figure 19.2 demonstrates the distortions that are caused by uncompensated surveillance bias. Using conventional case–control methods, the case group of women with endometrial cancer is selected in favor of estrogen exposure. The cell that represents women with endometrial cancer who used estrogens (a') is artefactually increased, because women who take estrogens are more likely to bleed and have an otherwise asymptomatic cancer detected. As a result, the ratio of diseased to non-diseased exposed patients is distorted, leading to a falsely elevated estimation of the odds ratio (a'/b ÷ c/d).

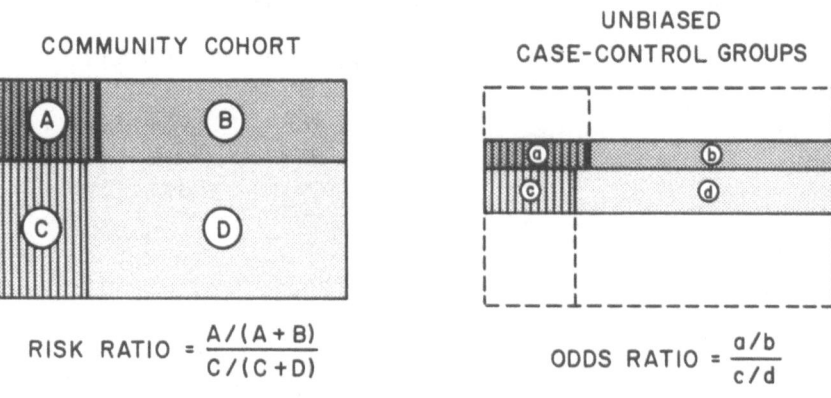

Figure 19.1   Upper-case letters refer to the cohort model, lower-case letters to the case–control model. The diseased (endometrial cancer) patients are located in cells A and C; the non-diseased (control) patients in cells B and D. Estrogen takers are represented by cells A and B; estrogen non-takers by cells C and D. In this diagram, the assembly of the case–control groups is unbiased, and the odds ratio is a valid approximation of the risk ratio (see text for detailed discussion)

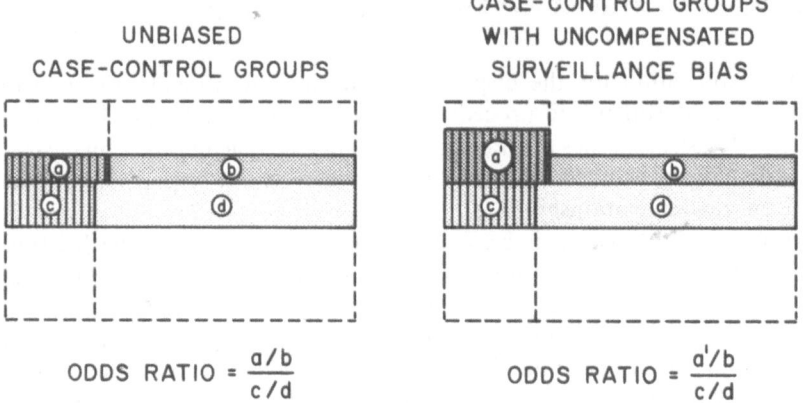

Figure 19.2   The patients with endometrial cancer are again represented in cells a and c; control patients in cells b and d. Exposed (estrogen users) women are in cells a and b; non-exposed in cells c and d. When case–control groups are assembled in a conventional manner, the cases are selected in favor of estrogen exposure. The cell that contains exposed and diseased patients (a') is augmented, and the odds ratio is artefactually elevated (a'/b ÷ c/d) (see text for detailed discussion)

Community surveillance bias, acting in this manner on conventional case–control studies, has led to an overestimation of the association between estrogens and endometrial cancer. Figure 19.3 demonstrates that the diagnostic-procedure method can substantially reduce this important source of bias by assembling as cases and controls women with an equal chance of having their endometrial cancer detected. Using this method, the ratio of diseased to non-diseased exposed women (a'/b') is adjusted, so that the resulting odds ratio may accurately represent the true risk ratio.

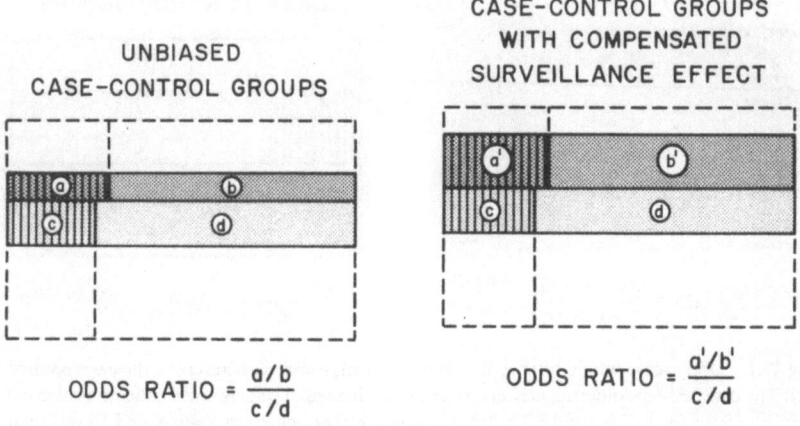

UNBIASED
CASE-CONTROL GROUPS

CASE-CONTROL GROUPS
WITH COMPENSATED
SURVEILLANCE EFFECT

$$\text{ODDS RATIO} = \frac{a/b}{c/d}$$

$$\text{ODDS RATIO} = \frac{a'/b'}{c/d}$$

Figure 19.3 The same notation is used as in Figure 19.2. Case–control groups are assembled using the diagnostic-procedure method, so that cases and controls are subject to 'equal forces of estrogen-related surveillance'. Thus, there is equal augmentation of exposed cases and controls, resulting in a more valid estimation of the odds ratio (see text for detailed discussion)

This explanation for the disparities between conventional case–control methods and the diagnostic procedure method has been challenged by several epidemiologists. Antunes *et al.*[7], using the data assembled in their own case–control study, concluded that surveillance bias was not responsible for the estrogen–cancer relationship.

Antunes *et al.* base their conclusion on observations that the lag-time between the onset of postmenopausal bleeding and contact with a physician was comparable for estrogen users and non-users. Thus, they argue, among women with uterine bleeding, estrogen usage does not advance the date of endometrial cancer detection. This interpretation is irrelevant to the issue of surveillance bias because the rapidity with which a bleeding woman goes to see her doctor has little to do with what makes her bleed. Surveillance bias results from the detection of endometrial cancer in otherwise asymptomatic women who were made symptomatic by estrogen-induced bleeding. The analysis by Antunes *et al.* did not measure the magnitude of surveillance bias, and their analytic procedures did nothing to reduce its effects.

The paper by Antunes *et al.* actually provides further evidence for the idea that surveillance bias is responsible for the observed association. When these authors selected controls from among women hospitalized on the gynecology service, the odds ratio declined to a value of only 2.1. This value is similar to the unstratified findings of our alternative series, and the odds ratio could be expected to drop even further if appropriate stratifications were made for uterine bleeding.

Other epidemiologists have criticized the selection of a control group that may include women with conditions that are possibly related to estrogen usage. However, the control group in the diagnostic procedure method is assembled in favor of estrogen usage in order to compensate for the selection bias that augments the proportion of estrogen users among the case group of endometrial cancer. Unless a control group is chosen with rates of diagnostic surveillance that are comparable to the case group, the odds ratio will be artificially elevated.

In summary, the association between estrogens and endometrial cancer appears to have been greatly overestimated because of the neglected effects of community surveillance bias. When cases and controls are selected to achieve comparable rates of diagnostic endometrial surveillance, the association between estrogens and endometrial cancer is substantially reduced.

ESTROGENS–BREAST CANCER

The question of a potential link between estrogen treatment and breast cancer is another important element in the analysis of risks and benefits associated with estrogen therapy. From physiologic evidence and animal studies, breast cancer has long been associated with reproductive hormones, but until recently no epidemiologic data in people had supported the idea of a causal relationship. In fact, several studies had even suggested that estrogens might protect against the development of breast tumors[11, 12].

In Table 19.3 are listed the results of cohort and case–control studies of estrogens and breast cancer. Among the cohort studies, both Wallach[11] and Wilson[12] concluded that estrogens protected against breast cancer[11–19]. In the report by Hoover, the authors concluded that estrogens possibly caused breast cancer, especially among long-term estrogen users. Among the case–control studies, all but one reported no statistically significant association. In the study by Casagrande *et al.*[19], two separate series of cases and controls were assembled. In one series, an apparent protective association was noted, while in the second series, a possibly causal association was observed.

The studies of estrogens and breast cancer have been affected by at least two important sources of bias. As in the studies of estrogens and endometrial cancer, community surveillance bias may play a prominent role. For example, in the study by Hoover *et al.*[14] that reported a causal association, the incidence

Table 19.3   Estrogens and breast cancer: conclusions and results

	Principal investigator	Risk ratio	Conclusion
Cohort studies	Wallach[11]	not available	protective
	Wilson[12]	0.03	protective
	Byrd[13]	1.38	no effect
	Hoover[14]	2.0 (15 y)	causal
Case–control studies	BCDSP[15]	0.96	no effect
	Wynder[16]	0.89	no effect
	Sartwell[17]	1.0	no effect
	Brinton[18]	0.97	no effect
	Casagrande[19]	0.47	protective
		2.15	causal

of breast cancer in women taking estrogens under the care of a single gynecologist was compared with the age-specific incidence rates derived from the Second and Third United States National Cancer Surveys. It has been repeatedly pointed out that these cancer survey incidence rates are likely to be falsely low because they are derived from a general population that does not receive the same careful surveillance provided to the patients followed by a gynecologist. This discrepancy would be increased in users of estrogens, since estrogen prescription leads to increased medical surveillance. Compared with a general population, the patients receiving such treatment under gynecologic supervision would be particularly likely to have increased rates of detection for breast cancer.

The second problem, protopathic bias, occurs when a pharmaceutical agent is inadvertently prescribed or withheld because of an early manifestation of a disease that has not yet been detected. When the disease is later discovered, a causal (or protective) relationship may be incorrectly inferred.

The problem arises when a patient has developed a target disease whose existence has not yet been suspected or diagnosed, and when that disease has an early (or protopathic) manifestation which becomes the stimulus for prescription of the alleged etiologic agent. Perhaps the best way to avoid protopathic bias in epidemiologic research is to determine why the alleged etiologic agent was prescribed, and to analyze the data according to the appropriate strata of the manifestations that evoked the prescription. Thus, in the studies of estrogens and endometrial cancer, if estrogen treatment was evoked by bleeding, the results should be analyzed for patients with and without bleeding.

If there is no association between estrogens and breast cancer, protopathic bias is a possible explanation for the 'protective' results found in several of the longitudinal epidemiologic studies. For example, if the signs or symptoms of breast disease were considered relative contraindications for estrogen use, the subsequent group of treated patients would have a low susceptibility for breast cancer. When the incidence rates of breast cancer for estrogen users and non-users is compared, the absence of estrogen use would appear to protect against breast cancer.

The problem could also occur in case–control studies. Patients with breast disease may discontinue the use of oral estrogens or may never receive them at all. When such a patient is later entered into a case–control study, she may be assigned to the case-group and is recorded as an estrogen non-user. Because of the protopathic discontinuation or avoidance of the agent, patients with breast disease may have a falsely low rate of estrogen usage. As a result of this bias the investigator may miss an association that is truly causal, or may erroneously conclude that the agent is protective.

The nine epidemiologic studies of estrogens and breast cancer are listed in Table 19.4, along with whether they avoided the problem of surveillance and protopathic bias. As demonstrated, only one study managed to adjust for the effects of surveillance bias, and no study attempted to minimize the effects of protopathic bias.

Table 19.4 Avoidance of surveillance bias and protopathic bias in studies of estrogens and breast cancer

| Investigator | Conclusion | Avoidance of | |
		Surveillance bias	Protopathic bias
Wallach[11]	protective	no	no
Wilson[12]	protective	no	no
Byrd[13]	no effect	no	no
Hoover[14]	causal	no	no
BCDSP[15]	no effect	no	no
Wynder[16]	no effect	no	no
Sartwell[17]	no effect	no	no
Brinton[18]	no effect	yes	no
Casagrande[19]	causal; protective	no	no

In summary, these are conflicting results in the studies associating estrogens and breast cancer. The contradiction may arise from inadequate attention to methodologic errors that result in important sources of bias. Consequently, the current literature cannot support either the causal or protective claims of opposing investigators.

CONCLUSIONS

Epidemiologic studies have assembled contradictory data on the association of exogenous estrogens to cancer of the breast and uterus. The conflicts appear to depend on the methodologic strategies that are used to perform observational cohort and case–control research. When important sources of surveillance and detection bias are removed or minimized in case–control studies of estrogens and endometrial cancer, the magnitude of the association is substantially reduced. For studies of estrogens and breast cancer, no conclusion is possible because of the methodologic deficiencies of the research.

Elucidating the relationship of pharmaceutical agents to cancer and other chronic diseases represents an important challenge in clinical epidemiologic research. The many conflicts and contradictions of the past indicate that we can no longer remain complacent about the absence of scientific standards for observational research. Future research will require adjustments for the problems of detection and protopathic bias, as well as the many other problems that distort the results of observational research.

References

1. Horwitz, R. I. and Feinstein, A. R. (1979). Methodologic standards and contradictory results in case–control research. *Am. J. Med.*, **66**, 556
2. Horwitz, R. I. and Feinstein, A. R. (1978). Alternative analytic methods for case–control studies of estrogens and endometrial cancer. *N. Engl. J. Med.*, **299**,1089
3. Smith, D. C., Prentice, R., Thompson, D. J. *et al.* (1975). Association of exogenous estrogens and endometrial carcinoma. *N. Engl. J. Med.*, **293**, 1164
4. Ziel, A. K. and Finkle, W. D. (1975). Increased risk of endometrial carcinoma among users of conjugated estrogens. *N. Engl. J. Med.*, **293**, 1167
5. Mack, T. M., Pike, M. C., Henderson, B. E. *et al.* (1976). Estrogens and endometrial cancer in a retirement community. *N. Engl. J. Med.*, **294**, 1262
6. McDonald, T. W., Annegers, J. F., O'Fallon, W. M. *et al.* (1977). Exogenous estrogen and endometrial carcinoma: case–control and incidence study. *Am. J. Obstet. Gynecol.*, **127**, 572
7. Antunes, C. M. F., Strolley, P. D., Rosenshein, N. B. *et al.* (1979). Endometrial cancer and estrogen use. *N. Engl. J. Med.*, **300**, 9
8. Gray, L. A., Christopherson, W. M. and Hoover, R. N. (1977). Estrogens and endometrial carcinoma. *Obstet. Gynecol.*, **49**, 385
9. Dunn, L. J. and Bradbury, J. T. (1967). Endocrine factors in endometrial carcinoma: a preliminary report. *Am. J. Obstet. Gynecol.*, **97**, 465
10. Pacheco, J. C. and Kempers, R. D. (1968). Etiology of post-menopausal bleeding. *Obstet. Gynecol.*, **32**, 40
11. Wallach, S. and Henneman, P. H. (1959). Prolonged estrogen therapy in postmenopausal women. *J. Am. Med. Assoc.*, **171**, 1637
12. Wilson, R. A. (1962). The roles of estrogen and progesterone in breast and genital cancer. *J. Am. Med. Assoc.*, **182**, 327
13. Byrd, B. F., Burch, J. C. and Vaughn, W. K. (1977). The impact of long-term estrogen support after hysterectomy: a report of 1016 cases. *Ann. Surg.*, **185**, 574
14. Hoover, R., Gray, L. A., Role, P. and McMahon, B. (1976). Menopausal estrogens and breast cancer. *N. Engl. J. Med.*, **295**, 401
15. Boston Collaborative Drug Surveillance Program (1974). Surgically confirmed gall-bladder disease, venous thromboembolism, and breast tumors in relation to postmenopausal estrogen therapy. *N. Engl. J. Med.*, **290**, 15
16. Wynder, E. L., MacCormack, F. A. and Stellman, S. D. (1978). The epidemiology of breast cancer in 785 United States caucasian women. *Cancer*, **41**, 2341

17. Sartwell, P. E., Arthes, F. G. and Tonascia, J. A. (1977). Exogenous hormones, reproductive history, and breast cancer. *J. Natl. Cancer Inst.*, **59**, 1589

18. Brinton, L. A., Williams, R. R., Hoover, R. N., Stegens, N. L., Feinleib, M. and Fraumeni, J. F. (1979). Breast cancer risk factors among screening program participants. *J. Natl. Cancer Inst.*, **62**, 37

19. Casagrande, J., Gerkins, V., Henderson, B. E., Mack, T. and Pike, M. C. (1976). Exogenous estrogens and breast canCer in women with natural menopause. *J. Natl. Cancer Inst.*, **56**, 839

20
Estrogens and Endometrial Cancer: A Pathologist's Perspective

S. J. ROBBOY and R. BRADLEY

INTRODUCTION

Recent investigations have implicated[1-6] and denied[7] the usage of exogenous estrogens in the two- to eight-fold increased risk in the development of endometrial carcinoma, the incidence of which in the general population is about one to three cases per 1000 postmenopausal women per year[8-11]. The occurrence of endometrial cancer with squamous components in young women with gonadal dysgenesis who had been treated for many years with estrogens[12] has also raised the possibility that the reported recent increase in frequency of adenosquamous carcinoma[13] may be a consequence of drug therapy. Since the cancer that occurs in most estrogen users is well differentiated and rarely invades deeply into the myometrium[14], the question has also arisen whether many of the lesions might in actuality be severe forms of atypical glandular hyperplasia that were overdiagnosed by the pathologist, or, if truly carcinoma, might be a unique form that behaves in a benign fashion.

To evaluate these questions, we reviewed, independently and in a random fashion, the slides from a cohort of patients who had received the diagnosis of endometrial carcinoma between 1940 and 1971 and correlated the micro-scopical findings with the clinical data that were subsequently obtained. The details of case selection, clinical and pathologic variables assessed, and ability to obtain follow-up data are presented elsewhere[15].

RESULTS

Estrogen usage

Information about estrogen usage was available for 190 of the 274 patients in this study; 32% had taken estrogen. Only three of the 61 estrogen users were under the age of 40 years (Figure 20.1). The drugs administered included Premarin (principally estrone sulfate) (30 patients), diethylstilbestrol (seven patients), Enovid (three patients) and, in one instance each, TACE, Ortho-novum and ethinyl estradiol; the drug administered to 17 patients was not recorded. Indications for therapy, recorded for 30 patients, were hot flushes (23 patients), osteoporosis (three patients) and postmenopausal spotting (four patients). No patient had received estrogen for purposes of contraception.

The percentage of patients with cancer who used estrogens during each 5-year interval may have risen during the 1940s and early 1950s, but has remained relatively constant since 1955 (average 32%) (Table 20.1). The average duration was 6.3 years (standard deviation 5.4 years).

Clinical comparison of estrogen users and non-users

Both groups were identical with respect to age at menarche (13 years) and age at menopause (48 years). The chief complaints in both groups were also similar: bleeding (85% in users and 91% in non-users), non-bloody discharge

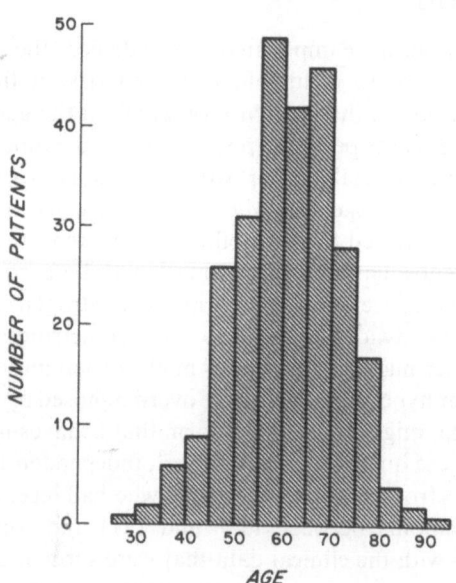

Figure 20.1   Age at diagnosis. (Reprinted from Robboy, S. J. and Bradley, R. (1979). *Obstet. Gynecol.*, **54**, 269)

Table 20.1   Estrogen usage

Year	No. of patients with cancer	No. of patients with positive or negative statement about estrogen history	% Estrogen users	Average duration in years ± std. deviation (number of patients)
1940–44	16	3	33%	2.0 ± N.A. (1)
1945–49	20	5	0%	N.A.
1950–54	36	17	18%	N.A.
1955–59	39	26	38%	8.8 ± 10.1 (3)
1960–64	66	55	29%	5.3 ± 5.6 (10)
1965–69	78	66	38%	7.1 ± 4.6 (13)
1970–71	18	18	33%	5.9 ± 4.4 (4)
Unknown	1	—	—	—
TOTAL	274	190	av. 32%	av. 6.3 ± 5.4

Reprinted from Robboy, S. J. and Bradley. R. (1979). *Obstet. Gynecol.*, **54**, 269

(8% and 6%), and incidental finding on pathologic examination of uterus (7% and 3%, respectively). The frequency of risk factors associated with endometrial carcinoma was also similar in both groups. The combined averages for both groups are: obesity 47%; nulliparity 41%; hypertension 26%; breast disorder 10%; thyroid disorder 8%; diabetes mellitus 8%; radiation-induced menopause 4%; Stein–Leventhal syndrome 2%.

The results of clinical staging are presented in Table 20.2. No differences between users and non-users were observed either when all cases were grouped or where each pattern of tumor was considered individually.

Table 20.2   Stage

Stage	Adenocarcinoma N = 168 %	Adenoacanthoma N = 49 %	Adenosquamous carcinoma N = 13 %	Undifferentiated carcinoma N = 9 %
1A	63	72	48	11
1B	24	20	26	33
2	5	6	22	22
3 and 4	8	2	4	33

Reprinted from Robboy, S. J. and Bradley. R. (1979). *Obstet. Gynecol.*, **54**, 269

Pathology

Endometrial cancers were defined as demonstrating characteristics of intra-glandular bridging (cribriform pattern), solid nests of cells, stromal invasion, or metastases (see Figures 20.2 and 20.3 for examples of histologic patterns and grades). Six histologic patterns of endometrial cancer were encountered

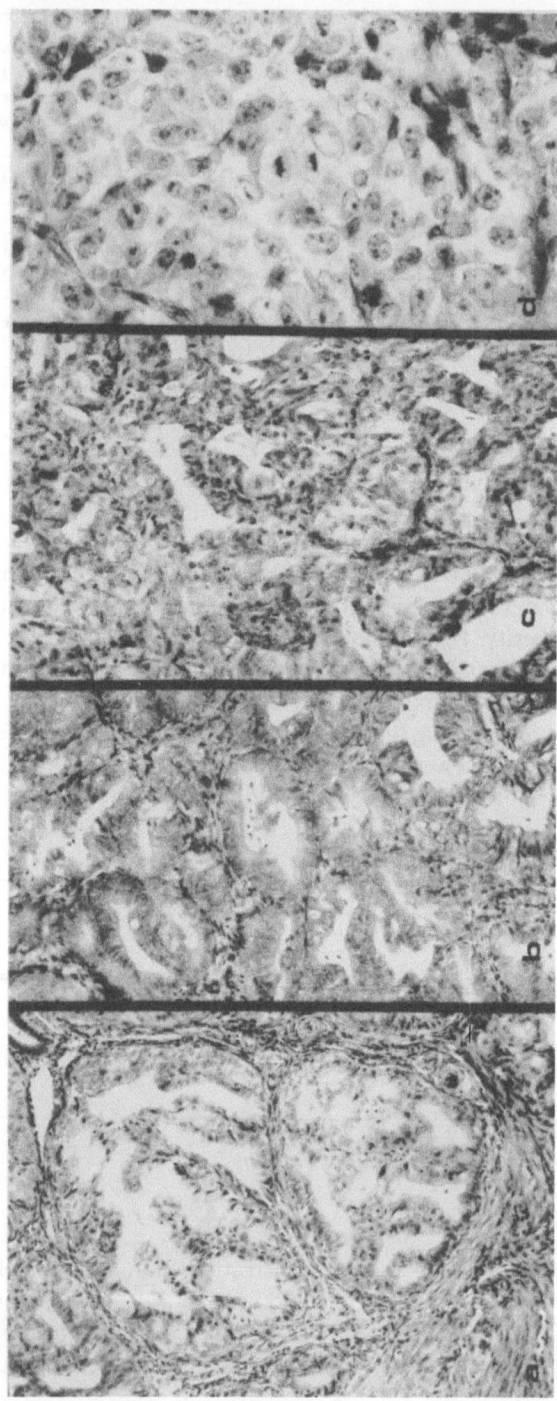

Figure 20.2 Glandular component of endometrial carcinoma. (a) Grade 1 – nests of tumor with intraglandular bridging (cribriform pattern) and highly differentiated cells with copious cytoplasm; (b) Grade 2 – extensive differentiation of tumor into glands composed of cells with large nuclei and small amounts of cytoplasm; (c) Grade 3 – mixture of focal glandular differentiation and solid sheets of tumor composed of cells with large nuclei and little cytoplasm; (d) Grade 4 – tumor composed of solid sheets of tumor devoid of glandular differentiation. (Reprinted from Robboy, S. J. and Bradley, R. (1979). *Obstet. Gynecol.*, **54**, 269) H & E, × 110 to 510

(Table 20.3). The most common was the typical pattern of adenocarcinoma (62%), which was composed entirely, or almost entirely, of glandular cells (Figure 20.2). A rare, tiny focus of squamous cells within the tumor or a cluster of squamous cells confined entirely to the surface was not considered sufficient to remove the neoplasm from the category of adenocarcinoma. The second most frequent pattern was adenoacanthoma (19%) (Figure 20.3). The squamous component consisted of morules of squamous cells within at least three separate neoplastic glands or as clusters of squamous cells with little or no cytologic atypia intermingled among glands. Adenosquamous

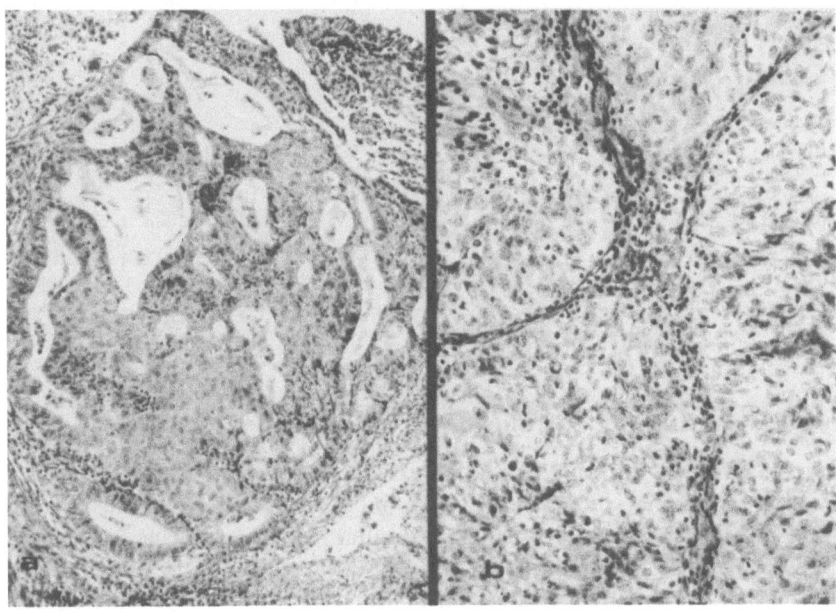

Figure 20.3 Adenocarcinomas with squamous cell component. (a) Adenoacanthoma characterized by a nest of adenocarcinoma within which are clusters of well differentiated squamous cells with uniform small nuclei and copious cytoplasm. (b) Adenosquamous carcinoma characterized by nests of poorly differentiated squamous cells with large pleomorphic nuclei and little cytoplasm. (Reprinted from Robboy, S. J. and Bradley, R. (1979). *Obstet. Gynecol.*, **54**, 269) H & E, × 110 to 200

carcinoma accounted for 11% of the tumors (Figure 20.3); by definition the squamous component displayed marked cytologic atypia and frequently invaded the endometrial stroma or myometrium. Several tumors with squamous components displayed features that were typical of neither the adeno-acanthoma nor adenosquamous tumor (4%) and were termed atypical adeno-acanthoma; in these instances the squamous cells in the morules exhibited moderate to marked degrees of cytologic atypia or cells invading the stroma appeared to be well differentiated. Clear cell adenocarcinoma, encountered in

1% of tumors, was composed of large cells with copious amounts of intracellular glycogen and 'hobnail' cells that lined glandular lumina. Undifferentiated carcinoma was encountered in 3% of cases; it was characterized by sheets of anaplastic epithelial cells that lacked obvious glandular or squamous differentiation and intracellular mucin.

Table 20.3 Histology

	Adeno-carcinoma %	Adeno-canthoma (typical) %	Atypical adeno-acanthoma %	Adeno-squamous %	Clear cell %	Undiffer-entiated %	Total cases %
1940–44	80	7	0	13	0	0	16
1945–49	60	25	10	5	0	0	20
1950–54	67	25	0	8	0	0	36
1955–59	59	26	3	5	0	8	39
1960–64	54	20	5	14	0	8	66
1965–69	70	12	3	13	3	1	78
1970–71	61	17	5	17	0	0	18
Unknown	—	—	—	—	—	—	1
TOTAL	62	19	4	11	3	1	274

Reprinted from Robboy, S. J. and Bradley, R. (1979). *Obstet. Gynecol.*, **54**, 1979

Clinicopathologic correlation

No statement is warranted about an absolute rise in the frequency of endometrial carcinoma, since the increased number of cases observed during recent years at the Massachusetts General Hospital may have reflected a changing utilization of the hospital for treatment of this disorder or the larger number of gynecologists in practice during the latter part of this study. The frequency of each microscopic pattern relative to the other five has changed only slightly

Table 20.4 Patterns of tumor, estrogen usage and age

	Estrogen history		Mean age in years	
	User	Non-user	User	Non-user
Adenoacanthoma	18 (51%)†	17†	57	55
Adenocarcinoma	33 (29%)	82	57*	60*
Adenosquamous carcinoma	6 (27%)	16	53	62
Atypical adenoacanthoma	3 (30%)	7	57	66
Clear cell adenocarcinoma	1	1	—	—
Undifferentiated	0 (0%)	6	—	67
			56*	60*

† Association with estrogens by χ^2, $p < 0.02$
* Difference of mean age, $p < 0.05$
Reprinted from Robboy, S. J. and Bradley, R. (1979). *Obstet. Gynecol.*, **54**, 269

during the study period (Table 20.3). The frequency of adenosquamous carcinoma rose from an average frequency of 7% during the interval 1940–59 to 14% during 1960–71, while the frequency of adenoacanthoma fell from 23% to 15% respectively. However, these changes are not statistically significant.

Comparisons of the histologic patterns of tumor, history of estrogen usage and the ages of the patients at the time of diagnosis indicated that the estrogen users were on the average 56 years of age (Table 20.4). The non-users with adenoacanthoma were also of similar age (55 years), in contrast to the significantly higher age of non-users with adenocarcinoma (60 years, $p < 0.05$), adenosquamous carcinoma (62 years) or undifferentiated carcinoma (67 years). These data also reveal distinct differences when the tumors were ranked by grade. Patients with grade 1 tumors were on the average 53 years of age and progressed to age 66 for those individuals with grade 4 tumors ($p < 0.001$) (Table 20.5). Although the data suggest that patients with higher stage (more widespread) tumor were older, insufficient numbers of cases were available to achieve statistical significance.

Table 20.5   Relation of grade, depth invasion, and stage to age

Grade	Age	Depth invasion	Age	Stage	Age
1	53	A	58	1A	60
2	60	B	61	1B	62
3	63	C	66	2	62
4	66	D	62	3	62
				4	67
p	<0.001		<0.01		NS

Reprinted from Robboy. S. J. and Bradley. R. (1979). *Obstet. Gynecol.*, **54**, 269

Two of the 19 microscopical features evaluated were associated with prior estrogen usage: histologic pattern and grade. Half of the patients with adeno-acanthomas (51%) had taken estrogens in contrast to one-fourth of the patients with other tumor patterns ($p < 0.02$) (Table 20.4). (Whether estrogen usage can be implicated in the development of any of these groups of tumors cannot be determined without appropriate controls.) Estrogen related tumors were more highly differentiated (lower grade) than those in non-users, even when segregated by microscopical pattern ($p < 0.005$) (Table 20.6). Among 156 hysterectomy specimens, the depth of myometrial invasion was associated with the age of the patients (Table 20.5), but not with a history of estrogen usage.

Survival

The cumulative survival rate from endometrial cancer alone for the entire study population was 80% after year 02, 73% after year 05 and 64% after year 10. Most deaths occurred within the first 2 years after the treatment of the primary tumor (48 of 87 deaths, 54%). Only 6% of the deaths (five of 87 cases) occurred after the tenth year. Grade and, to a lesser degree, histologic pattern, appeared to be the most discriminating prognostic features. Grade 1 neoplasms, regardless of histologic pattern and estrogen history, were associated with 5- and 10-year survivals of 100% (Tables 20.6–20.8). Patients with neoplasms graded 4 had poor survival rates. By histologic pattern, the adenoacanthoma had the best prognosis, ranging from 100% after 5 years if the

Table 20.6   Survival

Grade of tumor	Estrogen history		5-Year survival estrogen history		10-Year survival estrogen history	
	Yes	No	Yes	No	Yes	No
1	11	8	100%	100%	100%	100%
2	18	43	82%	81%	72%	70%
3	4	22	3/4	59%	1/3	59%
3	0	8	—	25%	—	25%
	$p < 0.005$					

Reprinted from Robboy. S. J. and Bradley. R. (1979). *Obstet. Gynecol.*, **54**, 269

glandular component was grade 1, to 89% if the grade of the glandular component was 3 (Table 20.8). Adenosquamous carcinomas with glandular components grade 2 or 3 also had favorable survival rates, which at 5 years were 100% and 83% respectively. The clinical stage also affected survival; the prognosis was poor (33% 5-year survival) when the stage was 3 or 4, whereas it was much higher for stage 1A neoplasms, even when the tumor was poorly differentiated (57% 5-year survival, Table 20.7). Although the overall survival in estrogen users was very high in general (only nine of 61 patients died during the entire study, five by year 5 and eight by year 10; five with adenocarcinoma, one with adenoacanthoma and three with adenosquamous carcinoma), it

Table 20.7   Stage, grade, and survival for all endometrial carcinomas

Stage	No. of patients* at grade				5-Year survival† at grade				10-Year survival† at grade			
	1	2	3	4	1	2	3	4	1	2	3	4
1A	23	84	42	11	100%	96%	66%	57%	100%	90%	63%	57%
1B	5	33	16	10	100%	74%	71%	44%	100%	43%	71%	16%
2	0	5	7	8	—	80%	42%	12%	—	—	—	—
3 and 4	0	8	6	6	—	25%	33%	17%	—	—	—	—
	$p < 0.001$											

— = inadequate sample
* = 264 patients with stage and grade recorded; 24 patients lack follow-up data
† = Based on 240 subjects. which includes the 228 listed in Table 20.8. and 12 with other histologic patterns not listed in Table 20.8
Reprinted from Robboy. S. J. and Bradley. R. (1979). *Obstet. Gynecol.*, **54**, 269

became similar to that of non-users once corrected for grade. Thus, 100% of patients with adenocarcinomas, grade 1, survived at both 5 and 10 years (Table 20.6). The survival in users and non-users with grade 2 tumors was identical (82% and 81%, respectively, at 5 years, and 72% and 70% at 10 years). Although there were too few estrogen users with adenocarcinoma, grade 3, to permit meaningful survival figures, three of four of the patients were alive at 5 years and one of three at 10 years, which approximated the rate for non-users (59% at both 5 and 10 years).

Table 20.8 Survival

Grade	Adenocarcinoma			Adenoacanthoma			Adenosquamous carcinoma			Undifferentiated carcinoma		
	N	Survival		N	Survival		N	Survival		N	Survival	
		5 y %	10 y %		5 y %	10 y %		5 y %	10 y %		5 y %	10 y %
1	22	100	100	5	100	100	0	—	—	0	—	—
2	76	79	66	27	96	84	5	100	—	0	—	—
3	41	49	46	9	89	89	12	83	83	0	—	—
4	13	45	32	0	—	—	9	33	22	9	22	11

Reprinted from Robboy, S. J. and Bradley, R. (1979). *Obstet. Gynecol.*, **54**, 269

Grade 1 neoplasms

As none of the 28 patients with grade 1 neoplasms died as a result of the cancer alone, the question was posed whether grade 1 lesions are in fact bona fide cancers, neoplasms of low malignant potential, or possibly markedly atypical forms of hyperplasia. At the time of diagnosis, every lesion was clinically confined to the corpus (stage 1). Although five of the 28 patients (18%) were asymptomatic or presented because of findings other than bleeding, almost all of the lesions tended to be small. At operation one of the tumors involved the surface of the ovary; the microscopical pattern was identical to that in the endometrium (adenoacanthoma). Although this lesion was felt to most likely represent a metastasis, the possibility of a second synchronous primary tumor of the ovary could not be excluded. The most convincing argument that grade 1 neoplasms are truly cancers, albeit of a low degree of aggressiveness, is that two of the 28 cancers had invaded into the myometrium and had penetrated up to half the thickness of the wall.

DISCUSSION

This study, which describes the clinicopathological characteristics of a cohort of patients treated and followed by five gynecologists during a span of four decades, suggests that (1) there has been relatively little change in the frequency of the adenosquamous carcinoma or any other histological pattern of tumor during this investigation, (2) that the adenoacanthoma is associated with estrogen usage more frequently than other patterns of tumor, (3) the more poorly differentiated neoplasms occur in older patients, and (4) the survival rates of patients with endometrial cancer who used estrogens are the same as for the non-users once the grade of the neoplasm is taken into consideration.

Thirty-two per cent of all subjects in the present study were estrogen users, and the average length of estrogen administration was 6.3 years. Whether several neoplasms might have been present before therapy is unknown, since asymptomatic endometrial cancers have been found in 1% of menopausal subjects who underwent diagnostic curettage prior to a consideration of commencing estrogen usage[16], in up to 3% of subjects shortly after therapy had been begun[17, 18] and in 20% of 84 patients in whom the cancer was observed at autopsy (Robboy, unpublished data). The requirements that estrogen users had received therapy for at least 6 months and the fact that all but four of the patients in whom the duration of usage was known had received the drug for 1 year or more should lessen the chance that the tumor had been present, but asymptomatic, prior to therapy.

In 1973, Ng et al. reported that the proportion of adenosquamous carcinoma had risen 20-fold, from 1.7% of all endometrial carcinomas observed during the years 1942–46 at the Case Western Reserve University to 32.8% during the interval 1967–71[13]. Others have reported a range of proportions between 1.9%[19] and 21%[20], but these studies have covered only short periods of times, usually the late 1960s or early 1970s. The average frequency in the present study was 11% (range 5 to 17%), which is similar to the frequency reported by several other investigators[21, 22]. The slight increase observed in the present study was not statistically significant.

Is the development of tumors with squamous components related to estrogen usage? The recent reports of adenosquamous carcinoma occurring in infantile uteri of young women with gonadal dysgenesis who had been treated with estrogens, usually for periods in excess of 6 years, has argued for a causal link; other of these women developed pure adenocarcinomas and rarely adenoacanthoma while on therapy. Although diethylstilbestrol has been the drug most frequently administered to these women, steroidal estrogens, e.g. ethinyl estradiol and conjugated estrogens, have also been used[23]. An intriguing finding in this study was recognition that each of the histologic patterns of tumor not associated with estrogen usage occurred in patients of different mean ages, ascending from adenoacanthoma (55 years) to adenocarcinoma (60 years), adenosquamous carcinoma (62 years) and undifferentiated carcinoma (67 years). This paralleled the ascending ages for higher grades of tumor, which ranged from age 53 for grade 1 tumors to age 66 for grade 4 tumors. Although this data is insufficient in itself to imply a progression of disease as patients age, it does suggest that each tumor is a unique form of cancer with its own biological characteristics and that the tumors in older patients are associated with progressively more lethal effects. The data may also be interpreted to suggest that the high frequency of estrogen usage in patients with adenoacanthoma may be coincidental and simply reflect the fact that estrogens may be frequently used by a high percentage of women for several years after the onset of menopause[24], but not later.

Some of the case–control studies on the topic of estrogen usage and endometrial cancer have been criticized on the ground that the authors' failure to review the slides inadvertently permitted inclusion of cases of atypical hyperplasia, which can be estrogen induced. It is well known that pathologists, even the experts in the field, differ in their criteria that distinguish advanced degrees of hyperplasia from adenocarcinoma[25–28]. Thus, concern has been raised that some cases of estrogen-related atypical hyperplasia have been falsely labelled as early carcinoma[29], which might account for a falsely strong association of estrogen usage with low-grade, low-stage lesions. The present study was conceived in a manner designed to overcome this objection; namely, features considered diagnostic of carcinoma were defined, the slides were reviewed by pathologists not aware of the clinical findings, and only those cases considered to be carcinoma were then analyzed from a clinical viewpoint. Notwithstanding the uniform method applied, users and non-users of estrogens differed significantly in several aspects, the most important being better differentiation of the tumor in estrogen users. In contrast to other reports, the clinical stage and depth of invasion were no different in estrogen users and non-users.

Although the rate of 5-year survival from endometrial cancer alone was higher for the entire cohort of estrogen users than non-users, the rates for both groups were equal once the grade of the tumor was considered. These data suggest that grade for grade, tumors that arise in the presence of exogenous estrogens are of about the same potential aggressiveness as those not associated with estrogens. Tumors that are of a high clinical stage, high grade (poorly differentiated) or penetrate deeply into the uterine wall are more likely to be fatal than those which are not, whether or not there is a history of estrogen usage.

One hypothesis that might explain the favorable prognosis for patients who had used estrogens is that their cancers may have been detected earlier, possibly because of better medical surveillance. In support are the observations that the users are younger[6] (4 years in this study and 5 years in postmenopausal women in another study) and experience shorter intervals between the onset of symptoms and detection of cancer[3, 30]. Thus Weiss[14] and Studd[31] have speculated that users are from a more privileged class of society that expects hormone replacement therapy, has greater access to care (as these women are already under the care of the physician who prescribed the drug), expects frequent follow-up, and has physicians who may be more conscious of the possibility of tumor development in estrogen users. Conversely, it is also possible that increasing age results in patients' responses that are less resistant to the effects of the cancer.

The findings in this study have several bearings on survival, and hence implications, regarding therapy, whether or not the patient has been an estrogen user. For stage 1 tumors, which comprise 84% of all neoplasms in this series (more than four-fifths in many series)[30, 32, 33], the grade of the tumor appears to be the single most important determinant of prognosis. Thus the 5-year survival rate for patients with grade 1 tumor is 100%, while it is less than 45% for tumors that are grade 4. The fact that a tumor also contains well differentiated squamous cells (adenoacanthoma) or poorly differentiated squamous cells (adenosquamous tumor) seems to be of less biologic consequence once the glandular portion of the tumor is evaluated for its grade. In general, the glandular cells in adenoacanthoma are grade 1–3, while the glandular cells in the adenosquamous carcinoma are grades 2–4. The fact that only five of 61 estrogen users died by the fifth year and that only three additional estrogen users died by the tenth year indicates that treatment can be satisfactory if the neoplasm is discovered at an early period in its development. From a practical viewpoint, tumors that develop in estrogen users are infrequently fatal.

References

1. Gray, L. A. Sr, Christopherson, W. M. and Hoover, R. N. (1977). Estrogens and endometrial carcinoma. *Obstet. Gynecol.*, **49**, 385
2. Hoogerland, D. L., Buchler, D. A., Crowley, J. J. *et al.* (1978). Estrogen use: risk of endometrial carcinoma. *Gynecol. Oncol.*, **6**, 451
3. Mack, T. M., Pike, M. C., Henderson, B. E. *et al.* (1976). Estrogens and endometrial cancer in a retirement community. *N. Engl. J. Med.*, **294**, 1262
4. McDonald, T. W., Annegers, J. F., O'Fallon, W. M. *et al.* (1977). Exogenous estrogen and endometrial carcinoma: case–control and incidence study. *Am. J. Obstet. Gynecol.*, **127**, 572
5. Smith, D. C., Prentice, R., Thompson, D. J. *et al.* (1975). Association of exogenous estrogen and endometrial carcinoma. *N. Engl. J. Med.*, **293**, 1164
6. Ziel, H. K. and Finkle, W. D. (1976). Association of estrone with the development of endometrial carcinoma. *Am. J. Obstet. Gynecol.*, **124**, 735
7. Horwitz, R. I. and Feinstein, A. R. (1978). Alternative analytic methods for case–control studies of estrogens and endometrial cancer. *N. Engl. J. Med.*, **299**, 1089
8. Elwood, J. M., Cole, P., Rothman, K. J. *et al.* (1977). Epidemiology of endometrial cancer. *J. Natl. Cancer Inst.*, **59**, 1055
9. Gambrell, R. D. Jr (1978). The prevention of endometrial cancer in postmenopausal women with progestogens. *Maturitas*, **1**, 107
10. Hulka, B. S., Hogue, C. J. R. and Greenberg, B. G. (1978). Methodologic issues in epidemiologic studies of endometrial cancer and exogenous estrogens. *Am. J. Epidemiol.*, **107**, 267
11. Kjellgren, O. (1977). Epidemiology and pathophysiology of corpus carcinoma. *Acta Obstet. Gynecol. Scand.*, Suppl. **65**, 77

12. Cutler, B. S., Forbes, A. B., Ingersoll, F. M. *et al.* (1972). Endometrial carcinoma after stilbestrol therapy in gonadal dysgenesis. *N. Engl. J. Med.*, **287**, 628
13. Ng, N. G., Reagan, J. W. and Storaagli, J. P. (1973). Mixed adenosquamous carcinoma of the endometrium. *Am. J. Clin. Pathol.*, **59**, 765
14. Weiss, N. S. (1978). Noncontraceptive estrogens and abnormalities of endometrial proliferation. *Ann. Intern. Med.*, **88**, 410
15. Robboy, S. J. and Bradley, R. (1979). Changing trends and prognostic features in endometrial cancer associated with exogenous estrogen therapy. *Obstet. Gynecol.*, **54**, 269
16. Whitehead, M. I., Minardi, J., McQueen, J. *et al.* (1978). Clinical considerations in the management of the menopause: the endometrium. *Postgrad. Med. J.*, **54** (Suppl. 2), 69
17. Suchman, M. I., Kramer, E. and Feldman, G. B. (1978). Aspiration curettage for asymptomatic patients receiving estrogen. *Obstet. Gynecol.*, **51**, 339
18. Sturdee, D. W., Wade-Evans, T., Paterson, M. E. L. *et al.* (1978). Relations between bleeding pattern, endometrial histology, and oestrogen treatment in menopausal women. *Br. Med. J.*, **1**, 1575
19. Greenwald, P., Caputo, T. A. and Wolfgang, P. E. (1977). Endometrial cancer after menopausal use of estrogen. *Obstet. Gynecol.*, **50**, 239
20. Underwood, P. B. Jr, Lutz, M. H., Kreutner, A. *et al.* (1977). Carcinoma of the endometrium: radiation followed immediately by operation. *Am. J. Obstet. Gynecol.*, **128**, 86
21. Salazar, O. M., DePapp, E. W., Bonfiglio, T. A. *et al.* (1977). Adenosquamous carcinoma of the endometrium. An entity with an inherent poor prognosis? *Cancer*, **40**, 119
22. Haqqani, M. T. and Fox, H. (1976). Adenosquamous carcinoma of the endometrium. *J. Clin. Pathol.*, **29**, 959
23. Benjamin, I. and Block, R. E. (1977). Endometrial response to estrogen and progesterone therapy in patients with gonadal dysgenesis. *Obstet. Gynecol.*, **50**, 136
24. Stadel, B. V. and Weiss, N. (1975). Characteristics of menopausal women: a survey of King and Pierce Counties in Washington, 1973–1974. *Am. J. Epidemiol.*, **102**, 209
25. Welch, W. R. and Scully, R. E. (1977). Precancerous lesions of the endometrium. *Hum. Pathol.*, **8**, 503
26. Gordon, J., Reagan, J. W., Finkle, W. D. *et al.* (1977). Estrogen and endometrial carcinoma. An independent pathology review supporting original risk estimate. *N. Engl. J. Med.*, **297**, 570
27. Szekely, D. R., Weiss, N. S. and Schweid, A. I. (1978). Incidence of endometrial carcinoma in King County, Washington: a standardized histologic review: brief communication. *J. Natl. Cancer Inst.*, **60**, 985
28. Muirhead, W. and Roberts, J. T. (1978). Selection of tumours with a poor prognosis in operable carcinoma of the endometrium. *Clin. Radiol.*, **29**, 17
29. Lauritzen, C. (1977). Oestrogens and endometrial cancer: a point of view. *Clin. Obstet. Gynaecol.*, **4**, 145
30. Miller, A., Mullen, D., Faraci, J. A. *et al.* (1978). Postmenopausal estrogens and endometrial cancer: clinico-pathologic correlations. In S. G. Silverberg and F. J. Major (eds), *Estrogens and Cancer*, pp. 35–43. (New York: John Wiley and Sons)
31. Studd, J. (1976). Oestrogens as a cause of endometrial carcinoma. *Br. Med. J.*, **1**, 1144
32. Lewis, B. V., Stallworthy, J. A. and Cowdell, R. (1970). Adenocarcinoma of the body of the uterus. *J. Obstet. Gynaecol. Br. Commonw.*, **77**, 343
33. Malkasian, G. D. Jr (1978). Carcinoma of the endometrium: effect of stage and grade on survival. *Cancer*, **41**, 996

21
Steroid-induced Changes in the Endometrium of Postmenopausal Women

R. J. B. KING, P. T. TOWNSEND and M. I. WHITEHEAD

INTRODUCTION

The controversy over the putative carcinogenic effects of estrogens on the human endometrium[1-3] can only be resolved by multidisciplinary studies which elucidate the effects of female sex hormones on the human endometrium. Retrospective analysis of epidemiologic data[4,5] has provided the basis for our current concern about the administration of estrogen to postmenopausal women. Histological and clinical observations from prospective studies have reinforced the view that estrogens should not be given alone over long periods and that for at least 7 and perhaps 10 days each month a progestin should be added to the estrogen therapy[6-8]. The third facet of such a multidisciplinary approach would be to study the biochemistry of endometria from women receiving different combinations of female sex hormones.

Our group has adopted the third approach and previous publications[6,9,10] have established the features shown in Table 21.1. The first conclusion is based on the observation that nuclear estrogen receptor levels (REN) and cytoplasmic progesterone receptor levels (RP, an index of estrogenic potency) were, for about 2 weeks of each 4-week treatment cycle, equivalent to those seen in endometrial samples obtained during the proliferative phase of the menstrual cycle from premenopausal women; no significant differences in receptor levels were observed with different dosages or type of estrogen preparation. Support for point two comes from the data showing that RP activity is lowered more effectively when a progestin is added to the treatment

221

schedule (i.e. combined estrogen/progestin therapy) than when unopposed estrogen therapy is cycled and the 3-week treatment cycles are interspaced by a treatment-free week (cyclical estrogen therapy). Justification of the third point comes from data showing that progestins induce the enzyme estradiol dehydrogenase. This enzyme, which markedly reduces the biological potency of estradiol by oxidizing it to estrone[9], can only be detected in reasonable quantities in endometria from postmenopausal women ingesting progestins; and progestogen ingestion coincides with a lowering of REN. The final point in Table 21.1 is intuitive. The quantitative effect of progestins in reducing estrogenic potency may be insufficient to account for the dramatic decrease in the incidence of both endometrial hyperplasia[6, 7] and carcinoma[8] in post-menopausal women receiving sequential estrogen/progestogen therapy as compared to women taking estrogen alone. Other progestin-mediated effects such as an increased efficiency of endometrial shedding[7, 11, 12] during sequential treatment may also be clinically important.

The present article will extend this general background and describe experiments aimed at clarifying four questions:

(1) What is the active intracellular estrogen in postmenopausal women?

(2) What is the role of estradiol dehydrogenase in mediating the anti-estrogenic effect of progestins?

(3) Are there important progestational effects other than those mediated via estradiol dehydrogenase?

(4) Can biochemical tests help to establish the form of progestin treatment that will be most efficacious in protecting the endometrium against adverse estrogenic effects?

Table 21.1

(1) All types of estrogen therapy subject the endometrium to a potent estrogenic stimulus for a long period.

(2) Cyclical estrogen treatment results in more prolonged stimulation of the endometrium than sequential estrogen/progestin therapy.

(3) The anti-estrogenic effect of progestins is, in part, mediated via the induction of estradiol dehydrogenase activity and alterations in intracellular estrogen receptor machinery.

(4) There may be additional effects of progestins that are clinically important.

Data in support of these conclusions will be found in refs. 6, 9 and 10

EXPERIMENTATION

Endometrial samples were obtained by Vabra suction curettage from women attending the menopause clinics at King's College Hospital and Chelsea Hospital for Women, London. Full details have been published elsewhere[9, 11, 13, 14]

The biochemical effects of different dosages of norethisterone were determined in endometrial samples obtained from postmenopausal women taking Premarin (conjugated equine estrogen) 1.25 mg daily continuously. In addition the patients ingested norethisterone daily for 7 days each calendar month and the dose of norethisterone was varied between patients. Curettage was performed on the sixth day of progestin administration. All patients had received at least 3 months therapy prior to curettage.

(1) WHAT IS THE ACTIVE, INTRACELLULAR ESTROGEN IN POSTMENOPAUSAL ENDOMETRIA?

It is currently believed that estrogens promote cell growth and proliferation by entering the cell nucleus in combination with a regulatory protein (the nuclear receptor); the estrogen-receptor protein complex then modifies transcription and translation. Estradiol has a greater affinity than estrone for this receptor and the former compound therefore has the greater biological activity[15]. This is in accordance with the observation that estradiol is the principal tissue estrogen in proliferative phase endometria from premenopausal women[16-18].

Table 21.2 Nuclear estradiol and estrone concentrations; and nuclear estrogen receptor levels during estrogen alone or estrogen plus progestin treatment. Results are expressed as mean ± SEM (no. observations)

	Estrogen	*Estrogen + progestin*
Nuclear concentration (pmole/mg DNA)		
Estrone	0.47 ± 0.01 (8)	0.46 ± 0.01 (8)
Estradiol	1.52 ± 0.06 (8)	0.66 ± 0.03 (8)
Receptor	1.40 ± 0.02 (9)	0.58 ± 0.01 (8)
Estradiol/estrone ratio		
Nucleus	3.60 ± 0.40 (11)	1.52 ± 0.11 (7)
Plasma	0.67 ± 0.02 (6)	0.41 ± 0.01 (7)

These results are apparently at variance with the hypothesis that estrone rather than estradiol is the predominant intracellular estrogen in postmenopausal women and that estrone may be involved in the genesis of endometrial cancer[19, 20]. The estrone hypothesis is based on the well-founded observations that estrone is the principal estrogen in plasma of postmenopausal women[21] and that estrone is biologically active in its own right, albeit only weakly so[22, 23]. Until now, however, no data on the identity of intracellular estrogens in endometria from postmenopausal women have been available.

It is possible to reconcile the pre- and postmenopausal models by postulating either selective uptake or retention of estradiol in postmenopausal endometria. Experimental proof of this supposition is available as we have assayed the concentrations of estrone and estradiol in endometrial nuclei from postmenopausal women taking oral estrogens. The results obtained (Table 21.2) show that estradiol is present in greater concentration than estrone[13, 24]. Endometrial nuclei from women taking estrogen alone have estradiol:estrone ratios of about 3:1 despite a plasma ratio of approximately 0.7:1. Furthermore, the nuclear estradiol levels are similar to the amounts of REN assayed independently (Table 21.2). Similar experiments on women taking both estrogen and norethisterone gave nuclear estradiol:estrone ratios approaching unity despite unchanged plasma values. Therefore norethisterone had inhibited to an appreciable extent the mechanism for selectively transferring estradiol and its receptor to the nucleus.

We have previously shown that norethisterone does not significantly decrease the total estrogen receptor content of the endometria. It thus seems unlikely that the nuclear inhibition is due to lack of sufficient receptors and the most probable explanation of the reduction in REN values is lack of suitable ligand. The presence of estradiol dehydrogenase in norethisterone-treated endometria therefore appears to provide the mechanism whereby the intracellular concentration of the effective ligand, estradiol, is lowered and this is discussed further in the following section.

These data on nuclear estradiol and estrone levels support a causal inter-relationship between dehydrogenase activity and REN concentrations.

(2) WHAT IS THE ROLE OF ESTRADIOL DEHYDROGENASE IN MEDIATING THE ANTIESTROGENIC EFFECTS OF PROGESTINS?

The original suggestion[25] that, in premenopausal human endometria, progestin-induced estradiol dehydrogenase has an important regulatory function has been amply substantiated[18, 26, 27]. For reasons stated previously, estradiol is appreciably more estrogenic than estrone and therefore is the more important intracellular estrogen. The cellular concentration of estradiol determines the mass bound to receptor and hence the biological effect. Estradiol dehydrogenase effectively decreases the concentration of estradiol by oxidizing it to estrone, and thus the overall estrogenic stimulus is diminished. As progestins induce estradiol dehydrogenase activity they effectively lower the intracellular concentration of estradiol.

Our data indicate that the above sequence of events, first proposed by

Gurpide, also occurs in the postmenopausal situation, and have important implications in the design of estrogen therapy. Currently, three general types of oral estrogen preparation are available based on estrone (Premarin, Harmogen), estradiol (Progynova, estradiol implants) and synthetic estrogens (Mestranol). The estrone and estradiol-type preparations give rise to similar plasma estrogen profiles, with estrone predominating over estradiol[11, 28]. Hence, the Gurpide model[26] would predict that comparable doses of the estrone and estradiol-type preparations would result in similar intracellular effects/stimulation. Furthermore, the detoxifying effect of effective levels of estradiol dehydrogenase would be of equal benefit to women taking either estrone or estradiol derivatives. Such logic would not apply to women taking compounds such as ethinylestradiol or diethylstilbestrol, as synthetic estrogens are not substrates for the enzyme.

It is clear from the above remarks that before better methods of protecting the postmenopausal endometrium against excessive estrogenization can be devised, more detailed information about estradiol dehydrogenase and the nature and concentrations of intracellular estrogens is required.

We have previously shown that the progestin, norethisterone, induces estradiol dehydrogenase in postmenopausal endometria with a concomitant decrease in REN[9]. These experiments neither defined the quantitative association between the enzyme and REN nor established whether or not the interrelationship was causal. The possibility that both parameters changed in response to another unknown alteration in cell biochemistry was not excluded.

Sufficient results have now been accumulated from women receiving Premarin plus different doses of progestin to show that a quantitative inverse relationship exists between estradiol dehydrogenase and REN[14]. Statistically, the best linear correlation is obtained by plotting log estradiol dehydrogenase against REN, although a double log representation would also fit the results. Whichever representation is correct, the implication is that relatively small increases above basal levels of dehydrogenase activity lead to disproportionately large falls in REN. Conversely, very high dehydrogenase activities are not required to reduce REN to low levels. In practice, 2.5 mg/day norethisterone for 6 days gives optimal suppression of REN.

(3) ARE THERE OTHER IMPORTANT PROGESTATIONAL EFFECTS?

The above arguments should not be interpreted as indicating that progestins only exert their biological effects by preventing accumulation of REN. Progestins also induce a secretory response that cannot be mimicked by antiestrogens such as Tamoxiphen. As discussed previously, efficiency of endometrial shedding may also have important implications in preventing the accumulation of potentially neoplastic cells. Certainly withdrawal bleeding occurs more regularly and completely in women taking estrogen and progestin than in those on estrogen alone[6-8]. A simple biochemical test for assessing the efficiency of endometrial shedding would be of value in quantifying this effect of progestins. In pursuit of such a test we have measured certain

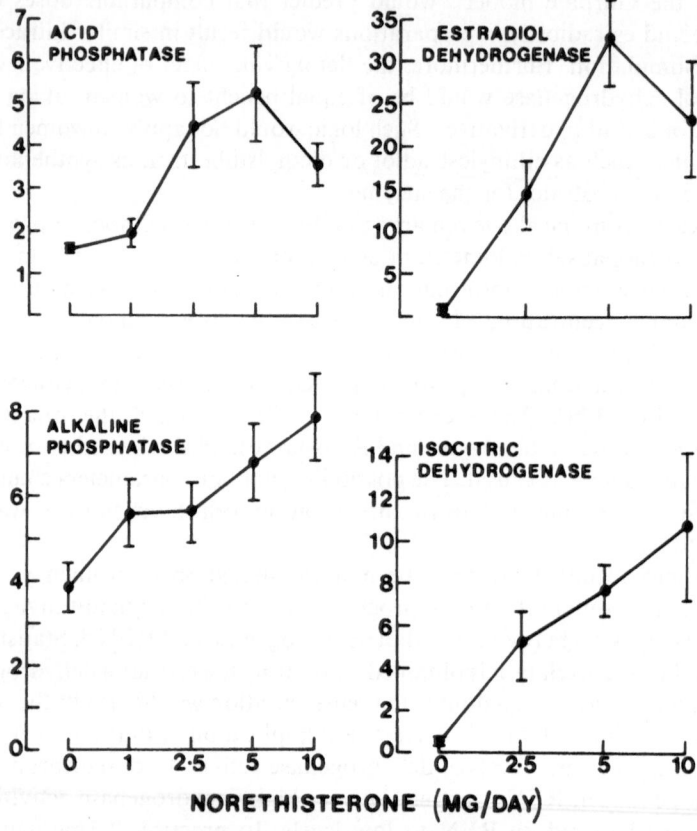

Figure 21.1 Endometrial enzyme levels after 6 days oral treatment with 1, 2.5, 5 or 10 mg daily of norethisterone. All the postmenopausal women were receiving Premarin continuously. Units of activity: acid phosphatase – mmol phosphate released/(mg protein h); alkaline phosphatase – mmol phosphate released/(10 mg protein h); estradiol dehydrogenase – nmol estrone formed/(mg protein h); isocitric dehydrogenase – mmol NADPH oxidized/(mg protein min). Results are expressed as mean ± SEM

enzymes that have been implicated in this process[29-31]. The concentrations of acid and alkaline phosphatases and isocitric dehydrogenase have been determined in endometrial samples (Figure 21.1) and the activities of these three enzymes are increased by norethisterone[14]. Additional effects of progestins are thus indicated.

(4) BIOCHEMICAL TESTS FOR DETERMINING THE OPTIMAL FORM OF PROTECTIVE PROGESTIN THERAPY

In a small percentage of patients, progestins cause unpleasant side-effects. Therefore it is important to establish the progestin treatment that will protect the endometrium against excessive estrogenization without negating the beneficial effects of estrogen therapy on the symptomatic and psychological status of climacteric women. The number of patients required to determine the minimal effective dose, duration and optimal type of progestin treatment by routine clinical trials would be large and therefore we are using biochemical methods. The aim is to monitor progestin-sensitive, biochemical parameters in endometria from women receiving Premarin plus graded doses of norethisterone as outlined at the beginning of this article. The parameters currently being investigated are thymidine labelling index, REN, estradiol dehydrogenase, acid and alkaline phosphatase, isocitric dehydrogenase and glucose-6-phosphate dehydrogenase[14]. Preliminary results indicate that acid phosphatase and estradiol dehydrogenase activities are particularly sensitive markers of progestin action and that maximum effects are obtained with between 2.5 and 5 mg norethisterone/day for 6 days; 1 mg/day is suboptimal, whilst 10 mg/day is no more effective than the 5 mg dose (Figure 21.1). These experiments are being extended to test different durations of norethisterone treatment.

Acknowledgments

We gratefully acknowledge the help of Jane Minardi and Osyth Young in obtaining the endometrial samples used in these studies. The technical help of Susan Leach and Gail Dyer in performing the enzyme and intracellular estrogen assays respectively is appreciated, as is the advice and help from W. P. Collins and S. Campbell.

References

1. Feinstein, A. R. and Horwitz, R. I. (1978). A critique of the statistical evidence associating estrogens with endometrial cancer. *Cancer Res.*, **38**, 4001
2. Mack, T. M. (1978). Exogenous oestrogens and endometrial carcinoma: studies, criticism and current status. *In:* M. G. Brush, R. J. B. King and R. W. Taylor (eds.). *Endometrial Cancer*, pp. 17–28. (London: Baillière Tindall)
3. Correspondence. *N. Engl. J. Med.*, **300**, 921
4. UICC Technical Report Series, Vol. 42, *Hormonal Biology of Endometrial Cancer*, G. S. Richardson and D. T. MacLaughlin (eds.). The patient with endometrial cancer, pp. 11–35. (Geneva: International Union Against Cancer)
5. Campbell, S. and Whitehead, M. I. (1979). The endometrium in the menopause. In P. A. van Keep, D. M. Serr and R. B. Greenblatt (eds.). *Female and Male Climacteric*, pp. 111–120. (Lancaster: MTP Press)

6. Whitehead, M. I., King, R. J. B., McQueen, J. and Campbell, S. (1979). Endometrial histology and biochemistry in climacteric women during oestrogen and oestrogen/progestogen therapy. *J. R. Soc. Med.*, **72**, 322

7. Sturdee, D. W., Wade-Evans, T., Paterson, M. E. L., Thom, M. and Studd, J. W. W. (1978). Relations between bleeding pattern, endometrial histology, and oestrogen treatment in menopausal women. *Br. Med. J.*, **1**, 1575

8. Gambrell, R. D. (1978). The prevention of endometrial cancer in postmenopausal women with progestogens. *Maturitas*, **1**, 107

9. King, R. J. B., Whitehead, M. I., Campbell, S. and Minardi, J. (1979). Effect of estrogen and progestin treatments on endometria from postmenopausal women. *Cancer Res.*, **39**, 1094

10. King, R. J. B., Whitehead, M. I., Campbell, S. and Minardi, J. (1978). Effects of estrogens and progestogens on the biochemistry of the post-menopausal endometrium. In I. D. Cooke (ed.). *The Role of Estrogen/Progestogen in the Management of the Menopause*, pp. 111–119. (Lancaster: MTP Press)

11. Whitehead, M. I. (1978). The effects of oestrogens and progestogens on the postmenopausal endometrium. *Maturitas*, **1**, 87

12. Gambrell, R. D., Castaneda, T. A. and Ricci, C. A. (1978). Management of postmenopausal bleeding to prevent endometrial cancer. *Maturitas*, **1**, 99

13. King, R. J. B., Dyer, G., Collins, W. P., Campbell, S. and Whitehead, M. I. (1979). Analysis of intracellular estradiol, estrone and estrogen receptor levels in endometria from postmenopausal women receiving estrogens and progestins. (In preparation)

14. King, R. J. B., Whitehead, M. I. and Townsend, P. (In preparation)

15. King, R. J. B. and Mainwaring, W. I. P. (1974). In *Steroid Cell Interactions*, pp. 288–378. (London: Butterworths)

16. Guerrero, R., Landgren, B. M., Monteil, R., Cekan, Z. and Diczfalusy, E. (1975). Unconjugated steroids in the human endometrium. *Contraception*, **11**, 169

17. Gurpide, E. and Tseng, L. (1974). Factors controlling intracellular levels of estrogens in human endometrium. *Gynecol. Oncol.* **2**, 221

18. Schmidt-Gollwitzer, M., Genz, T., Schmidt-Gollwitzer, K., Pollow, B. and Pollow, K. (1978). Correlation between oestradiol and progesterone receptor levels, 17β-hydroxy steroid dehydrogenase activity and endometrial tissue levels of oestradiol, oestrone and progesterone in women. In M. G. Brush, R. J. B. King and R. W. Taylor (eds.). *Endometrial Cancer*, pp. 227–241. (London: Baillière Tindall)

19. MacDonald, P. C. and Siiteri, P. K. (1974). The relationship between the extraglandular production of estrone and the occurrence of endometrial neoplasia. *Gynecol. Oncol.*, **2**, 259

20. Siiteri, P. K., Schwarz, B. E. and MacDonald, P. C. (1974). Estrogen receptors and the estrone hypothesis in relation to endometrial and breast cancer. *Gynecol. Oncol.*, **2**, 228

21. Baird, D. T. (1972). The secretion of estrogens from the ovary in normal and abnormal menstrual cycles. In O. Scow (ed.). *Endocrinology*, Excerpta Medica International Congress, Series No. 273, pp. 851–856. (Amsterdam: Excerpta Medica)

22. Emmens, C. W. and Martin, L. (1964). Estrogens. In R. I. Dorfman (ed.). *Methods in Hormone Research*, Vol. 3, pp. 1–75. (New York and London: Academic Press)

23. Ruh, T. S., Katzenellenbogen, B. S., Katzenellenbogen, J. A. and Gorski, J. (1973). Estrone interaction with the rat uterus: *in vitro* response and nuclear uptake. *Endocrinology*, **92**, 125

24. Whitehead, M. I., Dyer, G. and King, R. J. B. (In preparation)

25. Tseng, L. and Gurpide, E. (1973). Effect of estrone and progesterone on the nuclear uptake of estradiol by slices of human endometrium. *Endocrinology*, **93**, 245

26. Gurpide, E. (1978). Enzymatic modulation of hormonal action at the target tissue. *J. Toxicol. Environ. Health*, **4**, 249

27. Tseng, L., Gusberg, S. B. and Gurpide, E. (1977). Estradiol receptor and 17β-dehydrogenase in normal and abnormal human endometrium. *Ann. N.Y. Acad. Sci.*, **286**, 190

28. Hutton, J. D., Murray, M. A. F., Reed, M. J., Jacobs, J. S. and James, V. H. T. (1978).

Hormones after the menopause: levels, sources, effects of natural oestrogen therapy and possible relationship to endometrial carcinogenesis. In M. G. Brush, R. J. B. King and R. W. Taylor (eds.). *Endometrial Cancer*, pp. 363–374. (London: Baillière Tindall)

29. Henzl, M. R., Smith, R. E., Boost, G. and Tyler, E. T. (1972). Lysosomal concept of menstrual bleeding in humans. *J. Clin. Endocrinol.*, **34**, 860

30. McKay, D. G., Hertig, A. T., Barsawil, W. A. and Velardo, J. T. (1956). Histochemical observations on the endometrium. *Obstet. Gynecol.*, **8**, 22

31. Jelinek, J., Jelinkova, M., Hagenfeldt, K., Landgren, B. M. and Diczfalusy, E. (1978). Effect of two progestins on human endometrial enzymes and trace elements. *Acta Endocrinol.*, **88**, 580

22
Mutagenicity
and Estrogens

J. L. AMBRUS, C. M. AMBRUS, S. R. SIRIANNI, P. HALE,
M. BRAUN, C. C. HUANG and B. PAIGEN

INTRODUCTION

A number of recent papers suggested that estrogens, including conjugated estrogens, used for the treatment of menopausal symptoms and the prevention of postmenopausal osteoporosis, may cause uterine cancer and breast cancer[1-10]. On the other hand several investigators found no definite connection of estrogen therapy to uterine cancer or breast cancer[11-26]. Carcinogenicity of estrogens has been reported previously in experimental animals[27-30]. The question arises whether estrogens are indeed carcinogenic or mutagenic, and whether they act by altering the hormonal milieu or by increasing susceptibility of the host to other carcinogenic influences. For this reason, it appeared to be of interest to study the direct mutagenic effect of estrogens in bacterial and mammalian systems, including normal and neoplastic human cell lines. We investigated the most commonly used postmenopausal conjugated estrogen preparation: Premarin.

MATERIALS AND METHODS

The *Salmonella typhimurium* assay for mutagenicity was carried out as described by Ames *et al.*[31]. The TA 100 and TA 98 strains were used. Liver homogenates (9000 g supernatant, S-9) from polychlorinated biphenyl (PCB, Aroclor 1254) treated rats were prepared as described by Ames *et al.*[31] and used for exploring the possible production of mutagenically active metabolites.

A series of normal and neoplastic human and rodent cell lines were used to study potential induced chromosome changes in tissue culture and in diffusion chambers implanted into mice according to methods developed in this Institute[32-36]. The cytologic techniques were those described earlier[34]. The 'Jeff' lymphoid cell line was derived from a normal child and has a normal diploid constitution. The 'SP-163' lymphoid cell line was derived from the blood of a normal individual and is also diploid. The 'B-35 M' lymphoid cell line was derived from a patient with Burkitt's lymphoma and has a stemline chromosome number of $s = 47$. The 'HRIK' lymphoid cell line was derived from tumor tissue of a patient with Burkitt's lymphoma ($s = 47$–49). The 'Raji' lymphoid cell line is also from a patient with Burkitt's lymphoma with a hyperdiploid mode ($s = 47$–48). They were cultured in medium RPMI-1640 supplemented with 10% fetal calf serum without antibiotics. The 'V-79' cells of Chinese hamster origin were obtained from Dr C. C. Chang of Michigan State University, and maintained in Eagle's minimum essential medium with 10% fetal calf serum without antibiotics. It has a modal chromosome number of 21.

The experimental cell cultures were exposed continuously to estrogens at a concentration of 50 µg/ml. At various times after initiation of treatment, cell samples were withdrawn for viability counts (trypan blue exclusion) and chromosome study. Colcemid, 0.04 µg/ml, was added 2 hours before harvesting for chromosome preparations. Cells were then treated with 1% sodium citrate solution for 15 minutes and fixed in acetic acid : methanol (1 : 3). Flame-dried slides were stained with Giemsa stain. Metaphases were studied under oil objective for chromosome lesions, particularly gaps, breaks, exchanges, dicentrics, despiralization and pulverization. The results reported deal with 24-hour cultures.

Diffusion chamber cultures were established in dry sterilized chambers filled with 0.33 ml cell suspension containing 1×10^5 cells. They were implanted into the abdominal cavity of 6–8-week-old C_3H/St mice under ether anesthesia. Three days later, experimental animals were injected i.p. with 25–400 µg/g of estrogens. Twenty-four hours later 0.5 ml of 0.04% colchicine was injected i.p. and the chambers removed 2 hours later and treated with 0.5% Pronase in Hanks' balanced salt solution containing 5% Ficol for 90 minutes. Cell viability, number and cytogenetic characteristics were determined as described above. The validity of these methods to demonstrate known mutagenic and carcinogenic activity of chemicals and ionizing radiations has been demonstrated previously[32-36].

Commercial ampules of Premarin were used. This is a mixture of conjugated natural estrogens.

RESULTS AND DISCUSSION

Table 22.1 summarizes the results of the Ames test in two strains of *S. typhimurium*. The number of revertant–mutant colonies did not increase when exposed to 80–400 µg of Premarin per plate either with or without exposure to liver homogenates. Table 22.2 summarizes the results of *in vitro* cell culture studies. In the two normal and three neoplastic human lines, Premarin did not significantly increase chromosome aberrations as compared to controls. Table 22.3 summarizes the results of the diffusion chamber experiments. It appears

Table 22.1 Mutagenic activity of Premarin on *S. typhimurium* strains TA 98 and TA 100

Strain	µg Premarin/ plate	Incubation with hepatic enzyme preparation	No. revertants/ plate
TA 98	0	−	53
	0	+	49
	80	−	46
	80	+	47
	400	−	49
	400	+	65
TA 100	0	−	202
	0	+	202
	80	−	200
	80	+	200
	400	−	154
	400	+	218

that Premarin did not increase significantly the apparent chromosome aberrations. In neither of these experiments was there evidence of reduced cell viability or cell counts under the effect of Premarin as compared to controls.

In previous studies[37], a high correlation was shown between carcinogenicity and mutagenicity using the *Salmonella*/microsome test. It appears from the current studies that Premarin had no mutagenic or cytogenetic effect in either

Table 22.2 Induction of chromosome aberrations in five human lymphoid cell lines treated with 50 µg/ml Premarin*

Cell line	Treated or control	% gaps	Gaps/ cell	% breaks	Breaks/ cell	Total % aberrations
Jeff (normal)	control	4	0.04	—	—	4
	treated	2	0.02	—	—	2
SP-163 (normal)	control	2	0.02	—	—	2
	treated	—	—	2	0.02	2
B-35M (Burkitt)	control	2	0.02	—	—	2
	treated	2	0.02	4	0.04	6
Raji (Burkitt)	control	—	—	2	0.02	2
	treated	—	—	2	0.02	2
HRIK (Burkitt)	control	2	0.02	—	—	2
	treated	—	—	2	0.02	2

* Total of 100 metaphases were scored for control and treated cultures of the systems employed and therefore by implication is not likely to be carcinogenic in itself.

Table 22.3 Induction of chromosome aberrations in Chinese hamster V79 cells cultured in diffusion chambers in mice injected with various doses of Premarin

Premarin dose (μg/gm)	Meta-phases scored	% gaps	Gaps/ cell	% breaks	Breaks/ cell	Total % aberrations
control	50	0	0	2	0.02	2
25	50	2	0.02	0	0	2
50	50	2	0.02	0	0	2
100	50	2	0.02	4	0.04	6
200	50	0	0	0	0	0
400	50	0	0	0	0	0

References

1. Gambrell, R. D. (1977). Estrogens, progestogens and endometrial cancer. *J. Reprod. Med.*, **18**, 301
2. Gray, L. A., Christopherson, W. M. and Hoover, R. N. (1977). Estrogens and endometrial carcinoma. *Obstet. Gynecol.*, **49**, 385
3. Gordon, J., Reagan, J. W., Finkle, W. D and Ziel, H. K. (1977). Estrogen and endometrial carcinoma. *N. Engl. J. Med.*, **297**, 570
4. Hoover, R., Gray, L. A. and Cole, P. (1976). Menopausal estrogens and breast cancer. *N. Engl. J. Med.*, **295**, 401
5. Hoover, R., Fraumeni, J. F., Everson, R. and Myers, M. H. (1976). Cancer of the uterine corpus after hormonal treatment for breast cancer. *Lancet*, **1**, 885
6. MacMahon, B. (1974). Risk factors for endometrial cancer. *Gynecol. Oncol.*, **2**, 122
7. McDonald, T. W., Annegers, J. F., O'Fallon, W. M., Dockerty, M. B., Malkasian, G. D. and Kurland, L. T. (1977). Exogenous estrogen and endometrial carcinoma: case–control and incidence study. *Am. J. Obstet. Gynecol.*, **127**, 572
8. Siiteri, P. K., Schwartz, B. E. and MacDonald, P. C. (1974). Estrogen receptors and the estrone hypothesis in relation to endometrial and breast cancer. *Gynecol. Oncol.*, **2**, 228
9. Smith, D. C., Prentice, R., Thompson, D. J. and Hermann, W. L. (1975). Association of exogenous estrogen and endometrial carcinoma. *N. Engl. J. Med.*, **293**, 1164
10. Ziel, H. K. and Finkle, W. D. (1975). Increased risk of endometrial carcinoma among users of conjugated estrogen. *N. Engl. J. Med.*, **293**, 1167
11. Cooke, I. D. (1976). Estrogens as a cause of endometrial carcinoma. *Br. Med. J.*, **1**, 1209
12. Dunn, L. J. and Brandbury, J. T. (1967). Endocrine factors in endometrial carcinoma: a preliminary report. *Am. J. Obstet. Gynecol.*, **97**, 465
13. Gordan, G. S. and Greenberg, B. G. (1976). Exogenous estrogens and endometrial cancer. *Postgrad. Med.*, **59**, 66
14. Greenblatt, R. B. (1976). Oestrogens and endometrial cancer. In R. J. Beard (ed.). *The Menopause*, pp. 247–263. (Lancaster: MTP Press)
15. Horwitz, R. I. and Feinstein, A. R. (1977). New methods of sampling and analysis to remove bias in case–control research: no association found for estrogens and endometrial cancer. *Proc. Am. Soc. Clin. Invest.*
16. Lauritzen, C. (1976). Estrogens and *Corpus uteri* carcinoma. *Sexualmedizin*, **5**, 624

17. Malkasian, G. D., McDonald, T. W. and Pratt, J. H. (1977). Carcinoma of the endometrium. Mayo Clinic experience. *Mayo Clin. Proc.*, **52**, 175

18. Studd, J. W. W. (1976). Oestrogens as a cause of endometrial carcinoma. *Br. Med. J.*, **1**, 1144

19. Brezina, K., Janisch, H. and Muller-Tyl, E. (1973). Das Mammogramm unter Kontrazeptiva. *Wien Klin. Wochenschr.*, **85**, 785

20. Burch, J. C., Byrd, B. F. and Vaughn, W. K. (1975). Effects of long-term estrogen administration to women following hysterectomy. *Front. Hormone Res.*, **3**, 208

21. Drill, V. A. (1975). Oral contraceptives: relations to mammary cancer, benign breast lesions, and cervical cancer. *Ann. Rev. Pharmacol.*, **15**, 367

22. Fechner, R. E. (1970). Breast cancer during oral contraceptive therapy. *Cancer*, **26**, 1204

23. Gordan, G. S., Picchi, J. and Roof, B. S. (1973). Antifracture efficacy of long-term estrogens for osteoporosis. *Trans. Assoc. Am. Physicians*, **86**, 326

24. Henneman, P. H. and Wallach, S. (1957). A review of the prolonged use of estrogens and androgens in postmenopausal and senile osteoporosis. *Arch. Intern. Med.*, **100**, 715

25. Ostergaard, E. (1969). Oral anticonception: side effects and risks. *Acta Obstet. Gynecol.*, (Suppl. 1), **48**, 57

26. Wallach, S. and Henneman, P. H. (1959). Prolonged estrogen therapy in postmenopausal women. *J. Am. Med. Assoc.*, **171**, 1637

27. Cook, J. W. and Dodds, E. C. (1933). Sex hormones and cancer-producing compounds. *Nature*, **131**, 205

28. Gardner, W. U. (1944). Tumors in experimental animals receiving steroid hormones. *Surgery*, **16**, 8

29. Meissner, W. A., Sommers, S. C. and Sherman, G. (1957). Endometrial hyperplasia, endometrial carcinoma, and endometriosis produced experimentally by estrogen. *Cancer*, **10**, 500

30. Perry, I. H. and Ginzton, L. L. (1937). The development of tumors in female mice treated with 1:2:5:6-dibenzanthracene and Theclin. *Am. J. Cancer*, **29**, 680

31. Ames, B. N., McCann, J. and Yamasaki, E. (1975). Methods for detecting carcinogens and mutagens with the *Salmonella* mammalian-microsome mutagenicity test. *Mutat. Res.*, **31**, 347

32. Banerjee, A., Jung, O. and Huang, C. C. (1977). Response of hematopoietic cell lines derived from patients with Down's Syndrome and from normal individuals to mitomycin C and caffeine. *J. Natl. Cancer Inst.*, **59**, 37

33. Furukawa, M. and Huang, C. C. (1978). Sister chromatid exchanges induced by cyclophosphamide in V97 cells cultured in diffusion chambers in mice. *Mutat. Res.*, **57**, 233

34. Huang, C. C., Babbitt, H. and Ambrus, J. L. (1969). Chromosomes and DNA synthesis in the stumptailed monkey (*Macaca speciosa*), with special regard to marker and sex chromosomes. *Folia Primat.*, **11**, 28

35. Huang, C. C., Banerjee, A., Tan, J. C. and Hou, Y. (1977). Comparison of radiosensitivity between human hematopoietic cell lines derived from patients with Down's Syndrome and from normal persons. *J. Natl. Cancer Inst.*, **59**, 33

36. Huang, C. C. and Furukwa, M. (1978). Sister chromatid exchanges in human lymphoid cell lines cultured in diffusion chambers in mice. *Exp. Cell Res.*, **111**, 458

37. McCann, J., Choi, E., Yamasaki, E. and Ames, B. N. (1975). Detection of carcinogens as mutagens in the *Salmonella*/microsome test: assay of 300 chemicals. *Proc. Natl. Acad. Sci. USA*, **72**, 5135

23
Estrogens and Endometrial Cancer

A Preliminary Report

J. L. AMBRUS, M. GILETTE, C. NOLAN, O. JUNG,
S. REGALLA-SPAVENTO, P. SPAVENTO, A. NOVICK,
C. SUCHETZKY and C. M. AMBRUS

INTRODUCTION

The role of ovarian hormones in endometrial carcinoma was first suspected on the basis of observations of certain endocrine disorders, e.g. polycystic ovary syndrome and hormone secreting ovarian tumors[1,2]. Recently postmenopausal estrogen therapy became the center of controversy on possible endometrial carcinogenicity[3-50]. The possible effect of oral contraceptives in causing uterine cancer became equally debated[42,51-59]. Several other risk factors have been recognized, including diabetes, hypertension, obesity (possibly because of altered metabolism of steroids), advanced age, nulliparity, delayed menopause, lack of progesterone and family history of uterine cancer or other cancer[60-66].

During 1960-5 a study was undertaken by Graham[67,68] at this hospital on the value of total hysterectomy alone or with radium application in endometrial carcinoma. The data were analyzed from the point of view of estrogen use in 131 patients[68]. It appears that only 9% of the patients had estrogen treatment of any kind for any length of time prior to the diagnosis of endometrial carcinoma. Patient material from this same hospital was studied between 1970 and 1978 from this point of view and the results will be reported here.

PATIENTS AND METHODS

Between 1970 and 1978, 450 patients with biopsy-documented endometrial carcinoma were seen at this hospital. Of these adequate records were available, and further data could be obtained from the patient, her family, family doctor and referring gynecologist from 411 patients. A group of 450 female patients who came to the medical clinic of this hospital as diagnostic problems and were found to have no neoplastic disease or neoplasms other than of the female genital tract served as controls. Socio-economically and geographically this group was comparable to the study group. Of 450 control patients,

Table 23.1

	Control	Uterine cancer
Total number	450	450
Number with adequate data	421	411
Number with hysterectomy prior to uterine cancer diagnosis	83	0
Number finally evaluated	338	411
No estrogens used	246 (72.8%)	335 (81.5%)†
Oral contraceptives	24 (7.1%)	8 (1.9%)‡
Estrogens for menopausal or other gynecologic problems	49 (14.5%)	67 (16.5%)*
Estrogens for uncertain or unknown or other reasons	19 (5.6%)	1‡
Total number with estrogen history	92 (27.2%)	76 (18.5%)†
TYPE OF ESTROGEN USED		
Menopause or gynecologic problems		
Premarin	29	44
Other	3	12
Unknown	36	11
Oral contraceptives		
Various preparations	8	5
Unknown preparations or unknown dose schedules	16	4

Significance of difference from control group:
* = NS
† = $p \leqslant 0.006$
‡ = $p < 0.001$

adequate data became available of 421. Of these, 83 turned out to have had hysterectomies and were excluded for this reason. Thus the number of control patients evaluated was 338. All patients in this study were white females, their age distribution being shown in Figure 23.1. Since the largest group of estrogen-treated patients received Premarin as postmenopausal medication, we have also graphed the age distribution of this group (Figure 23.2).

Charts were carefully inspected for indications of estrogen use. Patients who were still coming to follow-up clinic were questioned personally. If not available they or their relatives were contacted by telephone and by letter. In addition, special questionnaires were sent to family physicians and referring gynecologists. Patients were included in the study only if adequate information was available from these sources. Minimal requirements for inclusion were (1) histologically proven diagnosis and (2) estrogen and other history from patient or family corresponding to history from one or more doctors who have treated the patient and who were contacted through this study. Data were less reliable on the exact duration of estrogen use, degree of compliance, and on onset of the menopause. For this reason, these were not included in the present analysis. Statistical evaluation was based on the ridit method of Bross[69].

Table 23.2 Risk factors

	All patients			Estrogen treated patients		
	Control	Uterine cancer	p	Control	Uterine cancer	p
Diabetes	9%	24%	<0.001	15%	12%	NS
Hypertension	18%	42%	<0.001	25%	30%	NS
Obesity	23%	47%	<0.001	20%	30%	NS
Nullipara	35%	30%	NS	37%	33%	NS
Family history of uterine cancer	3%	6%	NS	0%	5%	NS
Family history of other cancer	32%	41%	NS	15%	21%	NS

RESULTS AND DISCUSSION

Table 23.1 summarizes the results on the prevalence and type of estrogen use in the women in this study. Since most women in this study were of advanced age (see Figures 23.1 and 23.2), most completed their reproductive age before oral contraceptives became widely used; accordingly relatively few had this type of medication. Nevertheless, there was significantly more use of oral contraceptives in the control than in the uterine cancer group. Similarly, more patients used estrogens for uncertain, unknown, or other reasons (including discontinuation of breast feeding) in the control than in the uterine cancer group. Estrogens for menopausal or other gynecologic problems were used with about equal frequency (16.5% and 14.5% respectively) in both groups, the difference being not significant. This compares with a 9% estrogen use in uterine cancer patients found by Graham[68] in the same hospital between 1960 and 1965. Even though the use of estrogens increased somewhat between 1970 and 1978 it was still relatively modest and not apparently correlated with the incidence of uterine carcinoma. The total number of women who never used estrogens in our study was somewhat greater in the uterine cancer than in the control group.

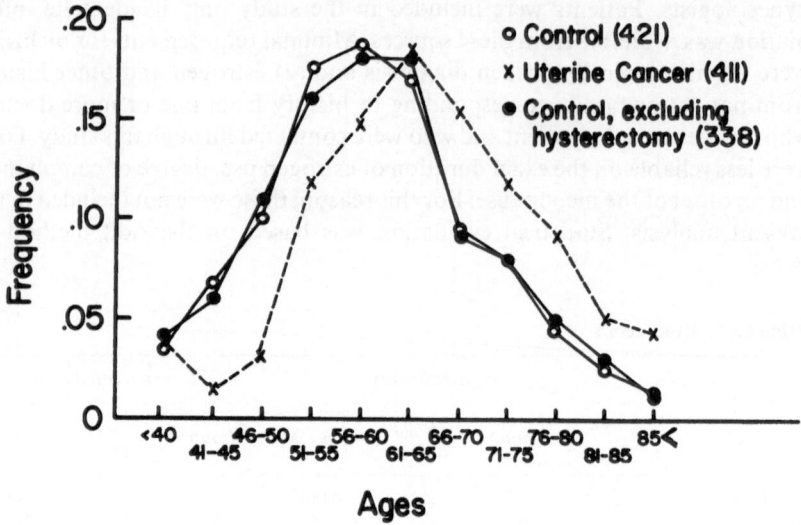

Figure 23.1   Age distribution of patients

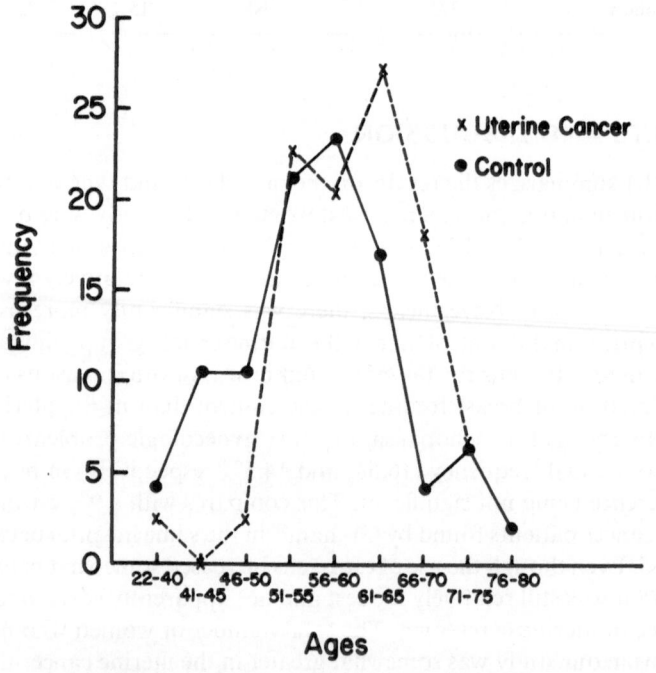

Figure 23.2   Age distribution of Premarin-treated patients

Table 23.2 summarizes the incidence of other recognized risk factors in the two groups under study. In all patients studied there was significantly more diabetes, hypertension and obesity in the uterine cancer patients than in the controls. On the other hand significant increase in uterine cancer risk with nulliparity, family history of uterine or other cancer could not be demonstrated in this patient group. When estrogen-treated patients were compared in the uterine cancer and control groups neither risk factor differed significantly in prevalence between these subgroups. This may be due in part to the lesser number of patients involved. It is interesting to note that in the study by Graham[68] there were relatively more patients with family history of uterine cancer in the estrogen treated than in the total patient group. However, this difference was statistically not significant in our study.

It appears that in the uterine cancer group there were a number of predisposing factors present at a higher level than in the controls (diabetes, hypertension, obesity). Family history may be a predisposing factor primarily in the estrogen-treated groups.

References

1. Speert, H. (1949). Cancer of the endometrium in young women. *Surg. Gynecol. Obstet.*, **88**, 332
2. Larson, J. A. (1954). Estrogen and endometrial carcinoma. *Obstet. Gynecol.*, **3**, 551
3. Greene, R. R., Roddick, J. W. Jr and Milligan M. (1959). Estrogens, endometrial hyperplasia and endometrial carcinoma. *Ann. New York Acad. Sci.*, **75**, 586
4. Gusberg, S. B. and Kaplan, A. A. (1963). Precursors of corpus cancer. *Am. J. Obstet. Gynecol.*, **87**, 667
5. Siiteri, P. K., Schwartz, B. E. and MacDonald, P. C. (1974). Estrogen receptors and the estrone hypothesis in relation to endometrial and breast cancer. *Gynecol. Oncol.*, **2**, 228
6. Quint, B. C. (1975). Changing patterns in endometrial adenocarcinoma. *Am. J. Obstet. Gynecol.*, **122**, 498
7. Ryan, K. J. (1975). Cancer risk and estrogen use in the menopause. *N. Engl. J. Med.*, **293**, 1199
8. Smith, D. C., Prentice, R., Thompson, D. J. and Herrmann, W. L. (1975). Association of exogenous estrogen and endometrial carcinoma. *N. Engl. J. Med.*, **293**, 1164
9. Weiss, N. S. (1975). Risks and benefit of estrogen use. *N. Engl. J. Med.*, **293**, 1200
10. Ziel, H. K. and Finkle, W. D. (1975). Increased risk of endometrial carcinoma among users of conjugated estrogens. *N. Engl. J. Med.*, **293**, 1167
11. Cooke, I. D. (1976). Estrogens as a cause of endometrial carcinoma. *Br. Med. J.*, **1**, 1209
12. Gambrell, R. D. Jr (1976). Estrogens, progestogens and endometrial cancer. In P. A. van Keep, R. B. Greenblatt and M. Albeaux-Fernet (eds), *Consensus on Menopause Research*, pp. 152–3. (Lancaster: MTP Press)
13. Gambrell, R. D. Jr (1977). Postmenopausal bleeding. *Clin. Obstet. Gynecol.*, **4**, 129
14. Gambrell, R. D. Jr (1977). Estrogens, progestogens and endometrial cancer. *J. Reprod. Med.*, **18**, 301
15. Gambrell, R. D. Jr (1978). The prevention of endometrial cancer in postmenopausal women with progestogens. *Maturitas*, **1**, 107
16. Gambrell, R. D. Jr (1978). The role of hormones in endometrial cancer. *South. Med. J.*, **71**, 1280

17. Gambrell, R. D. Jr, Castaneda, T. A. and Ricci, C. A. (1978). Management of post-menopausal bleeding to prevent endometrial cancer. *Maturitas*, 1, 99
18. Gambrell, R. D. Jr, Massey, F. M. and Castaneda, T. A. (1979). The reduction of endo-metrial cancer in postmenopausal women with progestogens. *J. Am. Geriatr. Soc.* (In press)
19. Gambrell, R. D. Jr, Massey, F. M. and Castaneda, T. A. (1979). Breast cancer and oral contraceptive therapy in premenopausal women. *J. Reprod. Med.* (In press)
20. Gordan, G. S. and Greenberg, B. G. (1976). Exogenous estrogens and endometrial cancer. *Postgrad. Med.*, **59** (6), 66
21. Greenblatt, R. B. (1976). Menopause. *Obstet. Gynecol. Digest*, **15**, 15
22. Hoover, R., Fraumeni, J. F. Jr, Everson, R. and Myers, M. H. (1976). Cancer of the uterine corpus after hormonal treatment for breast cancer. *Lancet*, 1, 885
23. Kistner, R. W. (1976). Estrogens and endometrial cancer. *Obstet. Gynecol.*, **48** (4), 479
24. Kohorn, E. I. (1976). Gestagens and endometrial carcinoma. *Gynecol. Oncol.*, **4** (4), 398
25. Lauritzen, C. (1976). Estrogens and corpus uteri carcinoma. *Sexualmedizin*, **5**, 624
26. Lilienfeld, A. M. (1976). Exogenous estrogens and endometrial cancer. *Postgrad. Med.*, **59** (6), 61
27. Mack, T. M., Pike, M. C., Henderson, B. E., Pfeffer, R. I., Gerkins, V. R., Arthur, M. and Brown, S. E. (1976). Estrogens and endometrial cancer in a retirement community. *N. Engl. J. Med.*, **294**, 1262
28. Nachtigall, L. E., Nachtigall, R. H., Nachtigall, R. B. and Beckman, E. M. (1976). Estrogens and endometrial carcinoma. *N. Engl. J. Med.*, **294**, 848
29. Sartwell, P. E. (1976). Estrogen replacement therapy and endometrial carcinoma: epidemio-logic evidence. *Clin. Obstet. Gynecol.*, **19** (4), 317
30. Studd, J. (1976). Oestrogens as a cause of endometrial carcinoma. *Br. Med. J.*, 1 (6018), 1144
31. Berger, G. S. and Fowler, W. C. Jr (1977). Exogenous estrogens and endometrial carcinoma: review and comments for the clinician. *J. Reprod. Med.*, **18** (4), 177
32. Casey, M. J. (1977). Estrogens, menopause and cancer. *Conn. Med.*, **41**, 776
33. Gordon, J., Reagan, J. W., Finkle, W. D. and Ziel, H. K. (1977). Estrogen and endometrial carcinoma. An independent pathology review supporting original risk estimate. *N. Engl. J. Med.*, **297** (11), 570
34. Gray, L. A. Sr, Christopherson, W. M. and Hoover, R. N. (1977). Estrogens and endometrial carcinoma. *Obstet. Gynecol.*, **49**, 385
35. Greenwald, P., Nasca, P. C., Caputo, T. A. and Janerich, D. T. (1977). Cancer risks from estrogen intake. *N.Y. State J. Med.*, **77** (7), 1069
36. Greenwald, P., Caputo, T. A. and Wolfgang, P. E. (1977a). Endometrial cancer after menopausal use of estrogens. *Obstet. Gynecol.*, **50** (2), 239
37. Horwitz, R. I. and Feinstein, A. R. (1977). New methods of sampling and analysis to remove bias in case–control research: no association found for estrogens and endometrial cancer. *Proc. Am. Soc. Clin. Invest.*
38. Horwitz, R. I. and Feinstein, A. R. (1978). Alternative analytic methods for case–control studies of estrogens and endometrial cancer. *N. Engl. J. Med.*, **299**, 1089
39. Knab, D. R. (1977). Estrogen and endometrial carcinoma. *Obstet. Gynecol.*, **32** (5), 267
40. Malkasian, G. D., McDonald, T. W. and Pratt, J. H. (1977). Carcinoma of the endo-metrium – Mayo Clinic experience. *Mayo Clin. Proc.*, **52**, 175
41. McDonald, T. W., Annegers, J. F., O'Fallow, W. M., Malkasian, G. D. and Kuland, L. T. (1977). Exogenous estrogen and endometrial carcinoma: case–control and incidence study. *Am. J. Obstet. Gynecol.*, **127**, 572
42. Reeves, K. O. and Kaufman, R. H. (1977). Exogenous estrogens and endometrial carcinoma. *J. Reprod. Med.*, **18**, 297
43. Rust, J. A., Langley, I. I., Hill, E. C. and Lamb, E. J. (1977). Estrogens: do the risks outweigh the benefits? *Am. J. Obstet. Gynecol.*, **128** (4), 431
44. Scully, R. E. (1977). Estrogens and endometrial carcinoma. *Hum. Pathol.*, **8** (5), 481

45. Whitehead, M. I., Campbell, S. C., King, R. J., McQueen, J. and Nordin, B. E. (1977). Oestrogen treatment and endometrial carcinoma. *Br. Med. J.*, **2** (6084), 453
46. Whitehead, M. I. (1978). The effects of oestrogens and progestogens on the postmenopausal endometrium. *Maturitas*, **1**, 87
47. Buchman, M. I., Kramer, E. and Feldman, G. B. (1978). Aspiration curettage for asymptomatic patients receiving estrogen. *Obstet. Gynecol.*, **51** (3), 339
48. Greenblatt, R. B. and Stoddard, L. D. (1978). The estrogen–cancer controversy. *J. Am. Geriatr. Soc.*, **26**, 1
49. Antunes, C. M. F., Stolley, P. D., Rosenshein, N. B., Davies, J. L., Tonascia, J. A., Brown, C., Burnett, L., Rutledge, A., Pokempner, M. and Garcia, R. (1979). Endometrial cancer and estrogen use. Report of a large case–control study. *N. Engl. J. Med.*, **300**, 9
50. Hammond, C. B., Jelovsek, F. R. and Lee, K. L. (1979). Effects of long-term estrogen replacement therapy. II. Neoplasia. *Am. J. Obstet. Gynecol.*, **133**, 537
51. Lyon, F. A. (1975). The development of adenocarcinoma of the endometrium in young women receiving long-term sequential oral contraception. Report of four cases. *Am. J. Obstet. Gynecol.*, **123**, 299
52. Lyon, F. A. and Frisch, M. J. (1976). Endometrial abnormalities occurring in young women on long-term sequential oral contraception. *Obstet. Gynecol.*, **47**, 639
53. Silverberg, S. G. and Makowski, E. L. (1975). Endometrial carcinoma in young women taking oral contraceptive agents. *Obstet. Gynecol.*, **46**, 503
54. Silverberg, S. G., Makowski, E. L. and Roche, W. D. (1977). Endometrial carcinoma in women under 40 years of age: comparison of cases in oral contraceptive users and non-users. *Cancer*, **39** (2), 592
55. Kelly, H. W., Miles, P. A., Buster, J. E. and Scragg, W. H. (1976). Adenocarcinoma of the endometrium in women taking sequential oral contraceptives. *Obstet. Gynecol.*, **47**, 200
56. Cohen, C. J. and Deppe, G. (1977). Endometrial carcinoma and oral contraceptive agents. *Obstet. Gynecol.*, **49**, 390
57. Hanson, F. W. (1977). Oral contraceptives: a possible association with liver tumors and endometrial carcinoma. *Adv. Planned Parent.*, **12** (2), 86
58. Moghissi, K. S. (1977). Oral contraceptives and endometrial and cervical cancer. *J. Toxicol. Environ. Health*, **3** (12), 243
59. Wigle, D. T. and Grace, M. (1977). Reproductive cancer and hormone use. *Am. J. Epidemiol.*, **106** (3), 233
60. MacMahon, B. (1974). Risk factors for endometrial cancer. *Gynecol. Oncol.*, **2** (2–3), 122
61. Aleem, F. A., Moukhtar, M. S., Hung, H. C. and Romney, S. L. (1976). Plasma estrogen in patients with endometrial hyperplasia and carcinoma. *Cancer*, **38** (5), 2101
62. Gusberg, S. B. (1976). The individual at high-risk for endometrial carcinoma. *Am. J. Obstet. Gynecol.*, **126**, 535
63. Schindler, A. E. (1976). Estrogens and endometrial cancer: aspects of etiology and survival rate. *Arch. Geschwulstforsch.*, **46** (5), 345
64. Shoemaker, E. S., Forney, J. P. and MacDonald, P. C. (1977). Estrogen treatment of post-menopausal women. Benefits and risks. *J. Am. Med. Assoc.*, **238**, 1524
65. MacDonald, P. C., Edman, C. D., Hemsell, D. L., Porter, J. C. and Siiteri, P. K. (1978). Effect of obesity on conversion of plasma androstenedione to estrone in postmenopausal women with and without endometrial cancer. *Am. J. Obstet. Gynecol.*, **130** (4), 448
66. Lachnit-Fixson, U. (1979). Oestrogens during the menopause and the risk of endometrial carcinoma. In O. Kraupp and E. Deutsch (eds), *Wiener Klinische Wochenschrift*, pp. 1–22. (Wien: Springer-Verlag)
67. Graham, J. (1971). The value of preoperative or postoperative treatment by radium for carcinoma of the uterine body. *Surg. Gynecol. Obstet.*, **132**, 855
68. Graham, R. M. (1976). Estrogens and endometrial carcinoma. *N. Engl. J. Med.*, **294** (15), 847
69. Bross, I. (1954). Is there an increased risk? *Fed. Proc.*, **13**, 818

70. Jick, H., Watkins, R. N., Hunter, J. R., Dinan, B. J., Madsen, S., Rotahman, K. J. and Walker, A. M. (1979). Replacement estrogens and endometrial cancer. *N. Engl. J. Med.*, **300**, 218
71. Kreuter, A. Jr, Johnson, D. and Williamson, H. O. (1976). Histology of the endometrium in long-term use of a sequential oral contraceptive. *Fertil. Steril.*, **27**, 905

24
Exogenous Estrogen Therapy in the Menopause: Influence on Mammary Cancer Risk

K. I. BLAND, J. B. BUCHANAN, B. F. WEISBERG
and L. A. GRAY, Sr.

With the introduction of estrogen replacement therapy for menopausal symptoms in the early 1930s came the concern of neoplasia risk for target organs subject to the endocrine influence of estrogenic steroids and their analogues. It is currently estimated that the use of exogenous female hormone therapy for spontaneous or surgical menopausal symptoms has increased two- to three-fold since the early 1960s[1]. Thus, the epidemiologic association of endogenous and exogenous estrogens and their metabolites with regard to breast carcinogenesis emerged as an issue of considerable controversy, as mammary parenchyma is subject to the physiologic perturbations of various hormone sites. Endocrine regulation of breast tissue development and neoplastic alteration is complex, involving a variety of hormones, including estrogen and progesterone, prolactin, growth hormone, adrenal steroids and thyroxin[2-7]. Estrogenic steroids promote the growth of mammary ducts and periductal stroma, while progesterone influences the structural development of acini and lobules[8]. Progesterone is not carcinogenic to breast parenchyma in man or animals, and investigators[9-11] suggest a direct antagonistic effect on the potentially hyperplastic and/or carcinogenic effect produced by estrogens. Additionally, Huggins and Yang[12] demonstrated a decrease in the incidence and rate of growth of mammary carcinomas with the addition of progesterone to estrogens in their experimental tumor–host system.

Premarin[R] (conjugated estrogens, USP), the most commonly used estrogen replacement therapy, was introduced in the United States in the 1930s. This preparation is a mixture of estrogens obtained exclusively from natural equine sources and contains equilin, estrone and 17α-estradiol. Of the three estrogen fractions, estrone is the stronger carcinogen and estradiol the more active symptomatic estrogen, whereas estriol has minimal estrogen activity and no carcinogenic potential. Indeed, estriol may serve as an antagonist to the potential carcinogenic activity of estrone and estradiol[3, 13–17]. Thus, the physiologic administration of Premarin and related compounds on a cyclic basis has emerged as a potential neoplastic role deserving study.

The role of environmental factors (including hormonal usage and chemical carcinogens) as explicit contributors to breast neoplasia is difficult to evaluate, as a definition of the cause–effect relationship must also include reproductive, socio-economic and familial history. Few antecedent studies have allowed for consideration of these interrelated risk-factors and their contributions to breast neoplasia in the female receiving exogenous estrogens for the menopause. The authors were interested in evaluating the effect of long-term, cyclic, therapeutic estrogens on breast parenchyma and the resultant carcinogenic risk with such therapy.

CLINIC POPULATION: MATERIAL AND METHODS

The clinical data available from the records of 14023 patients were reviewed in order to gather case material for this pilot study. The patient data sources used for analysis of evaluable patients treated with exogenous estrogens for spontaneous or surgical menopausal symptoms were obtained from three sources: (1) the private gynecologic office practice of one author (L.A.G., Sr.); (2) the Louisville Breast Cancer Detection Demonstration Project (BCDDP); and (3) the Louisville Breast Diagnostic Center (BDC). All patients classified as symptomatic with breast disease and 'users' of estrogens were derived from the above private office source. Both users and non-users of estrogens were classified as having symptomatic mammary disease if (1) mass lesion or thickening, (2) mastalgia, (3) macrocystic changes, and (4) nipple discharge were evident at clinical examination. Patients subsequently classified as asymptomatic were essentially all evaluated from case history and records of the Louisville Breast Cancer Detection Demonstration Project (BCDDP), while symptomatic non-users were patients previously treated in the Louisville Breast Diagnostic Center (BDC). Figure 24.1 documents the patient data distribution with regard to estrogen history and clinical presentation. Ninety-three postmenopausal patients were identified initially as symptomatic users of estrogens, in whom case-matching for the risk factors of age and parity to the remaining categories was possible in 54 women. These 54 symptomatic patients were long-term users of Premarin in therapeutic ranges (0.3–1.25 mg per day) who had been referred for serial xeromammography at the Louisville BCDDP or BDC. To allow a large sample population for matching analysis, multiple case-matches for symptomatic users were available in subsequent categories. Patients were categorized as follows: Asymptomatic, user of estrogens (152); Asymptomatic, non-user of estrogens (124); Symptomatic, user of estrogens (54); and Symptomatic, non-user of estrogens (75). Thus, 405 postmenopausal patients were considered evaluable as to their exact hormone history and mammary neoplasia risk. The population was predominantly (>96%) Caucasian, of whom 242 women (60%) were exactly matched for for the parameters of age, parity, race and the additional risk-factor of age at birth of first child.

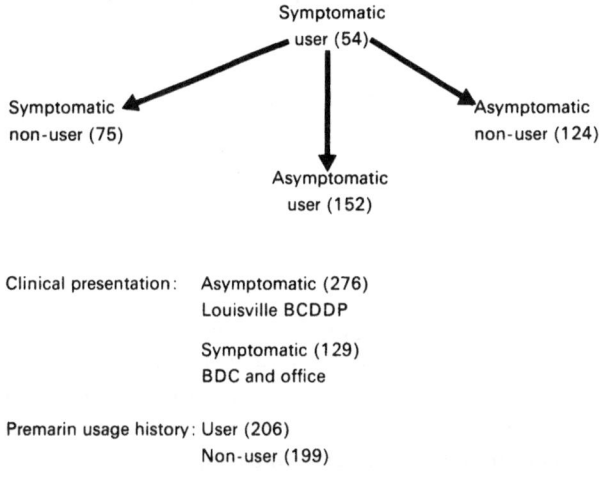

Figure 24.1   Matching distribution of 405 patients for age and parity

Patients were considered estrogen users if (1) Premarin usage was equal to or exceeded 18 consecutive months of therapy, (2) Premarin Vaginal Cream or an analogue was not the sole estrogen therapy, (3) oral contraceptive medication had never been used on a cyclic basis, and (4) precise documentation of exogenous estrogen dosage and duration of therapy was available for analysis.

Ages of evaluable patients ranged from 37 to 84 years (mean 59.7, median 60.0). The median Premarin dosage in users was 0.625 mg per day (range 0.3–1.25 mg per day). The intervals of estrogen replacement for the 206 users (asymptomatic and symptomatic) of Premarin ranged from 19 to 233 months (mean = 79 months). The 54 symptomatic patients on estrogens had an interval of replacement of 18–220 months (mean = 91 months). Patients considered evaluable were included only if complete follow-up was available to allow documentation and reporting of end results. Follow-up was defined as the period from start of estrogen replacement therapy to present and ranged from 39 to 344 months (mean = 133.3 months).

RESULTS

The interval follow-up of these 405 patients allowed the identification of 13 cancers (10.1%) in 129 patients symptomatic with breast disease (Table 24.1). Eleven carcinomas (14.7%) were identified in the symptomatic group of non-users of estrogens, whereas only two cancers (3.7%) were identified in the symptomatic patients considered to be users of Premarin in therapeutic doses.

Table 24.1   Cancer detection results in patients symptomatic with breast disease

Estrogen (Premarin) history	Total patients no. (%)	Biopsies no. (%)	Cancers detected no. (%)
User*	54 (41.9)	45 (34.9)	2 (3.7)
Non-user	75 (58.1)	45 (34.9)	11 (14.7)
Total	129 (100.0)	90 (69.8)	13 (10.1)

*Premarin user–therapeutic dose of conjugated equine estrogens (median 0.625 mg) ≥ 18 consecutive months

Of 276 asymptomatic screenees in the Louisville BCDDP matched to the risk factors of age and parity, 12 patients (4.3%) were found to have mammary carcinoma on screening (clinical history, physical examination, two-view xeromammography and thermography). No significant difference in the occurrence of cancer was noted between asymptomatic non-users who were screened (seven cancers, 5.6%) and asymptomatic users of estrogens (five cancers, 3.3%) in these therapeutic dosages (Table 24.2).

Table 24.2   Cancer detection results in patients asymptomatic with breast disease

Estrogen (Premarin) history	Total %	Cancers detected %
User*	152 (55.1)	5 (3.3)
Non-user	124 (44.9)	7 (5.6)
Total	276 (100.0)	12 (4.3)

*Premarin user–therapeutic dose of conjugated equine estrogens (median 0.625 mg) ≥ 18 consecutive months

Table 24.3 shows the correlation in these matched subgroups between estrogen usage history and the occurrence of cancer by clinical presentation.

In the population of 199 non-users of estrogens, a total of 18 cancers (9.0%) was identified in the symptomatic and asymptomatic subgroups. The 206 women considered to be users of therapeutic doses of Premarin were observed to have seven cancers (3.4%). Clearly, the higher incidence of carcinoma was noted in the non-user group of matched patients. Interestingly, the highest

Table 24.3 Occurrence of cancer: correlation of Premarin usage history and clinical presentation

| Clinical presentation | Premarin therapy | | | |
| | Non-user | | User* | |
	No. (%)	No. cancers (%)	No. (%)	No. cancers (%)
Asymptomatic	124 (62.3)	7 (3.5)	152 (73.8)	5 (2.4)
Symptomatic	75 (37.7)	11 (5.5)	54 (26.2)	2 (1.0)
Total	199 (100.0)	18 (9.0)	206 (100.0)	7 (3.4)

* Premarin user – therapeutic dose of conjugated equine estrogens (median 0.625 mg) ≥ 18 consecutive months

incidence of carcinoma was detected in symptomatic non-users of estrogens (11 cancers, 5.5%). The collective series of 405 patients was observed to have 25 cancers (6.2%). Again, the occurrence of carcinoma was observed to be greatest in women considered to be non-users of replacement estrogens in whom no regard is made for their clinical presentation (Table 24.4).

Table 24.4 Frequency of breast carcinoma with regard to Premarin usage history

Premarin replacement history	No.	Cancers	(%)
User*	206	7	(3.4)
Non-user	199	18	(9.0)
Total	405	25	(6.2)

* User – Premarin therapeutic dose (median 0.625 mg) of conjugated equine estrogens ≥ 18 consecutive months

DISCUSSION

A review of the literature on the relationship between estrogen therapy in the human female and mammary carcinoma reveals conflicting argument and conclusion. Many studies of postmenopausal women treated for varying intervals with estrogens have been reviewed for the incidence of cancer developing during or subsequent to therapy. Regrettably, these patient populations were drawn from various socio-economic sectors without attempting

Table 24.5 Studies of the relationship of non-contraceptive estrogens to the risk of breast cancer*

Type of study	First author	Type of controls	No. of cases	Year during which breast cancer was diagnosed	Measure of estrogen use	Relative risk
Hospital-based Case–control	Sartwell[25]	hospital	284	1969–1972	ever	0.82
	Boston Collaborative Drug Surveillance Program[26]	hospital	51	1972	ever	1.0
	Ravnihar[27]	clinic	374	1972–1974	ever	0.78
Population-based Case–control	Henderson[28]	office	100	1969–1972	ever	0.75
	Casagrande[10]	neighborhood	47	1972–1973	ever	3.1
	Craig[20]	population and neighborhood	134	1949–1967	ever	1.0
	Mack[30]	population	111	1971–1975	ever	1.6
Practice-based	Burch[31]	none	19	1948–1973	≥5 y	1.2
Prospective	Hoover[21]	none	49	1939–1972	≥6 months	1.3

* Reproduced with permission from Thomas, D. B. (1978), *Cancer Res.*, **38**, 3997

to make correlations among subsets with similar risk-factors. Often these studies added bias as there was no similar untreated group for comparison and the expected frequency in women of similar age had to be computed. Further complicating the issue is the fact that many series have reported varying results in women treated with a variety of estrogens alone, and in others with combination estrogen and progesterone or androgens with no distinction of dosage and therapy duration. An objective consideration of estrogen dose-relationship and therapy interval must be allowed in the evaluation of any study.

Thomas[18], in a recent review of the role of exogenous hormones in human neoplasms, noted seven case–control studies of non-contraceptive estrogens to breast cancer risk (Table 24.5). This author comprehensively reviewed case–control data and suggested that no significant association existed between mammary carcinogenesis and exogenous estrogen therapy for the menopause. Analysis of these case–control studies shows that the relative-risk ratio ranges from 0.75 to 3.1. Casagrande et al.[19] were at variance with the remaining investigators and observed a relative risk of 3.1 in this small series of women with natural menopause treated with estrogen replacement. With the exception of the studies by Burch et al.[20] and Hoover et al.[21], and the authors of this study, the measure of estrogen therapy was indeterminate, with a classification as 'ever-user' in instances of short and prolonged interval therapy. Additionally, few antecedent epidemiologic surveys, as well as these studies, have provided analysis for the confounding variables of risk-factors such as age, parity, race, family history and age at birth of first child.

The thorough study by Hoover et al.[21] of menopausal estrogens and breast cancer overlaps this current study in that our symptomatic estrogen-user population was gathered from the same data source. These investigators acknowledge that the relative risk of 1.3 after 10–14 years therapy was not attributable simply to prolonged estrogen therapy, as there was no clear dose–response relationship to accumulated years of use. This study suggested a higher risk accrued to women using higher-dose therapy and in circumstances where the medication was taken other than daily.

The observed occurrence of breast cancer in this predominantly Caucasian series of 405 patients (users and non-users of estrogens) matched to the risk factors of age and parity was 6.2% – that expected in the female population. The therapeutic dose range for the symptomatic user of our study was 0.3–1.25 mg and the therapeutic interval of this subset was 18–220 months. This group of patients was acknowledged as having the highest expected incidence of carcinoma as they presented with breast symptoms highly suggestive of cancer to the examining physician. Additionally, this patient group had a mean therapeutic interval (mean = 91 months), which was 12 months longer than the asymptomatic user subset (79 months). Despite a longer therapeutic interval with estrogen therapy in this symptomatic user group, there were similar incidences of carcinoma in the asymptomatic (5/152 or 2.4%) and symptomatic (2/54 or 1.0%) categories, whereas the non-user groups (regardless of clinical presentations) had the higher incidence of breast carcinoma. This would suggest no added risk for breast cancer with the use of Premarin for menopausal symptoms in daily therapeutic doses (median 0.625 mg). The conclusions of our study are supported by antecedent studies of breast cancer risk with postmenopausal estrogen therapy. Two recent publications by Burch, Byrd and Vaughn[22, 23], as well as a review on neoplasia following estrogen therapy by Greenblatt[24], strengthen these opinions.

We consider our data to be a pilot study which we hope will stimulate further investigations to elucidate the physiologic effects of estrogens and hormone analogues on breast parenchyma. Future epidemiologic and clinical analyses conducted in a prospective, randomized fashion are encouraged to document the benefit and risk to patient subgroups using estrogens.

CONCLUSIONS

This retrospective pilot analysis is of 206 postmenopausal (spontaneous and surgical) patients (mean age 59.7 years) treated with therapeutic doses of Premarin conjugated estrogens for 19–233 months (mean 6.6 years) who were matched to 199 postmenopausal non-users of estrogen for the risk-factors of age and parity. This predominantly Caucasian population was observed to have 25 breast cancers (6.2%), of which 18 (9.0%) were detected in the non-user group and seven (3.4%) in the user category. These data suggest:

(1) The greatest observed incidence of mammary cancer was found in the symptomatic non-users of estrogens (11/75 = 5.5%).

(2) No significant difference in the occurrence of breast carcinoma was noted in symptomatic (2/54) and asymptomatic (5/152) Premarin users, despite longer (mean 12 months) therapy in the symptomatic category.

(3) The use of Premarin conjugated estrogens in therapeutic daily doses (median 0.625 mg) did not increase the risk for breast cancer in follow-up (mean > 11 years).

(4) There is a need for further epidemiologic case–control data studies incorporating risk-factor analyses.

Acknowledgments

This work was supported in part by the American Cancer Society and the National Cancer Institute, Grant No. NOI-CN-55307; and the American Cancer Society Junior Faculty Clinical Fellowship No. 436 (Dr Bland).

References

1. U.S. Bureau of the Census (1962–73). *Current Industrial Reports: Pharmaceutical Preparations, Except Biologicals.* (Washington, D.C.: Government Printing Office)
2. Kapdi, C. C. and Wolfe, J. N. (1976). Breast cancer: relationship to thyroid supplements for hypothyroidism. *J. Am. Med. Assoc.*, **236**, 1124
3. Leis, H. P. Jr. (1976). Hormones in the epidemiology of breast cancer. *Breast Dis. Breast*, **2**, 7
4. Lipschutz, A. and Varga, L. Jr. (1940). Tumorgenic powers of stilbestrol and follicular hormone. *Lancet*, **1**, 541
5. Mustacchi, P. and Greenspan, R. (1977). Thyroid supplementation for hypothyroidism: an iatrogenic cause of breast cancer? *J. Am. Med. Assoc.*, **237**, 1446
6. Siiteri, P. (1974). Endocrine aspects of breast cancer. In J. R. Castro, T. S. Meyler and D. G. Baker (eds.). *Current Concepts in Breast Cancer.* (Flushing, N.J.: Medical Examination Publishing Co. Inc.)
7. Wallace, R. B., Sherman, B. M., Bean, J. A. and Leeper, J. (1978). Thyroid hormone use in patients with breast cancer: absence of an association. *J. Am. Med. Assoc.*, **239**, 958
8. Lipsett, M. D. (1977). Estrogens use and cancer risk. *J. Am. Med. Assoc.*, **237**, 1112
9. Leis, H. P. Jr. (1970). *Diagnosis and Treatment of Breast Lesions.* (Flushing, N.Y.: Medical Examination Publishing Co. Inc.)
10. Leis, H. P. Jr. and Raciti, A. (1975). The search for the high-risk patient. In B. A. Stoll (ed.). *New Aspects of Breast Cancer – Patients at High Risk.* (London: Heinemann Medical Books Ltd.)
11. Papaioannou, A. N. (1974). Etiologic factors in cancer of the breast in humans. *Surg. Gynecol. Obstet.*, **138**, 257
12. Huggins, C. and Yang, N. C. (1962). Induction and extinction of mammary cancer. *Science*, **137**, 257
13. Cole, P. and MacMahon, B. (1969). Hypothesis: oestrogen fractions during early reproductive life in the etiology of breast cancer. *Lancet*, **1**, 605
14. Lemon, H. M. (1969). Endocrine influence upon human breast cancer formation. *Cancer*, **23**, 781
15. Lemon, H. M. (1970). Abnormal estrogen metabolism and tissue estrogen receptor proteins in breast cancer. *Cancer*, **25**, 423
16. MacMahon, B. and Cole, P. (1969). Endocrinology and epidemiology of breast cancer. *Cancer*, **24**, 1146
17. MacMahon, B., Cole, P. and Brown, J. B. (1971). Oestrogen profiles of Asian and North American women. *Lancet*, **2**, 900
18. Thomas, D. B. (1978). Role of exogenous female hormones in altering the risk of benign and malignant neoplasms in humans. *Cancer Res.*, **38**, 3991
19. Casagrande, J., Gerkins, V., Henderson, B. E., Mack, T. and Pike, M. C. (1976). Exogenous estrogens and breast cancer in women with natural menopause. *J. Natl. Cancer Inst.*, **56**, 839
20. Burch, J. C., Byrd, B. F. and Vaughn, W. K. (1974). The effects of long-term estrogen on hysterectomized women. *Am. J. Obstet. Gynecol.*, **118**, 778
21. Hoover, R., Gray, L. A. Sr., Cole, P. and MacMahon, B. (1976). Menopausal estrogens and breast cancer. *N. Engl. J. Med.*, **295**, 401
22. Burch, J. C., Byrd, B. F. and Vaughn, W. K. (1975). The effects of long-term estrogen administration to women following hysterectomy. In P. A. van Keep and C. Lauritzen (eds.). *Estrogens in the Post-Menopause. Front. Hormone Res.*, Vol. 3, pp. 208–214. (Basel: Karger)
23. Burch, J. C., Byrd, B. F. and Vaughn, W. K. (1976). Results of estrogen treatment in one thousand hysterectomized women for 14,318 years. In P. A. van Keep, R. B. Greenblatt and M. Albeaux-Fernet (eds.). *Consensus on Menopause Research*, pp. 164–169. (Baltimore: University Park Press)
24. Greenblatt, R. B. (1974). Reprise: complications of hormone replacement therapy. In R. B.

Greenblatt, V. B. Mahesh and P. G. McDonough (eds.). *The Menopausal Syndrome*, pp. 222–231. (New York: Medcom Press)

25. Sartwell, P. E., Arthes, F. G. and Tonascia, J. A. (1977). Exogenous hormones, reproductive history and breast cancer. *J. Natl. Cancer Inst.*, **59**, 1589

26. Boston Collaborative Drug Surveillance Program (1973). Oral contraceptives and venous thromboembolic disease, surgically confirmed gall-bladder disease, and breast tumors. *Lancet*, **1**, 1399

27. Ravnihar, B., Seigel, D. G. and Lindtner, J. (1978). An epidemiologic study of breast cancer and benign breast neoplasias in relation to the oral contraceptive and estrogen use. *Eur. J. Cancer.* (In press)

28. Henderson, B. E., Powell, D., Rosario, I., Keys, C., Hanisch, R., Young, M., Casagrande, J., Gerkins, V. and Pike, M. C. (1974). An epidemiologic study of breast cancer. *J. Natl. Cancer Inst.*, **53**, 609

29. Craig, M. J., Comstock, G. W. and Geiser, P. B. (1974). Epidemiologic comparison of breast cancer patients with early and late onset of malignancy and general population controls. *J. Natl. Cancer Inst.*, **53**, 1577

30. Mack, T. M., Henderson, B. E., Gerkins, V. R., Arthur, M., Baptista, J. and Pike, M. C. (1975). Reserpine and breast cancer in a retirement community. *N. Engl. J. Med.*, **29**, 1366

31. Burch, J. C. and Byrd, B. F. (1971). Effects of long-term administration of estrogen on the occurrence of mammary cancer in women. *Ann. Surg.*, **174**, 414

25
The Effects of Exogenous Estrogen Replacement on Breast Parenchymal Patterns

J. B. BUCHANAN, K. I. BLAND, B. F. WEISBERG
and L. A. GRAY, Sr.

Mammary ducts and lobules are subject to the physiological influence of pituitary, adrenal and ovarian hormones. The association of these hormones as well as exogenous steroids with breast maturation and neoplasia is complex and the subject of great debate[1–10].

The association of certain morphologic characteristics of benign proliferative breast lesions with subsequent breast cancer risk has been aptly described. Atypical epithelial hyperplasia of terminal ducts is considered a likely pre-cancerous lesion[1–3, 8, 11–26]. The development of *in situ* carcinoma in an area of duct hyperplasia[21] and the five-fold increase in risk of invasive breast cancer[11] have been reported in patients with these pre-cancerous aberrations.

Because of the widespread use of mammography, breast parenchymal patterns can be observed, classified[27, 28] and followed. A recent study[29] suggests a strong correlation between the parenchymal patterns as reflected on the mammogram and the morphologic characteristics viewed microscopically. The direct relationship of an increasing number of atypical lobules with a more severe classification suggests that the risk of breast cancer can be predicted with considerable accuracy using xeromammographic criteria[27].

While it has been reported that age, parity, age at first childbirth and probably family history of breast cancer influence breast parenchymal patterns[30-32], the effects of exogenous estrogens on parenchymal pattern classifications have not been reported. A single report[33] of a small number of cases suggested that postmenopausal estrogens produced characteristic benign changes on the mammogram which regressed on discontinuation of therapy. Others[12, 34-36] have suggested an increase in breast cancer risk with prolonged use of exogenous estrogens.

Although the significance of using the breast parenchymal patterns as a relative-risk indicator remains unproven, mammographic evaluation of parenchymal pattern changes as a reflection of the use of exogenous estrogens can be studied. If women with a more severe classification are at a significantly higher risk than those women in a less severe classification, and if exogenous estrogens add to this risk, then an analysis of mammograms from this population should show a shift toward the more severe classification.

MATERIALS AND METHODS

Case material was derived from three sources: (1) Louisville Breast Cancer Detection Demonstration Project; (2) Breast Diagnostic Center; and (3) office practice of one author (L.A.G.). The collaborative review of the data on 14 023 patients was available from the combined sources. Patients were classified as symptomatic with breast cancer if they presented with (1) mass or thickening, (2) mastodynia, (3) macrocystic changes, and (4) nipple discharge. Patients subsequently classified as asymptomatic were essentially all evaluated from records and case history at the Louisville Breast Cancer Detection Demonstration Project.

Eighty-three symptomatic women were initially identified from among 1891 long-term users of therapeutic estrogens[35] who recently (within 2 years) had been referred for xeromammography. Historically, this physician (L.A.G.) referred for mammography those patients who presented diagnostic problems clinically. This patient selection bias should weight this group in the direction of increasing numbers of breast dysplasias (P_2DY) as well as breast cancers. As breast parenchymal patterns and cancer incidence are both influenced by age and parity, these women were precisely matched for these two factors with varying numbers of women in three additional categories. These three categories include symptomatic non-users of estrogens and asymptomatic users and non-users of estrogens. The additional factor of age at birth of first child was matched in 62% of these populations. Over 96% of the entire study group were Caucasian. With the above population base, 535 patients in whom an exact history was available were identified, analyzed and compared.

All patient mammograms had previously been assigned to a specific pattern according to the Wolfe classification[27, 28]. This was completed prior to the initiation of the study. All mammograms were subsequently classified as follows:

N_1 – a breast composed mainly of fat;
P_1 – prominent ducts in the subareolar area involving less than one-fourth of the breast;
P_2 – prominent duct pattern with more severe breast involvement;
DY – severe involvement with coalescent density coexistent with areas of nodularity.

Mammograms were read sequentially at annual and semi-annual screenings by two different persons and then re-reviewed to insure final pattern classification for reporting of end results. The mammographic interpretations were performed by individuals unaware of the current patient history as to whether the individuals were symptomatic or asymptomatic with breast disease and users or non-users of exogenous estrogens.

An additional subset of patients was identified among the 10 130 asymptomatic patients screened annually in the Breast Cancer Demonstration Project. This study involved the observed changes in parenchymal patterns in 250 patients in whom exogenous estrogens were begun or halted during their 5 years of follow-up in the Breast Cancer Demonstration Project. Two criteria had to be met. Xeromammograms had to be available before and after estrogen manipulation. In addition, there should have been a minimum 24-month interval between mammographic examinations.

RESULTS

The four population groups in our initial study, which include symptomatic and asymptomatic users and non-users of exogenous hormones, are compared in Table 25.1 with a random normal population with regard to parenchymal pattern classifications. These subgroups can also be compared with populations from other reported series (Table 25.2). It is noted that patients on exogenous hormones in both symptomatic and asymptomatic categories do not reflect a shift to a more severe or higher classification. The percentage of patients that fall into the P_2–DY category is similar in all groups and parallels that seen in random populations.

Table 25.1 The four population study groups are compared with a random normal population. No significant shift to the P_2–DY classification is noted in the users of exogenous estrogens

	Random normal population (%)	(Symptomatic) no exogenous hormones (%)	(Asymptomatic) no exogenous hormones (%)	(Symptomatic) exogenous hormones (%)	(Asymptomatic) exogenous hormones (%)
N_1	10.0	12.7	10.6	9.6	9.8
P_1	38.4	36.5	29.2	30.8	33.6
P_2	35.0 ⎱ 51.6	31.8 ⎱ 50.8	43.4 ⎱ 60.2	32.7 ⎱ 59.6	35.0 ⎱ 56.6
DY	16.6 ⎰	19.0 ⎰	16.8 ⎰	26.9 ⎰	21.6 ⎰

Table 25.2 Parenchymal pattern classification from other reported series are compared with our total population. It is most important to compare percentage totals combining N_1-P_1 and P_2-DY

	% of population (all ages)		
	Krook/Carlisle (BCDP-screening) asymptomatic	Wolfe (Diagnostic Center) symptomatic	Buchanan (BCDP screening and diagnostic) asymptomatic and symptomatic
N_1	21.6 ⎫ 45.7	29.1 ⎫ 53.2	10.0 ⎫ 48.4
P_1	24.1 ⎭	24.1 ⎭	38.4 ⎭
P_2	32.2 ⎫ 54.3	29.7 ⎫ 46.8	35.0 ⎫ 51.6
DY	22.1 ⎭	17.1 ⎭	16.6 ⎭
Total	100.0	100.0	100.0

In addition, 250 cases were available for review in which the screened patient had been 'placed on' or 'removed from' exogenous estrogens during her 5 years of follow-up in the Louisville Breast Cancer Demonstration Project. A 24-month interval was selected as a satisfactory time span to reflect progressive or regressive changes in the breast parenchyma. Double-blind readings by an experienced mammographer and an experienced screening technologist resulted in no classification changes (Figures 25.1 and 25.2).

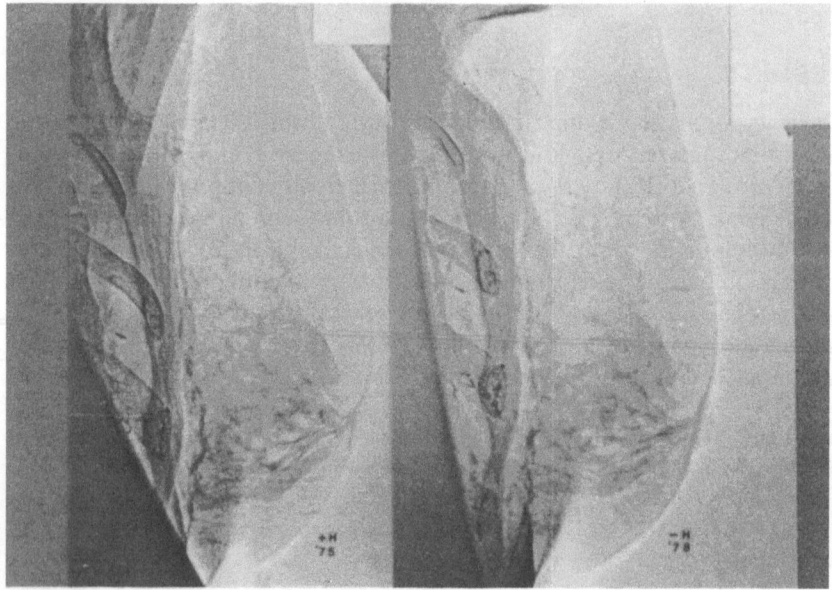

Figure 25.1 Similar xeromammographic images of the right breast of a screenee. The image on the left was taken in 1975 while the screened patient was on exogenous estrogen. No exogenous estrogen was given in the 3-year interval prior to the image on the right. Note no change in the DY classification

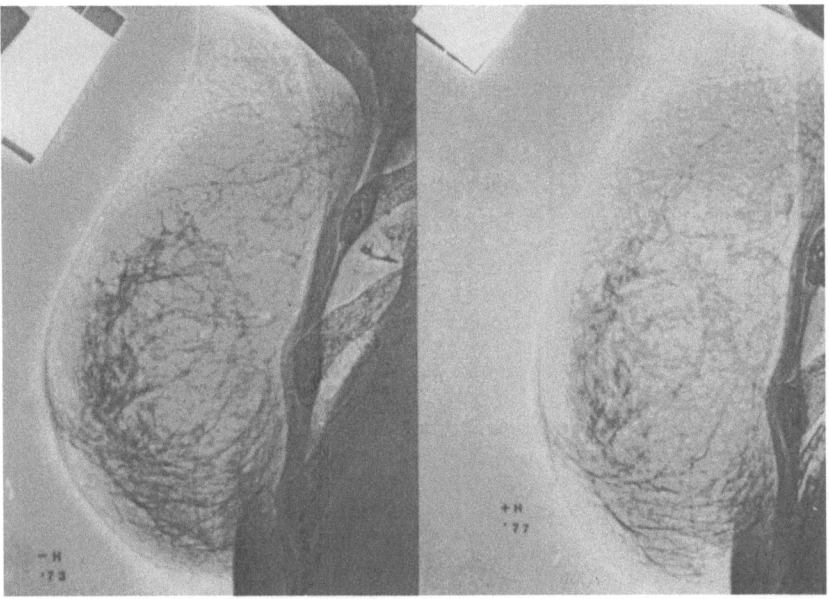

Figure 25.2 Similar images of the left breast of another screened patient. During the time interval between these images, the screenee was placed on exogenous estrogens for 4 years. Note no change in the P_2 classification

DISCUSSION

Breast carcinomas arise from ductal and lobular parenchymal cells, the growth and function of which are subject to influences of estrogen and a host of endogenous hormones. Although using proven excess cancer development as the end point for analyzing what might be the most severe effect of estrogen replacement therapy, we chose first to look at the influence of replacement estrogens on the breast parenchymal patterns as reflected on high quality xeromammograms.

Based on the mammographic characteristics of breast parenchyma, four major groups of patients can be identified. Wolfe[27] first described these groups and classified them as N_1, P_1, P_2 and DY based on the ratio of fat to connective tissue densities (Figure 25.3). Using the classification and applying it to 7214 symptomatic patients followed for $2\frac{1}{2}$ years, the authors found women classified as DY had a 21–37 times greater risk of developing breast cancer than women with an N_1 classification. The combined P_2–DY group had a 9.5 times greater risk than the N_1–P_1 group. Other retrospective studies[4, 32, 37] have sided with Wolfe's conclusions, although with less enthusiasm and lower risk ratios. Others[38, 39] have shown little, if any, correlation between progressing classification and increasing risk (Table 25.3). Still others can demonstrate no

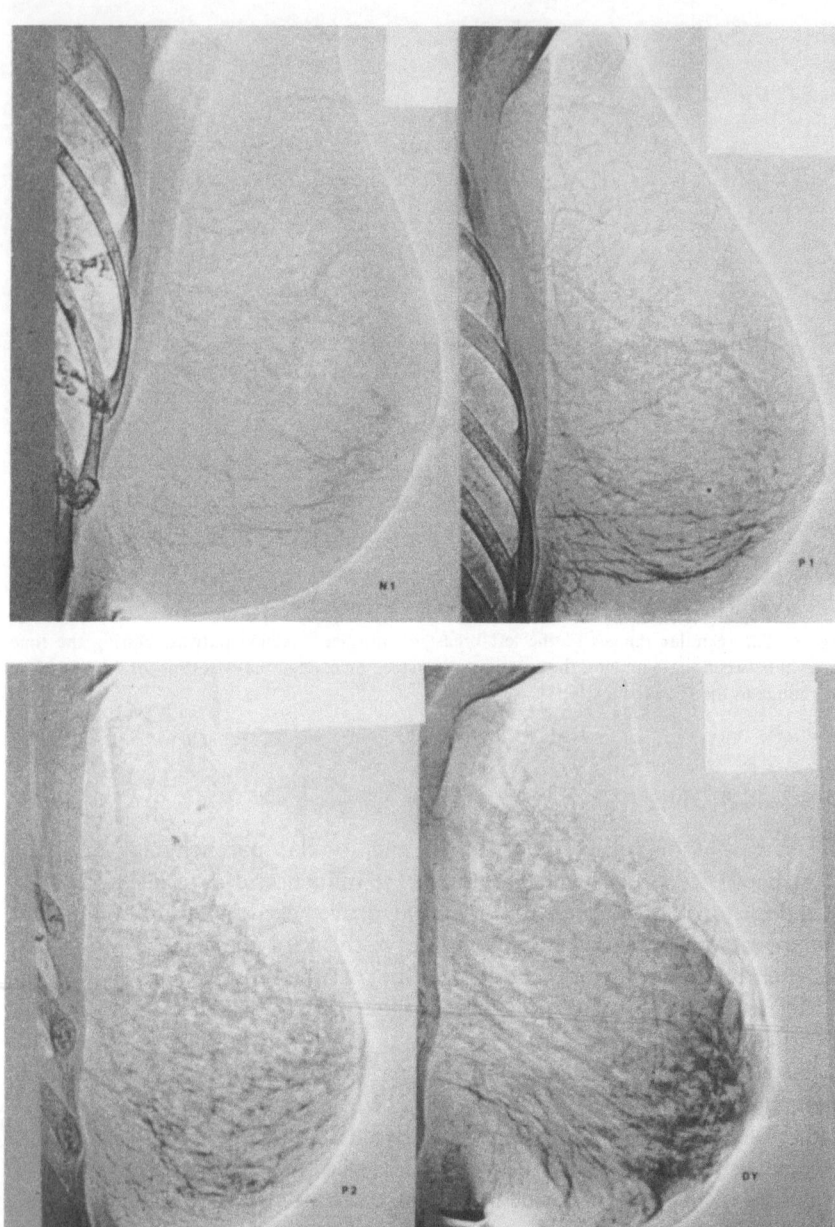

Figure 25.3 The classification system is based on duct response and the relative amount of fat to parenchymal or connective tissue elements. The combined N_1–P_1 group (A and B) represents a very low risk population, while the P_2–DY group (C and D) is at a significantly higher risk for having or developing breast cancer

correlation in prospective studies and insist that the classification is much too simple and true risk can only be predicted using a combination of factors[40].

Anatomically and biologically, the Wolfe classification of the female breast into four parenchymal patterns seems credible. Nevertheless, the feasibility of using it to predict breast cancer risk remains in question. The wide-ranging results noted by various investigators employing different study designs may result from one of many factors. Wolfe's original classifications and risk predictions are based on a population of referred symptomatic patients. Applying this classification to a self-referred asymptomatic population might well result in a different risk prediction. The wide variation in xeromammographic techniques combined with differing interpretative abilities will contribute to varying results. Because of the subjective nature of the classification, each category overlaps with the next, contributing further to discrepancies in end results. Certain studies have combined existing or prevalent cancers with developing incident cancers, while others have attempted to separate them. Most cancers that become clinically or mammographically detectable within 24 months of a negative examination are, in this author's opinion (J.B.B.), 'missed prevalent' cancers and not 'interval' cancers. Unanimous agreement with this does not exist, which can account for a sizeable error in reporting results.

While using breast parenchymal patterns as a means of predicting breast cancer risk remains controversial, the influence of exogenous estrogen use on these patterns can be studied. Group matching to eliminate other factors which might affect parenchymal patterns adds validity to these data.

Table 25.3 Breast cancer risk ratio. Various studies to date have shown a wide variation in breast cancer risk related to parenchymal patterns

	Wolfe symptomatic	Krook asymptomatic	Wilkinson asymptomatic	Mendel symptomatic
N_1	1.0	1.0	1.0	1.0
P_1	4.0	2.5	2.1	1.0
P_2	17.0	4.0	2.1	1.23
DY	22.0	6.8	5.8	1.23

SUMMARY

Although using excess cancer development as the end point for analyzing what might be the most severe effect of estrogen replacement therapy, we chose first to look at the possible stimulation of proliferative benign disorders by exogenous estrogens as reflected on high quality xeromammograms. Our studies indicate no alteration of breast parenchymal patterns with either long-term or short-term replacement estrogens. These findings seem to corroborate the finding of no alteration in breast cancer risk in these populations.

References

1. Gullino, P. M. (1977). Natural history of breast cancer. Progression from hyperplasia to neoplasia as predicted by angiogenesis. *Cancer*, **39** (6 Suppl.), 2697

2. Humphrey, L. J. and Swerdlow, M. (1962). Relationship of benign breast disease to carcinoma of the breast. *Surgery*, **52**, 841

3. Kodlin, D., Winger, E. E. and Morgenstern, N. L. *et al.* (1977). Chronic mastopathy and breast cancer. A follow-up study. *Cancer*, **39**, 2603

4. Krook, P. M., Carlile, T., Bush, W. and Hall, M. (1978). Mammographic parenchymal patterns as a risk indicator for prevalent and incident cancer. *Cancer*, **41**, 1093

5. Leis, H. P. Jr. (1976). Hormones in the epidemiology of breast cancer. *Breast – Dis. Breast*, **2**, 7

6. Lipsett, M. D. (1977). Estrogens use and cancer risk. *J. Am. Med. Assoc.*, **237**, 1112

7. Lipschutz, A. and Varga, L. Jr. (1940). Tumorgenic powers of stilbestrol and follicular hormone. *Lancet*, **1**, 541

8. Muir, R. (1941). The evolution of carcinoma of the mamma. *J. Pathol. Bacteriol.*, **52**, 155

9. Siiteri, P. (1974). Endocrine aspects of breast cancer. In J. R. Castro, T. S. Meyler and D. G. Baker (eds.). *Current Concepts in Breast Cancer*. (Flushing: Medical Examination Publishing Co. Inc.)

10. Wallace, R. B., Sherman, B. M., Bean, J. A. and Leeper, J. (1978). Thyroid hormone use in patients with breast cancer: absence of an association. *J. Am. Med. Assoc.*, **239**, 958

11. Black, M. M., Barclay, T. H. and Cutler, S. J. *et al.* (1972). Association of atypical characteristics of benign breast lesions with subsequent risk of breast cancer. *Cancer*, **29**, 339

12. Black, M. D. and Leis, H. P. Jr. (1972). Mammary carcinogenesis: influence of parity and estrogens. *N.Y. State J. Med.*, **72**, 1601

13. Carter, D. (1977). Intraductal papillary tumors of the breast. A study of 78 cases. *Cancer*, **39**, 1689

14. Cheatle, G. L. (1926). Desquamative and dysgenetic epithelial hyperplasia in breast: their situation and characteristics: their likeness to lesions induced by tar. *Br. J. Surg.*, **13**, 509

15. Dao, T. L. (1972). The question of 'preneoplastic' lesions. *J. Surg. Oncol.*, **4**, 397

16. Dawson, E. K. (1933). Carcinoma in mammary lobule and its origin. *Edinburgh Med. J.*, **40**, 57

17. Fisher, E. R., Shoemaker, R. H. and Sabnis, A. (1975). Relationship of hyperplasia to cancer in 3-methylocholanthrene-induced mammary tumorgenesis. *Lab. Invest.*, **33**, 33

18. Jensen, H. M., Rice, J. R. and Wellings, S. R. (1976). Preneoplastic lesions in the human breast. *Science*, **191**, 295

19. Kern, W. H. and Brooks, R. N. (1969). A typical epithelial hyperplasia associated with breast cancer and fibrocystic disease. *Cancer*, **24**, 668

20. Medina, D. and Warner, M. R. (1976). Mammary tumorgenesis in chemical carcinogen-treated mice. Induction of mammary ductal hyperplasias. *J. Natl. Cancer Inst.*, **57**, 57

21. Moskowitz, M. and Wirman, J. (1976). Proliferative mammary dysplasia with subsequent development of in situ cancer. *Breast*, **2**, 34

22. Ryan, J. A. and Coady, C. J. (1952). Ductal proliferation in breast cancer. *Canad. J. Surg.*, **5**, 12

23. Sinha, D. and Dao, T. L. (1977). Hyperplastic alveolar nodules of the rat mammary gland: tumor-producing capability in vivo and vitro. *Cancer Lett.*, **2**, 153

24. Slemmer, G. (1972). Host response to premalignant mammary tissues. *Natl. Cancer Inst. Monogr.*, **35**, 57

25. Wellings, S. R. and Jensen, H. M. (1975). An atlas of subgross pathology of the human breast with special reference to possible precancerous lesions. *J. Natl. Cancer Inst.*, **55**, 231

26. Welsch, C. W. (1976). Prophylaxis of early preneoplastic lesions of the mammary gland. *Cancer Res.*, **36**, 2621

27. Wolfe, J. N. (1976). Risk of breast cancer development determined by mammographic parenchymal pattern. *Cancer*, **37**, 2486

28. Wolfe, J. N. (1976). Breast patterns as an index of risk for developing cancer. *Am. J. Roentgenol.*, **126**, 1130

29. Wellings, S. R. and Wolfe, J. N. (1978). Correlative studies of the histological and radiographic appearance of the breast parenchyma. *Radiology*, **129**, 299

30. Anderson, I., Andren, L. and Petterson, H. (1978). Influence of age at first pregnancy on breast parenchymal pattern: a preliminary report. *Radiology*, **126**, 675

31. Ernster, V. L., Sacks, S. T. and Peterson, C. (1979). Mammographic parenchymal patterns and risk factors for breast cancer. Paper presented to the *Third Annual Meeting of the American Society for Preventive Oncology*, New York, March 8–9

32. Wilkinson, E., Clopton, C., Gordonson, J., Green, R., Hill, A. and Pike, M. C. (1978). Mammographic parenchymal pattern and the risk of breast cancer. *Am. J. Roentgenol.*, **130**, 1157

33. Peck, D. P. and Lowman, R. M. (1978). Estrogen and the postmenopausal breast: mammographic considerations. *J. Am. Med. Assoc.*, **240**, 1733

34. Casagrande, J., Gerkins, V., Henderson, B. E., Mack, T. and Pike, M. C. (1976). Exogenous estrogens and breast cancer in women with natural menopause. *J. Natl. Cancer Inst.*, **56**, 839

35. Hoover, R., Gray, L. A. Sr., Cole, P. and MacMahon, B. (1976). Menopausal estrogens and breast cancer. *N. Engl. J. Med.*, **295**, 401

36. Thomas, D. B. (1978). Role of exogenous female hormones in altering the risk of benign and malignant neoplasms in humans. *Cancer Res.*, **38**, 3991

37. Hainline, S., Myers, L., McLelland, R., Newell, J., Grufferman, S. and Shingleton, W. (1978). Mammographic patterns and risk of breast cancer. *Am. J. Roentgenol.*, **130**, 1157

38. Mendell, L., Rosenbloom, M. and Naimark, A. (1977). Are breast patterns a risk index for breast cancer? A reappraisal. *Am. J. Roentgenol.*, **128**, 547

39. Peyster, R. G., Kalisher, L. and Cole, P. (1977). Mammographic parenchymal patterns and prevalence of breast cancer. *Radiology*, **125**, 387

40. Egan, R. L. (1979). Estimated risk and occurrence of breast cancer in asymptomatic and minimally symptomatic patients. *Cancer*, **43**, 871

41. Foote, F. W. and Stewart, F. W. (1945). Comparative studies of cancerous versus noncancerous breasts. *Ann. Surg.*, **121**, 6, 197

42. Hertz, R. (1976). The estrogen–cancer hypothesis. *Cancer*, **38**, 534

43. Kapdi, C. C. and Wolfe, J. N. (1976). Breast cancer: relationship to thyroid supplements for hypothyroidism. *J. Am. Med. Assoc.*, **236**, 1124

44. Mustacchi, P. and Greenspan, R. (1977). Thyroid supplementation of hypothyroidism: an iatrogenic cause of breast cancer? *J. Am. Med. Assoc.*, **237**, 1446

26
Replacement Therapy of the Menopause and Breast Cancer

R. VOKAER and J. P. THOMAS

It is estimated that, in order to relieve their symptoms of menopause, more than two million American women are presently taking estrogens for more or less extended periods of time. In spite of this large number and in spite of the abundance of literature on the use of estrogens during this period of their lives, only seven cases of mammary cancer have been reported in patients undergoing estrogen therapy[1-4]. These reports extend from 1939 through 1945, a period when synthetic estrogens (diethylstilbestrol) were at their peak volume of use. Also, these were isolated cases, wherein the cause and effect relationship was not clearly established by statistical comparison with control groups.

These past few years, the use of natural, sulfo- and glucurono-conjugated estrogens has increased throughout the population. Most of the latest appearing articles concern this type of estrogen.

The present authors, by the selection of six of the more recent, better conducted *retrospective studies*[5-10], analyzed a number of cases of breast cancer. The authors attempted to find a relationship between the estrogen treatment for menopausal symptoms and the occurrence of cancer in these patients (Table 26.1).

None of these studies reveal a significant relationship between estrogen therapy and the appearance of breast cancer. The risk (being $\rho = 1.0$ in a control population) these authors observed varied between 0.75 and 1.0, with a single exception[9], where it was 3.1. In this one isolated study, however, the sample is rather small (47 cases), resulting in this risk not being statistically different from the risk observed in the control group.

Table 26.1 Studies of the relationship of non-contraceptive estrogens to the risk of breast cancer

Type of study	Reference	Type of controls	No. of cases	Year during which breast cancer was diagnosed	Measure of estrogen use	Relative risk
Hospital-based case–control	Sartwell et al.[5] Boston Collaborative Drug Surveillance	hospital	284	1969–1972	ever	0.82
	Program[6]	hospital	51	1972	ever	1.0
	Ravnihar et al.[7]	clinic	374	1972–1974	ever	0.78
Population-based case–control	Henderson et al.[8]	office	100	1969–1972	ever	0.75
	Casagrande et al.[9]	neighborhood	47	1972–1973	ever	3.1
	Craig et al.[10]	population and neighborhood	134	1949–1967	ever	1.0
	Mack	population	111	1971–1975	ever	1.6
Practice-based prospective	Burch et al.[11]	none	19	1948–1973	≥5 y	1.2
	Hoover et al.[15]	none	49	1939–1972	≥6 months	1.3

From Thomas[19]

Among these retrospective studies, that of the Boston Collaborative Drug Surveillance Program[6] is particularly interesting. Among its 5339 post-menopausal women studied there occured 51 cases of breast cancer and 52 benign breast lesions (fibroadenomas and fibrocystic disease). Here again, there was no statistically significant correlation between conjugated estrogen therapy and the advent of these lesions.

As well as these retrospective studies, two *prospective studies* cover this problem. A study by Burch *et al.*, resulting in three publications[11-13], analyzed the results of long-term follow-up of hysterectomized women for whom estrogen treatment started, either when menopausal symptoms appeared spontaneously a few years postoperatively, or immediately, when a castration accompanied hysterectomy. In this series of 735 women treated by conjugated estrogens during a minimum of 5 years, 21 breast cancers were observed. Epidemiologic studies would have led one to expect 18 cases in this group of patients had they not been under estrogen therapy. In conclusion, here, there is not significant difference between the frequencies of the appearance of breast cancer in the treated and untreated groups (relative risk $\rho = 1.2$) (Table 26.2).

Table 26.2   Anticipated and realized incidence of various types of cancer

Type of cancer	Number anticipated	Number realized
Breast	18.1	21
Colon	5.8	3
Skin	7.8	3
Lung	1.5	1
Other	32.1	16
Total	65.3	44

From Burch *et al.*[13]

It is interesting to note that the Burch studies showed that despite the fact that there was no difference in the probability of occurence of breast cancer, there was a significant reduction in the frequency of a number of other cancers (colon, skin, lungs)[14], as well as a reduction in the occurence of cerebro-vascular accidents and bone fractures in patients taking estrogens[13]. It should be noted that all the subjects in this study had undergone hysterectomies and as a consequence the possibility of cancer of the endometrium was eliminated as well.

The second prospective study is that of Hoover *et al.*[15]. It concerns 1891 women taking conjugated estrogens for a minimum of 6 months, who were followed for an average of 12 years during the period 1939–72. This study is by far the most complete (Table 26.3). Epidemiologic data would predict 39 cases of breast cancer in this group. The authors observed 49 cases, resulting in a

Table 26.3 Observed and expected numbers of cases of breast cancer according to follow-up duration

Follow-up duration (y)	Cases of breast cancer		Relative risk	95% Confidence interval
	Observed	Expected		
<5	13	13.9	0.9	0.5–1.5
5–9	13	11.1	1.2	0.6–2.0
10–14	10	7.5	1.3	0.6–2.4
15+	13	6.6	2.0	1.1–3.4
Totals	49	39.1	1.3	1.0–1.7

From Hoover *et al.*[15]

relative risk of 1.3, at the limit of statistical significance ($p = 0.06$). A number of conclusions resulted from this study:

(1) The relative risk increases progressively as the years of follow-up go by. It reaches 2.0 after 15 years ($p = 0.01$). Therefore, it seems that, after 10 years of surveillance, two 'protective' factors (multiparity and castration) do not play a significant role.

(2) In comparing those women who discontinued their therapy (but not after less than 6 months of therapy) and those who continued it, it was observed that this progressive increase in risk over time was equal in the two groups. Therefore, it may be concluded that neither the duration nor the total quantity of estrogen administered seems to modify the risk.

Table 26.4 Observed and expected cases of breast cancer according to follow-up duration and strength and frequency of estrogen used*

Follow-up duration (y)	Strength			Frequency	
	0.3 mg (873)†	0.625 mg (1262)	>0.625 mg (246)	Daily (1830)	Other (278)
<10:					
Observed	13.0	17.0	4.0	25.0	5.0
Expected	13.8	16.5	3.2	25.4	4.1
Relative risk	0.9	1.0	1.3	1.0	1.2
95% confidence interval	0.5–1.5	0.6–1.6	0.4–3.3	0.7–1.5	0.4–2.8
10+:					
Observed	14.0	11.0	8.0	20.0	9.0
Expected	8.5	9.8	3.0	14.8	3.9
Relative risk	1.6	1.1	2.7	1.4	2.3
95% confidence interval	0.9–2.7	0.5–2.0	1.2–5.3	0.9–2.2	1.1–4.4

* Tabulated according to whether ever used a particular type of therapy. Number of women > total in study since in this classification a woman could be in > 1 category
† Figures in parentheses denote number of women
From Hoover *et al.*[15]

(3) The relative risk went up to 2.7 for those who took 1.25 mg tablets of Premarin, whereas doses of 0.625 mg or 0.3 mg resulted in a 1.1 relative risk (Table 26.4). Therefore, although the total quantity of estrogen does not influence the frequency of breast cancer, it seems that the strength of the dose may play a crucial role.

(4) Curiously, the risk of developing breast cancer was found to be higher in patients who took Premarin tablets every other day rather than in those who took a daily dose. The relative risk increased to 4.7 for those who took 0.625 mg every other day (Table 26.5).

Table 26.5 Observed and expected cases of breast cancer cross-tabulated according to follow-up duration, whether > 0.625 mg of medication ever used and whether it was ever taken daily

Use of estrogen	Women who ever used ≤0.625 mg Follow-up duration (y)		Women who ever used >0.625 mg Follow-up duration (y)	
	<10	10+	<10	10+
Ever used daily:				
Observed	24.0	20.0	4.0	6.0
Expected	24.8	14.1	2.8	2.8
Relative risk	1.0	1.4	1.4	2.1
95% confidence interval	0.6–1.5	0.9–2.2	0.4–3.6	0.8–4.6
Ever used on other than daily basis:				
Observed	5.0	7.0	2.0	7.0
Expected	3.5	3.5	1.5	1.5
Relative risk	1.4	2.0	1.3	4.7
95% confidence interval	0.5–3.3	0.8–4.1	0.2–4.7	1.9–9.7

From Hoover et al.[15]

From these last two observations, it would seem to follow that it is better to prescribe weaker doses (≤0.625 mg) of Premarin every day rather than stronger doses administered two or three times per week.

(5) An observation of perhaps even greater interest concerned the appearance of benign breast lesions during conjugated estrogen therapy. In the patients in whom a benign lesion was diagnosed *during* their period of treatment (and histologically confirmed), the relative risk of appearance of breast cancer reaches the astonishing value of 6.7. On the other hand, if a benign lesion of the breast was diagnosed *before* the start of treatment, the relative risk was only 2.1, which, in itself, is also very high.

It seems well-established that conjugated estrogens are not implicated in the etiology of benign breast disease[6, 7, 16]. What is more, a pathologic study by Fechner[17], who followed fibroadenomas and fibrocystic sclerosis in a group of

43 women taking conjugated estrogens, estradiol valerianate and diethyl-stilbestrol showed no qualitative difference (as judged by the degree of epithelial hyperplasia) as compared to slides from women not taking estrogens.

In conclusion, the Hoover et al.[15] study has drawn attention to the fact that there exists a latent period of 10 to 15 years before a statistically significant rise in the risk of cancer appeared. This long latent period is comparable to that observed in the appearance of the 'protective' effect of certain hormonal situations (such as oophorectomy or early natural menopause).

The debate over the carcinogenic potential of estrogens, in particular for the mammary glands, was opened in 1932 by Lacassagne[20], who demonstrated that folliculine injections to male mice, who never show breast cancer spontaneously, led to their malignant transformation.

Of an opposing opinion were Huggins and Yang, who, in a study[21] published in 1962, showed that estradiol had a protective effect on the development of breast cancer induced by dimethylbenzanthracene in Sprague–Dawley rats. Huggins and Yang underlined the fact that this observation was in contradiction with human clinical experiences.

As we have seen, the problem is not simple, since different responses exist between different types of laboratory animals studied, and especially since the animal model cannot be extrapolated to apply to human species.

There exists today a wide consensus that menopausal women who show the distressing symptoms of this period should be treated. However, it must be emphasized that a strict surveillance is in order for these women, especially for those who have a family history of breast cancer or who, themselves, have benign breast changes.

References

1. Allaben, G. R. and Owen, S. E. (1939). Adenocarcinoma of the breast coincidental with strenuous endocrine therapy. *J. Am. Med. Assoc.*, **112**, 1933
2. Auchincloss, H. and Haagensen, C. D. (1940). Cancer of breast possibly induced by estrogenic substance. *J. Am. Med. Assoc.*, **114**, 1517
3. Foote, F. W. and Stewart, F. W. (1945). Comparative studies of cancerous versus non-cancerous breasts. *Ann. Surg.*, **121**, 197
4. Parsons, W. H. and McCall, E. F. (1941). The role of estrogenic substances in the production of malignant mammary lesions with report of a case of adenocarcinoma of the breast. *Surgery*, **9**, 780
5. Sartwell, P. E., Arthes, F. G. and Tonascia, J. A. (1977). Exogenous hormones, reproductive history and breast cancer. *J. Natl. Cancer Inst.*, **59**, 1589
6. Boston Collaborative Drug Surveillance Program (1974). Surgically confirmed gallbladder disease, venous thromboembolism and breast tumor in relation to postmenopausal estrogen therapy. *N. Engl. J. Med.*, **290**, 15
7. Ravnihar, B., Seigel, D. G. and Lindtner, J. *Eur. J. Cancer.* (In press)
8. Henderson, B. E., Powell, D., Rosario, I., Keys, C., Hamisch, R., Young, M., Casagrande, J.,

Gerkins, V. and Pike, M. C. (1974). An epidemiologic study of breast cancer. *J. Natl. Cancer Inst.*, **53**, 609

9. Casagrande, J., Gerkins, J., Henderson, B. E., Mack, T. and Pike, M. C. (1976). Exogenous estrogens and breast cancer in women with natural menopause. *J. Natl. Cancer Inst.*, **56**, 839

10. Craig, M. J., Comstock, G. W. and Geiser, P. B. (1974). Epidemiologic comparison of breast cancer patients with early and late onset of malignancy and general population controls. *J. Natl. Cancer Inst.*, **53**, 1577

11. Burch, J. C. and Byrd, B. F. (1971). The effects of long-term administration of estrogen on the occurence of mammary cancer in women. *Ann. Surg.*, **174**, 415

12. Burch, J. C., Byrd, B. F. and Vaughn, W. K. (1974). The effects of long-term estrogen on hysterectomized women. *Am. J. Obstet. Gynecol.*, **118**, 778

13. Burch, J. C., Byrd, B. F. and Vaughn, W. K. (1975). The effects of long-term estrogen administration to women following hysterectomy. In *Estrogens in the Post-Menopause. Frontiers of Hormone Research*, Vol. 3, pp. 208–214. (Basel: Karger)

14. Byrd, B. F., Burch, J. C. and Vaughn, W. K. (1973). Significance of post-operative estrogen therapy on the occurence and clinical course of cancer. *Ann. Surg.*, **177**, 626

15. Hoover, R., Gray, L. A., Cole, P. and MacMahon, B. (1976). Menopausal estrogens and breast cancer. *N. Engl. J. Med.*, **295**, 401

16. Nomura, A. and Comstock, G. W. (1976). Benign breast tumor and estrogenic hormones: a population-based retrospective study. *Am. J. Epidemiol.*, **103**, 439

17. Fechner, R. E. (1972). Benign breast disease in women on estrogen therapy. *Cancer*, **29**, 273

18. MacMahon, B., Cole, P. and Brown, J. (1973). Etiology of human breast cancer: a review. *J. Natl. Cancer Inst.*, **50**, 21

19. Thomas, D. B. (1978). Role of exogenous female hormones in altering the risk of benign and malignant neoplasms in humans. *Cancer Res.*, **38**, 3991

20. Lacassagne, A. (1932). Apparition des cancers de la mamelle chez la souris mâle soumise à des injections de folliculine. *C.R. Acad. Sci.*, **195**, 630

21. Huggins, C. and Yang, N. C. (1962). Induction and extinction of mammary cancer. *Science*, **137**, 257

27
Estrogen and Estrogen–Progestogen Compounds. Is there a Risk for the Development of Endometrial and Breast Cancer in the Perimenopausal Woman?

W. VÖLKER

Morbidity of endometrial cancer as well as breast cancer has considerably increased. In Germany, breast cancer has lately become the number one cancer disease of women[1–4], a development leading to a variety of multi-pronged studies designed to pinpoint possible genetic, endocrine, immunologic, chemical and viral contributory factors. Inasmuch as the endometrium no less than the mammary glands are target organs for hormones, much discussion in recent years has centered on possible syncarcinogenetic effects of estrogen therapy.

On the other hand, the favorable effects of estrogen therapy on climacteric disturbances are incontestable, not forgetting the effects on trophic diseases and osteoporosis. By sophisticated diagnostic methods[5], i.e. X-ray of the corticalis, we are able now to quantify the favorable effects of estrogen therapy on osteoporosis. Estrogen therapy reduces calcium loss and reduction of bone mass, which is due to an exaggerated response to parate hormone in estrogen deficiency, and by this means is able to stop osteoporosis. Prophylactic therapy is able to prevent serious forms. Nordin and his group[6] even lay stress upon a long-term prophylactic estrogen or estrogen–progestogen therapy as soon as higher values of calcium and hydroxyproline can be found in the morning urine of climacteric women.

But however great the benefits of a therapy may be, they must also be safe; first, the old question, which has been cropping up periodically for decades, has to be answered: whether estrogen therapy increases the risk for endometrial cancer. In particular, the studies of Smith *et al.*[7], Ziel and Finkle[8] and Mack *et al.*[9] aroused the attention of the scientific community. They calculated a 4.5- to 8-fold higher relative risk of the development of endometrial carcinoma after estrogen treatment. These studies, as well as a number of others striking the same note which appeared in the aftermath[10–15, 67], set off a discussion, initially among the profession, but then among the general public as well.

For decades, but most particularly since 1975, the warning that estrogens may contribute to endometrial carcinoma has been disputed by a number of authors[16–28, 30]. The high point so far of the debate was reached in the hearings of the American Food and Drug Administration in December 1975, followed by an equally significant official statement of the Drug Commission of the German Medical Society in January 1976. Both boards denied any demonstrable connection between estrogen therapy and endometrial carcinoma. The opposition voices in the debate took their cues primarily from the following points:

(a) Statistical comparative studies stand or fall with the comparability of the groups. Control groups should at least not differ from the case group in regard to factors which are known promoters of endometrial carcinoma. It is claimed that this point has not been taken into account in studies so far.

(b) Observations. Without exception, all those studies in which an increased risk of endometrial carcinoma has been found were retrospective studies with all the well known potential sources of error they contain.

(c) Means of obtaining data. In some studies[7, 8, 10, 11, 13], data – especially with regard to estrogen therapy – have been gleaned from patient files. As a point of criticism, it may be mentioned that the potential sources of error in such instances are great, since often it is neglected to record estrogen therapy[22, 23]. Conversely, it is very likely that a woman with endometrial cancer will be asked if she has had estrogen treatment.

   It must also be borne in mind in this connection that women of high social status usually are more concerned about their health, visit their doctor more frequently, and hence are more often asked specifically and thus are more often scraped.

(d) Histological diagnostics. Most of the cases studied have been in the preliminary stages or have been cases without infiltrative growth[22]. As is known, even experienced pathologists interpret a finding as incipient carcinoma where others will see only atypical hyperplasia. A diagnosis of cancer is made more often in borderline cases for forensic reasons, especially in the USA[19]. In most of the studies discussed[7, 9, 13, 31], no independent check was made of the histological findings.

Quite possibly, studies which have found an increased risk included cases in which estrogens had been taken for a previous endometrial carcinoma. In such cases, atypical bleeding would generally occur earlier[19].

In view of the close correlation between endometrial cancer and breast cancer the question has to be answered whether estrogen therapy is without any danger of breast cancer. Even though many project teams have failed to find in recent years any evidence of increased breast cancer risk[32–46, 58], nevertheless reports to the contrary[47–49], isolated observations[50–52] and animal experiments[53, 54] keep raising the issue again and again.

Similarly for endometrial carcinoma, risk factors have been found for breast cancer as well. In the discussion of a possible triggering or synergetic role of estrogen therapy in endometrial cancer, it has become apparent that any study of this nature will stand – or fall – on the accuracy of the statistical material; in other words, the validity of any study is predicated on the exact comparability of the major risk factors[17, 30]. The same is true of breast cancer[1, 55–57].

With all the caution in assessing the validity of risk factors, and cognizant of other, as yet unknown, variables capable of promoting cancer, it is nevertheless essential even in breast cancer to strive for the greatest possible comparability of control groups. To our knowledge, such a statistical comparison has not yet been undertaken in relation to breast cancer.

The reports cited so far for both cancers lack a strict classification of control groups in relation to known risk factors. This is what our study attempted to accomplish.

CASE MATERIAL AND METHODS

One hundred and thirty patients with endometrial cancer in FIGO stages I–III over the period from 1966 to 1976 were compared with an equal number of matched control subjects within the same period with regard to estrogen treatment. An effort was made to select control subjects from the same year of treatment.

The following stages were represented:

FIGO stage I: 118 cases = 90.8%
FIGO stage II: 9 cases = 6.9%
FIGO stage III: 3 cases = 2.3%

Cases in stage 0 were omitted from consideration. All of the patients in the control group had undergone hysterectomies or curettage on account of menstrual disorders.

Each of the patients with endometrial carcinoma was matched with a control subject with regard to the following points. If it proved impossible to achieve an exact correspondence in all points, the control subject was included in the comparison group only if there was nothing contradictory in terms of the criterion used for comparison. The criteria applied in the comparison and the range of tolerance were as follows:

Age at time of diagnosis – tolerance 6 years.

Age at menopause – tolerance 6 years.

Childbirths: barrenness, nulliparous, 1–2 children, 3–4 children, more than 4 children.

Abortions and miscarriages: barren, 1–2 miscarriages, 3–4 miscarriages, more than 4 miscarriages.

Body-weight and height: obesity/no obesity (tolerance: normal weight + 10%).

Carbohydrate metabolism: diabetes/no diabetes.

Blood pressure: limiting value 160/95 mmHg.

Histological findings in addition to the endometrial carcinoma: adenomatous hyperplasia, glandular hyperplasia, polyps, myomas.

Income group: very high, high, satisfactory, sufficient, low, no data.

Schooling: university level, gymnasium level, junior high equivalent, elementary school equivalent, no data.

Cancer check-up: yearly, every 2 years, every 3 years, irregular.

Drug therapy: cardiac agents, antihypertensives, sedatives.

The data were obtained from the patient's files and from standardized questionnaires.

For diabetes and hypertension, five cases were matched in the former case and 46 in the latter. The question concerning intake of estrogens was excluded from this comparison.

After the comparison groups were finally put together, in the next step the respective numbers of subjects who had received estrogens were determined from the questionnaires and patient files.

The relative risk was calculated (RR) for:

Estrogen intake in general.

Various estrogen preparations (conjugated estrogens, estriol, estradiol compounds, ovulation inhibitors, 'estrogens', more precise description not obtainable).

Duration of estrogen intake: ≤ 1 year, > 1 year and ≤ 3 years, > 3 years and ≤ 5 years, > 5 years and ≤ 10 years, > 10 years.

Estrogen ingestion in coincidence with known risk factors for endometrial carcinoma.

Because of the relatively extensive use, in addition the relative risk for conjugated estrogens was determined depending on the duration of ingestion.

Using the same schedule, 120 women with histologic evidence of breast cancer in the years between 1969 and 1974 were matched with the same number of controls[58]. In selecting the control group, each cancer patient was matched with a control presenting an overlapping picture of risk factors, as follows:

Age at time of diagnosis – tolerance 6 years.

Age at the time of menopause – tolerance 6 years.

Number of births: barrenness, nulliparous, one–two children, three–four children, more than four children.

Abortions and miscarriages: barren, one–two miscarriages, three–four miscarriages, more than four miscarriages.

Body-weight and height: obesity/no obesity (tolerance normal weight + 10%).

Carbohydrate metabolism: diabetes/no diabetes.

Blood pressure: limiting value 160/95 mmHg.

Income group: very high, high, satisfactory, sufficient, low, no data.

Schooling: university level, gymnasium level, junior high equivalent, elementary school equivalent, no data.

Record of lactation.

Age at first pregnancy.

In the case of diabetes and hypertension, the number of cases matched, that is, there were no diabetics and 19 hypertensives in each group.

Statistical procedures and calculation of relative risk (RR) for different estrogen and estrogen–progestogen compounds and duration of use were identical to the procedure described above.

Based on TNM classification, the staging of cancer was as follows:

T_1N_0 . . . . 60 cases
T_2N_0 . . . . 18 cases
T_3N_0 . . . . 4 cases
T_1N_1 . . . . 13 cases
T_2N_1 . . . . 14 cases
T_2N_2 . . . . 5 cases
T_3N_1 . . . . 4 cases
T_3N_2 . . . . 1 case
$T_2N_2M_1$ . . . 1 case

The histological classification according to Jagla's simplified scheme[59] was as follows:

Non-invasive carcinoma of mammary duct . . . 21
Invasive carcinoma of mammary duct 11

```
Solid carcinoma . . . . . . . . . . . . . . . .  26
Solid scirrhous carcinoma . . . . . . . . . .  40
Adenocarcinoma . . . . . . . . . . . . . . . .   6
Paget's disease. . . . . . . . . . . . . . . .   2
Gelatinous carcinoma . . . . . . . . . . . .   4
Lobular carcinoma . . . . . . . . . . . . . .   1
Lobular carcinoma in situ . . . . . . . . .   4
Others . . . . . . . . . . . . . . . . . . . .   5
```

The relative risk was calculated by the method of Mantel and Haenszel[60]. For expected values equal or less than 2, Yates correction and Fisher test were applied.

RESULTS

(1) Endometrial carcinoma

Taking all estrogen preparations together we find that the number of those taking estrogens was smaller in the cancer group than in the control group ($p < 0.01$). Thus, the relative risk (RR) for endometrial carcinoma is not elevated (RR = 0.44) (Table 27.1).

Table 27.1   Relative risk (RR) of endometrial cancer for estrogen ingestion in general and for different estrogen preparations

	Endometrial carcinoma n	Control n	RR	χ^2	p
Conjugated estrogens	12	21	0.44	4.56	<0.05
Estriol	1	6	0.13	4.86	<0.05
Estrogen–androgen combinations	10	6	1.28	0.21	>0.05
Estradiol	5	6	0.64	0.52	>0.05
Oral contraceptives	1	8	0.1	7.13	<0.01
'Estrogens'; type not specified	7	16	0.34	5.58	<0.05
Totals	31	54	0.44	9.25	<0.01

Considered separately, estrogens (conjugated), estriol, ovulation inhibitors, and estrogen compounds, for which a more precise description could not be obtained, showed the same trend ($p < 0.01$–0.05) (Table 27.1). No difference was noted in the case of estrogen–androgen compounds or of estradiol compounds.

There is no statistical evidence that the risk of endometrial carcinoma increases with increase in the duration of ingestion of estrogens (Table 27.2). The same holds if conjugated estrogens are considered separately (Table 27.3).

Interestingly, a significantly lower relative risk was calculated in those cases where there was a coincidence with known risk factors such as barrenness, hypertension and obesity. When the factors of obesity and estrogen intake were taken together there was even a highly significant reduction in relative risk for the cancer group ($p < 0.001$, $RR = 0.3$, Table 27.4).

Table 27.2 Duration of ingestion for estrogen intake in general and relative risk (RR) of endometrial cancer

Duration of use	Carcinoma n	Control n	RR	χ^2	p
≤ 1 y	12	20	0.46	3.96	<0.05
> 1 y, < 3 y	4	13	0.24	6.80	<0.01
> 3 y, < 5 y	4	9	0.34	3.25	>0.05
> 5 y, < 10 y	5	4	0.96	0.004	>0.05
> 10 y	3	2	1.15	0.02	>0.05

Table 27.3 Duration of ingestion of conjugated estrogens and relative risk (RR) of endometrial cancer

Duration of use	Endometrial carcinoma n	Control n	RR	χ^2	p
≤ 1 y	3	5	0.46	1.13	>0.05
> 1 y, ≤ 3 y	2	9	0.17	6.15	<0.05
> 3 y, ≤ 5 y	3	3	0.77	0.10	>0.05
> 5 y, ≤ 10 y	2	1	1.54	0.06	>0.05
> 10 y	1	1	0.77	0.28	>0.05

Table 27.4 Relative risk (RR) for estrogen ingestion in coincidence with risk factors

	Endometrial carcinoma n	Control n	RR	χ^2	p
Nulligravidity	5	10	0.34	4.1	<0.05
Hypertension	5	16	0.23	7.47	<0.01
Obesity	13	35	0.30	11.1	<0.001

(2) Breast cancer

For estrogen therapy as a whole, no increase was found in the relative risk ratios (RR). Thirty-nine women with breast cancer took estrogens compared with 42 in the control group who did not take estrogens, for a risk ratio $RR = 0.89$ ($p > 0.05$) (Table 27.5). No indication of any increased risk could be found in the estradiol, estrogen–androgen combination and oral contraceptive users ($RR = 0.77–1.11$; $p > 0.05$).

Table 27.5   Relative risk (RR) of breast cancer for estrogen ingestion in general and for different estrogen preparations. Several patients took different preparations at various times. The total number of specific drug users, therefore, differs from and is larger than, the number of actual cases (39 and 42)

	Breast cancer n	Control n	RR	χ^2	p
Conjugated estrogens	6	18	0.32	5.63	<0.05
Estriol	1	4	0.24	1.86	>0.05
Estrogen–androgen combinations	4	4	0.96	0.003	>0.05
Estradiol	4	5	0.77	0.14	>0.05
Oral contraceptives	15	13	1.11	0.06	>0.05
'Estrogens'; type not specified	14	12	1.12	0.08	>0.05
Totals	39	42	0.89	0.17	>0.05

For conjugated estrogens and estriol users, there was a consistently larger percentage of cases in the control group ($RR = 0.32$ and 0.24). The difference in the reduced risk ratio for patients taking conjugated estrogens is statistically significant ($p < 0.05$). In the control group, 18 patients had taken estrogens, compared to six.

Furthermore, increasing duration of therapy for all estrogen preparations did not show any increase in the risk ratio ($RR = 0.36-1.36$; $p > 0.05$) (Table

Table 27.6   Duration of ingestion for estrogen intake in general and relative risk (RR) of breast cancer

Duration of use	Breast cancer n	Control n	RR	χ^2	p
≤1 y	17	12	1.36	0.58	>0.05
>1 y, ≤3 y	7	10	0.67	0.59	>0.05
>3 y, ≤5 y	3	4	0.72	0.18	>0.05
>5 y	3	8	0.36	2.31	<0.05

Table 27.7   Duration of ingestion of conjugated estrogens and relative risk (RR) of breast cancer. Two patients in the control group were unably to give clear information; they were eliminated from this table

Duration of use	Breast cancer n	Control n	RR	χ^2	p
≤1 y	3	6	0.48	1.06	>0.05
>1 y, ≤3 y	2	4	0.48	0.72	>0.05
>3 y, ≤5 y	1	4	0.24	1.86	>0.05
>5 y	0	2	0	4.6	<0.05

27.6). The same trend was observed when conjugated estrogens were segregated for assessment of the length-of-use factor ($RR = 0$–0.48; $p > 0.05$) (Table 27.7).

The calculations also failed to disclose any heightened risk in relation to such factors as nulligravidity ($RR = 0.58$; $p > 0.05$), hypertension ($RR = 1.48$; $p > 0.05$) and obesity ($RR = 0.68$; $p > 0.05$) (Table 27.8).

Table 27.8   Relative risk (RR) of estrogen ingestion in coincidence with risk factors for breast cancer

	Breast cancer n	Control n	RR	χ^2	p
Nulligravidity	7	10	0.58	0.82	>0.05
Hypertension	8	5	1.48	0.31	>0.05
Obesity	12	19	0.68	0.76	>0.05

DISCUSSION

In contrast to a number of Anglo-American publications which have disturbed the medical world over the last 4 years, the present statistical study provides no evidence that estrogen therapy increases the risk of endometrial cancer in the climacteric. Even in those cases where estrogen therapy was received over a relatively long period, no evidence of an elevated risk was found either for estrogens as a whole or for conjugated estrogens, regarded by other investigators as especially dangerous[8, 9, 11, 12, 61]. The finding of a distinct decrease in the relative risk in the case of a coincidence of barrenness, hypertension and obesity with estrogen ingestion, which we obtained in agreement with Smith et al.[7], was, however, interesting.

What is the reason for the discrepancy between this study and the preceding ones? The greatest potential source of error is to be found in the selection of the control group of subjects. In the preceding studies, there is a strict correspondence between the groups with regard to general epidemiologic data, not to speak of the known risk factors.

On the other hand, our results showed quite broad agreement with those of Dunn and Bradbury[62] (1967), who found no increase in risk. In cases, however, where the control group and case group differed on essential points, the relative risk figures are falsely high. This is the case, for example, with the study by Smith et al.[7]. These investigators compared a group comprising cases of cervical, ovarian and vulval cancer for which the risk factors did not agree. On the other hand, Dunn and Bradbury had matched quite carefully.

The recently published reports of Antunes et al.[14] and Jick et al.[15] give no further concern in this aspect. Horwitz and Feinstein[17] recently furnished statistical proof that the relative risk of endometrial cancer decreased for subjects receiving estrogens in proportion to the increase in the degree of agreement between the groups. The relative risk was 9.8 for groups for which equivalence was not certain. As agreement increased, this figure fell to 1.2. Exact agreement appears to be important, especially with regard to obesity. More recent studies[63, 64] have shown a significantly greater rate of conversion of androstenedione to estrone with increase in body-weight. In turn, since the study of Siiteri[65], estrone is discussed as being a potential carcinogen.

It is interesting enough that in 1974, Siiteri et al.[65] and MacDonald and Siiteri[87] reported that in patients with endometrial carcinoma the conversion to estrone would be increased. The authors had to withdraw this statement after further studies in 1978[66].

All these facts lead to the conclusion that studies without careful matching give no further elucidation. It is, therefore, astonishing that Hammond et al.[67] recently reported an increased risk after estrogen therapy, but set forth with the most striking differences in the compared groups: in a follow-up study the authors observed cases and controls for 5 years. Strikingly, in the control group, nine patients entered the observation period with a manifest endometrial carcinoma, while in the estrogen group only one patient had to be treated at the beginning.

A survey of Anglo-American publications, as well as of the discussion among the public and the profession, leads to an astonishing fact: all European epidemiologic studies on this matter are not known and/or not mentioned. All these studies come to a negative result[36, 68–73]. The diametrical antithesis of some of the American studies and the European results leads to the following conclusion: that in the United States, indications, contraindications and basic rules for estrogen therapy have not been observed as carefully as in Europe.

The problem of estrogens and endometrial carcinoma is not denied, but the fact that for the last 50 years this matter has been discussed makes it unlikely that there is a simple connection of causes and effects.

What are the conclusions for therapy which follow from the above-mentioned results? These rules have usually been observed in Europe for the last decades:

Individual prescription.
Lowest effective dose.
Cyclical substitution, i.e. every 4 weeks an interval of 7 days, or biphasic
    substitution.
Gynecologic controls every 6 months.
In case of atypical bleeding curettage.

Special attention should be called to the fact that primary risk groups are not excluded.

In view of the conflicting results, and in view of the close correlation of the two forms of cancer, urgent elucidation becomes necessary, whether or not restraint in prescribing estrogens out of fear of promoting breast cancer is justified.

Outside the period of pregnancy, the most important hormonal factors involving the mammary gland are the sex hormones and prolactin. At the moment there is no established correlation between serum prolactin levels and breast cancer[74-76]. On the other hand, it would be of interest to corroborate Henderson's findings[78] to the effect that daughters of breast cancer patients had elevated serum prolactin and estradiol levels. After all, there can be little doubt that endogenous estrogens are a factor contributing to breast cancer:

The condition is a hundred times more frequent in women than in men.
Breast cancer invariably occurs after puberty.
There is a correlation between the length of sexual maturity and the incidence of breast cancer.
Ovarian dysgenesis and breast cancer are mutually exclusive.
The incidence of breast cancer is reduced after oophorectomy[77].

Sherman and Koreman[79] found increased incidence of breast cancer among women exposed to the influence of endogenous estrogens over many years in the face of corpus luteum insufficiency, though this conflicts with the fact that victims of breast cancer are seldom suffering from a progesterone deficiency[77]. Much has been said about the special significance of the interrelationship among different endogenous estrogens; thus MacMahon et al.[80] and Lemon et al.[81] found in breast cancer patients a lower urinary fraction of estriol as compared to estradiol and estrone. This gave rise to the since disputed theory that an increase in this quotient implied a certain protective action[82, 83].

At the moment, the existence of a characteristic hormonal profile has not been established. Further concern was aroused by the report of Hoover et al.[49] (1976) to the effect that women initially responding to estrogen therapy with benign changes eventually constituted a heightened risk. Beyond that, increased risks ($RR = 2.0$) were reported after estrogen therapy lasting more than 15 years and under higher doses (in excess of 0.625 mg conjugated estrogens). This study, however, lacked a closely comparable group. One can only guess to what extent the growing restraint in the use of oral contraceptives is also conditioned by the resultant fear of cancer.

The comparative study described here shows no increased risk of breast cancer in the wake of estrogen therapy, and this is true of the test compounds as a whole, as well as individual products. A breakdown based on the length of use similarly failed to disclose any heightened risk, although contrary to Hoover's series we had only three patients taking estrogens in excess of 10 years. In our country, it is not at all customary to take estrogens for nearly as long as in the United States. Interestingly enough, in the case of conjugated estrogens the risk actually proved to be statistically reduced. Even though we applied the Yates correction and the Fisher test to these readings, the modest number of cases counsels discretion in assessing this finding.

Remarkably enough, Gambrell and his associates came to much the same conclusions in a newly published, partly prospective study[43] involving 123 cases of breast cancer, which indicated that women with no history of estrogen therapy have a three times higher incidence of breast cancer. Just as in our study, no difference emerged from a comparison of combined estrogen–progestin therapy vs. estrogen therapy alone. Nevertheless, Gambrell and his associates also do not go as far as claiming any protective action of estrogens in relation to breast cancer. Similar figures are reported by Nachtigall[46] in a long-term prospective study involving 168 women over a 10-year span, leading the author to the assumption that estrogen therapy 'may have protected these women against it'. She found in her control group four cases of breast cancer, compared to none among the estrogen users. A number of authors found no enhanced risk in recent years[33-41, 43-46, 58].

Extensive studies support the view that oral contraceptives afford protection against benign changes[84, 85].

In conclusion, it must be said that with estrogens used for periods below 15 years – a span seldom exceeded in Europe – and at dosage levels customary in our country, there is no demonstrable increase of risk. Our study, along with a number of recent American reports[43, 46] in fact suggest a mild protective action. For this reason, one should avoid alarming physicians and the public in regard to an otherwise indicated estrogen therapy[86].

References

1. Sachs, H. and Maas, H. (1969). Neuere epidemiologische Gesichtspunkte zum Brustdrüsenkreks der Frau. *Geburtsch. Frauenheilk.*, **29**, 932
2. Maas, H., Trams, G. and Sachs, H. (1970). Das Mammacarcinom, Epidemiologie und Endokrinologie. *Gynäkologe*, **3**, 2
3. *Krebsregister Hamburg*, FRG, 1969–1977
4. *Krebsdokumentation Saarland*, FRG, 1972–1974
5. Hermanutz, K. D.. Beck, K. J. and Franken, Th. (1977). Radiologischer Nachweis von Knochenveränderungen bei beidseitig ovariektomierten Frauen mit und ohne Östrogenprophylaxe. *Fortschr. Röntgenstr.*, **126**, 546
6. Nordin, B. E. C. (1976). Hormonal control of calcium metabolism. Presented at *V. International Congress of Endocrinology*, 13 November, Hamburg
7. Smith, D. C., Prentice, R., Thompson, D. C. and Herrmann, W. L. (1975). Association of exogenous estrogen and endometrial carcinoma. *N. Engl. J. Med.*, **293**, 1164
8. Ziel, H. K. and Finkle, W. D. (1975). Increased risk of endometrial carcinoma among users of conjugated estrogens. *N. Engl. J. Med.*, **293**, 1167
9. Mack, Th. M., Pike, M. P. H., Henderson, B. E., Pfeffer, R. J., Gerkins, V. R., Arthur, M. and Brown, S. E. (1976). Estrogens and endometrial cancer in a retirement community. *N. Engl. J. Med.*, **294**, 1262
10. Ziel, H. K. and Finkle, W. D. (1976). Association of estrone with the development of endometrial carcinoma. *Am. J. Obstet. Gynecol.*, **124**, 735
11. McDonald, Th. W., Annegers, J. F., O'Fallon, W. M., Dockerty, M. B., Malkasian, G. D. and Kurland, L. T. (1977). Exogenous estrogen and endometrial carcinoma: case control and incidence study. *Am. J. Obstet. Gynecol.*, **127**, 572

12. Gordon, J., Reagan, J. W., Finkle, W. D. and Ziel, H. K. (1977). Estrogen and endometrial carcinoma. *N. Engl. J. Med.*, **297**, 570

13. Cohen, C. J. and Deppe, G. (1977). Endometrial carcinoma and oral contraceptive agents. *Obstet. Gynecol.*, **49**, 390

14. Antunes, C. M. F., Stolley, P. D., Rosenhein, N. B., Davies, J. L., Toascia, J. A., Brown, C., Burnett, L., Rutledge, A., Pokempner, M. and Garcia, R. (1979). Endometrial cancer and estrogen use. *N. Engl. J. Med.*, **300**, 9

15. Jick, H., Watkins, R. N., Hunter, J. R., Dinau, B. J., Madsen, S., Rothman, K. J. and Walker, A. M. (1979). Replacement estrogens and endometrial cancer. *N. Engl. J. Med.*, **300**, 218

16. Wynder, E. L., Escher, G. H. and Mantel, N. (1966). An epidemiologic investigation of cancer of the endometrium. *Cancer*, **19**, 489

17. Horwitz, R. I. and Feinstein, A. R. (1977). New methods of sampling and analysis to remove bias in case–control research: no association found for estrogens and endometrial cancer. Presented at the *Meeting of the Am. Soc. for Clin. Invest.*, 1 May, Washington DC

18. Wallach, S. and Hennemann, P. H. (1959). Prolonged estrogen therapy in postmenopausal women. *J. Am. Med. Assoc.*, **171**, 1637

19. Lauritzen, Ch. (1976). Ostrogene und Korpuskarzinom. *Dtsch. Med. Wochenschr.*, **43**, 1581

20. Schleyer-Saunders, E. (1960). The management of the menopause. *Med. Press*, **244**, 337

21. Schleyer-Saunders, E. (1971). Results of hormone implants in the treatment of the climacteric. *J. Am. Geriatr. Soc.*, **19**, 114

22. Lauritzen, Ch. (1976). Gestagene, Östrogene und fakultative Synkarzinogenese. *Dtsch. Ärztebl.*, **43**, 2715

23. Cyran, W. (1976). Östrogene und Endometriumkarzinom. *Fortschr. Med.*, **34**, 2001

24. Lau, H.-U., Petschelt, E., Poehls, H., Pollex, G., Unger, H.-H. and Zegenhagen, V. (1975). Epidemiologische Aspekte beim Korpuskarzinom. *Zbl. Gynäk.*, **97**, 1025

25. Geist, S. H. and Salmon, U. J. (1941). Are estrogens carcinogenic in the human female? The effect of long continuated estrogen administration upon the uterine and vaginal mucosa of the human female. *Zbl. Gynäk.*, **41**, 29

26. Bishop, P. M. (1960). Hormones and cancer. *Clin. Obstet. Gynecol.*, **3**, 1109

27. Herrenberg, C. A. (1960). Treatment of postmenopausal osteoporosis with estrogens and androgens. *Acta Endocrinol.*, **34**, 51

28. Dibbelt, L., Müller, H. G. and Ehlers, F. (1962). Die Häufigkeit konstitutioneller und exogener Faktoren bei Kranken mit einem Karzinom des Corpus uteri. *Z. Geburtsh. Gynäk.*, **160**, 1

29. Greenberg, B. G. (1975). Testimony regarding presumed relationship between use of conjugated estrogens and endometrial carcinoma. Presented at the *Hearing of the Obstetrics and Gynecology Advisatory Committee, FDH, DHEW*, 16 December, Boston

30. Völker, W., Kannengiesser, U., Majewski, A. and Vasterling, H. W. (1978). Östrogentherapie und Endometriumkarzinom. *Geburtsh. Frauenheilk.*, **38**, 735

31. Gray, L. H., Christopherson, W. M. and Hoover, R. N. (1977). Estrogens and endometrial carcinoma. *Obstet. Gynecol.*, **49**, 385

32. Wynder, E. L., MacCornack, F. A. and Stellmann, S. D. (1978). The epidemiology of breast cancer in 785 United States Caucasian women. *Cancer*, **41**, 2341

33. Vessey, M. P., Doll, R. and Sutton, P. M. (1971). Investigation of the possible relationship between oral contraceptives and benign and malignant breast disease. *Cancer*, **28**, 1395

34. Arthes, F. G., Sartwell, Ph. E. and Lewison, E. F. (1971). The pill, estrogen and the breast. Epidemiologic aspects. *Cancer*, **28**, 1392

35. Burch, J. C. and Byrd, B. F. (1971). Effects of long-term administration of estrogen on the occurence of mammary cancer in women. *Ann. Surg.*, **174**, 414

36. Burch, J. C. and Byrd, B. F. (1974). The effects of long-term estrogen on hysterectomized women. *Am. J. Obstet. Gynecol.*, **118**, 788

37. Wilson, R. (1962). The role of estrogen and progesterone in breast and genital cancer. *J. Am. Med. Assoc.*, **182**, 327
38. Boston Collaborative Drug Surveillance Program (1973). *Cancer*, **1**, 1399
39. Gray, L. A. and Barnes, M. L. (1871). Effects of estrogenic therapy of the breast. *South. Med. J.*, **64**, 835
40. Henderson, B. E., Powell, D., Rosario, I., Keys, C., Hanisch, R., Young, M., Casagrande, J., Gerkins, V. and Pike, M. C. (1974). An epidemiologic study of breast cancer. *J. Natl. Cancer Inst.*, **53**, 609
41. Leis, H. P. (1970). The pill and the breast. *NY State J. Med.*, **70**, 2911
42. Royal College of General Practitioners. *Oral Contraceptives and Health: an Interim Report*, p. 98. (London: Pitman Medical)
43. Gambrell, R. D., Massey, F. M., Castaneda, T. A. and Boddie, A. W. (1978). Estrogen therapy and breast cancer in postmenopausal women. Presented at the *Armed Forces District Meeting, American College of Obstetricians and Gynecologists*, 15–19 October, Washington DC
44. Gordon, G. S., Picchi, J. and Roof, B. S. (1973). Anti-fracture efficacy of long-term estrogen for osteoporosis. *Clin. Res.*, **21**, 733
45. Vessey, M. P., Doll, R. and Jones, K. (1775). Oral contraceptives and breast cancer. *Lancet*, **1**, 941
46. Nachtigall, L. (1977). *The Nachtigall Report*. (New York: Putnam)
47. Hertz, R. (1969). The problem of possible effects of oral contraceptives in breast cancer. *Cancer*, **23**, 1140
48. Dallenbach-Hellweg, G. and Dallenbach, F. D. (1970). Besteht ein morphologisch faßbarer Zusammenhang zwischen Oestrogen und Karzinogenese? Presented at *70. Tagung der Dtsch. Ges. Gynäkologie, 1970, Hamburg*
49. Hoover, R., Gray, L. A., Cole, Ph. and MacMahon, B. (1976). Menopausal estrogens and breast cancer. *N. Engl. J. Med.*, **295**, 401
50. Izsak, F. G. and Mauldin, W. P. (1968). Cancer of the breast in an adolescent girl. *Harefuah*, **75**, 464
51. Goldenberg, V. E., Mothet, N. K. and Wolff, M. (1968). Atypical features in breast carcinoma in patients on oral contraceptives. *Am. J. Clin. Pathol.*, **506**, 635
52. Fechner, R. E. (1970). Breast cancer during oral contraceptive therapy. *Cancer*, **26**, 1204
53. Kirschstein, R. L., Rabson, A. S. and Rusten, G. W. (1972). Infiltrating duct carcinoma of the mammary gland of a rhesus monkey after administration of an oral contraceptive: a preliminary report. *J. Natl. Cancer Inst.*, **48**, 551
54. Clayson, D. B. (1970). Tumors induced by hormones without added carcinogenic stimuli. *Chemical Carcinogenesis*, p. 315. (London: Churchill)
55. Bamber, M. and Sachs, H. (1976). Epidemiologische und ätiologische Faktoren beim Mammakarzinom. Katamnestische Untersuchungen an 742 Patientinnen der Strahlenklinik Essen. *Röntgen-Bl.*, **29**, 55
56. Stoll, B. A. (1976). *Risk Factors in Breast Cancer. New Aspects of Breast Cancer*, 2nd ed. (London: Heinemann)
57. Anderson, D. E. (1971). Some characteristics of familial breast cancer. Presented at the *2nd Nat. Conf. on Breast Cancer, 1971, Los Angeles*
58. Völker, W., Kannengiesser, U. and Majewski, A. (1979). Östrogentherapie und Mammakarzinom. *Geburtsh. Frauenheilk.* (In press)
59. Jagla, K. L. (1977). Multizentrische Carcinome und atypische Epithelproliferationen der weiblichen Brustdrüse. *Dissertation*, Hannover
60. Mantel, N. and Haenszel, W. (1959). Statistical aspects of the analysis of data from retrospective studies of disease. *J. Natl. Cancer Inst.*, **22**, 719
61. Greenblatt, R. B. (1963). The menopause and its management. In R. J. Dorfman and M. Nevese (eds.). *Pituitary Ovarian Endocrinology*. (San Francisco: Castro Edit., Holden Day Inc.)

62. Dunn, L. J. and Bradbury, J. T. (1967). Endocrine factors in endometrial carcinoma. *Am. J. Obstet. Gynecol.*, **97**, 465

63. Hensell, P. L., Grodin, J. M., Brenner, P. F., Siiteri, P. K. and MacDonald, P. C. (1974). Plasma precursors of estrogen. II. Correlation of the extent of conversion of plasma androstendione to estrone with age. *J. Clin. Endocrinol.*, **38**, 476

64. Siiteri, P. K. and MacDonald, P. C. (1973). Role of extraglandular estrogen in human endocrinology. In R. O. Greep and E. B. Astwood (eds.). *Handbook of Physiology, Section 7, Endocrinology. Vol. II. Female Reproductive System, Part 1.* (Washington DC: Am. Physiol. Soc.)

65. Siiteri, P. K., Schwarz, B. E. and MacDonald, P. C. (1974). Estrogen receptors and the estrone hypothesis in relation to endometrial and breast cancer. *Gynecol. Oncol.*, **2**, 228

66. MacDonald, P. C., Edman, C. D., Hemsell, D. L., Porter, J. C. and Siiteri, P. K. (1978). Effect of obesity on conversion of plasma androstendione to estrone in postmenopausal women with and without endometrial carcinoma. *Am. J. Obstet. Gynecol.*, **130**, 448

67. Hammond, C. B., Jelovsek, F. R., Lee, K. C., Creasman, W. T. and Parker, R. T. (1979). Effects of long-term estrogen replacement therapy. *Am. J. Obstet. Gynecol.*, **133**, 525

68. Smartzis, S. and Hauser, G. A. (1976). Die Postmenopausenblutung. *Geburtsh. Frauenheilk.*, **36**, 326

69. Uyttenbroeck, F. and Wauters, H. (1978). L'influence des contraceptives oraux, des progestagénes et des oestrogénes dans la genèse des lesions precancéreuses et cancéreuses de l'appareil genital et du sein. Presented at *Soc. Belge-Pay-Bas d'Obstet. Gynecol.*, 13 November, Antwerpen.

71. Lauritzen, Ch. (1977). A retrospective study concerning postmenopausal estrogen therapy and endometrial cancer. Presented at the *Second International Meeting on Endometrial Cancer and Related Topics*, 30–31 March, London

72. Pfleiderer, A. (1977). Risk for endometrial cancer. Presented at the *Second International Meeting on Endometrial Cancer and Related Topics*, 30–31 March, London

73. Rauramo, L. (1977). Estrogen therapy and endometrial cancer. Presented at the *Second International Meeting on Endometrial Cancer and Related Topics*, 30–31 March, London

74. Boyns, A. R., Cole, E. N., Griffiths, K., Roberts, M. M., Buchan, R., Wilson, R. G. and Forrest, A. P. M. (1973). Prolactin in breast cancer. *Eur. J. Cancer*, **9**, 99

75. Franks, S., Ralphs, D. N. L., Seegroat, V. and Jacobs, H. S. (1974). Prolactin concentrations in patients with breast cancer. *Br. Med. J.*, **2**, 320

76. Kwa, H. G., Engelsman, H., DeJong-Bakken, R. and Cuton, F. J. (1974). Plasma prolactin in human breast cancer. *Lancet*, **1**, 433

77. Kirschner, M. A. (1977). The role of hormones in the etiology of human breast cancer. *Cancer*, **39**, 2716

78. Henderson, B. E., Gerkins, V., Rosario, R., Casagrande, J. and Pike, M. C. (1975). Serum levels of estrogen and prolactin in daughters of patients with breast cancer. *N. Engl. J. Med.*, **293**, 790

79. Sherman, B. M. and Koreman, S. C. (1974). Inadequate corpus luteum function: a pathophysiological interpretation of human breast cancer epidemiology. *Cancer*, **33**, 1306

80. MacMahon, B., Cole, P., Brown, J. B., Aoki, K., Lin, T. M., Morgan, R. W. and Woo, N. Ch. (1974). Urine estrogen profiles of Asian and North American women. *Int. J. Cancer*, **14**, 161

81. Lemon, H. M., Wotiz, H. H., Parsons, L. and Mozden, P. J. (1966). Reduced estriol excretion in patients with breast cancer prior to endocrine therapy. *J. Am. Med. Assoc.*, **196**, 112

82. Hellmann, L., Zunoff, B., Fishman, J. and Gallagher, T. F. (1971). Peripheral metabolism of ^{3}H-estradiol and the excretion of endogenous estrone and estriol glucosiduronate in women with breast cancer. *J. Clin. Endocrinol. Metab.*, **33**, 138

83. Flood, C., Pratt, J. H. and Longcope, C. (1976). The metabolic clearance and blood production rates of estriol in normal, non-pregnant women. *J. Clin. Endocrinol. Metab.*, **45**, 1

84. Ory, H., Cole, Th., MacMahon, B. and Hoover, R. (1976). Oral contraceptives and reduced risk of benign breast diseases. *N. Engl. J. Med.*, **294**, 419
85. Tapia, J. E. and Mall-Haefeli, I. (1978). Verändern hormonale Kontrazeptiva die Brust. *Der Informierte Arzt*, **2**, 102
86. Kubli, F. (1978). Hormonsubstitution der Frau. *Sexualmedizin*, **12**, 1006
87. MacDonald, P. C. and Siiteri, P. K. (1974). The relationship between the extraglandular production of estrone and the occurence of endometrial neoplasia. *Gynecol. Oncol.*, **2**, 259

28
Role of Estrogens and Progestogens in the Etiology of Breast and Endometrial Neoplasia

R. DON GAMBRELL, Jr

Attempts have been made for many years to associate hormones, particularly estrogens, with endometrial and breast cancer. Some of the early reports were based on a higher incidence of endometrial cancer in young women with the polycystic ovary syndrome[1]. Other studies associated adenocarcinoma of the endometrium in postmenopausal women with estrogen-secreting ovarian tumors[2]. Interest was renewed in the mid-1970s when several reports implicated estrogen replacement therapy for postmenopausal women with an increased risk of endometrial cancer[3-11]. Even the sequential oral contraceptives have been suggested as a cause of uterine malignancy in young women[12-16]. Whether estrogen is causally related to breast cancer has been debated for many years. However, recent reports have not been able to incriminate estrogen replacement therapy for postmenopausal women as a cause of breast cancer[17, 18]. It has been speculated for many years that oral contraceptives might cause breast cancer[19]. However, efforts to link birth control pills to mammary malignancy have been totally unsuccessful[20-25]. Because of the estrogen–cancer controversy that arose in 1975, retrospective data concerning estrogen use was obtained for that year at Wilford Hall USAF Medical Center and a prospective estrogen survey was initiated early in 1976. Information obtained from these continuing studies for the 4 years 1975–8 is reviewed in this report[26-34].

ROLE OF EXOGENOUS ESTROGENS IN ENDOMETRIAL CANCER

Studies were performed at Wilford Hall USAF Medical Center during 1975–8 to determine the incidence of endometrial cancer in postmenopausal women using various hormone therapies. During 10 872 patient-years of observation in women with intact uteri, 17 endometrial malignancies were diagnosed during these 4 years for an annual incidence rate of 1.6:1000 women (Table 28.1). Adenocarcinoma of the endometrium was detected in eight estrogen users during 2228 patient-years of observation for an incidence of 3.6:1000 women per year. Among the estrogen–progestogen users, three endometrial cancers were discovered; so during 5323 patient-years of observation the incidence of cancer was 0.6:1000. The difference between the estrogen users and the estrogen–progestogen users was statistically significant with $p < 0.01$. The next lowest incidence of endometrial carcinoma was found in the estrogen vaginal cream users, with one malignancy during 910 patient-years, for an incidence of 1.1:1000. No adenocarcinomas of the endometrium were observed in either the progestogen or androgen users. This included 182 postmenopausal women who by 1978 were being treated with monthly progestogen only because they had withdrawal bleeding each time they were challenged with the progestogen. Adenocarcinoma of the endometrium was diagnosed in five of the untreated women for an incidence of 3.5:1000 women per year. The difference between the estrogen–progestogen users (0.6:1000) was also significantly lower than the untreated women (2.5:1000) with $p < 0.05$.

Table 28.1 Incidence of endometrial cancer: 1975–1978

Therapy group	Patient-years of observation	Patients with cancer	Incidence
Estrogen users	2228	8	3.6:1000
Estrogen–progestogen users	5323	3	0.6:1000
Estrogen vaginal cream users	910	1	1.1:1000
Other hormones*	397	0	—
Untreated women	2014	5	2.5:1000
TOTAL	10 872	17	1.6:1000

* Progestogens – 354, androgens – 43

The time relationship of hormone therapy to endometrial cancer is demonstrated in Figure 28.1. Duration of estrogen therapy varied from 2½ to 12 years. All but one of these eight women (Case No. 7) were on cyclic estrogen therapy from the first to the 25th of the month. All three of the estrogen–progestogen users had used estrogens only for 2–7 years before the progestogen was added the last 1–2 years before diagnosis of endometrial cancer. The three estrogen–progestogen users were prescribed only 5–8 days of the progestogen each month. No adenocarcinomas of the endometrium have been found to date in women using at least 10 days of progestogen each month. In case number 9, adenomatous hyperplasia of the endometrium was diagnosed after 5 years of estrogen therapy, at age 56. A progestogen was added to the estrogen for only 5 days each month and 2 years later adeno-carcinoma of the endometrium was detected. This indicates that 5 days of progestogen is insufficient to halt the progression of hyperplasia to cancer. The mean age and standard deviation at diagnosis of endometrial cancer was 55.8 ± 6.36 years for the hormone users and 60.2 ± 7.02 years for the untreated women.

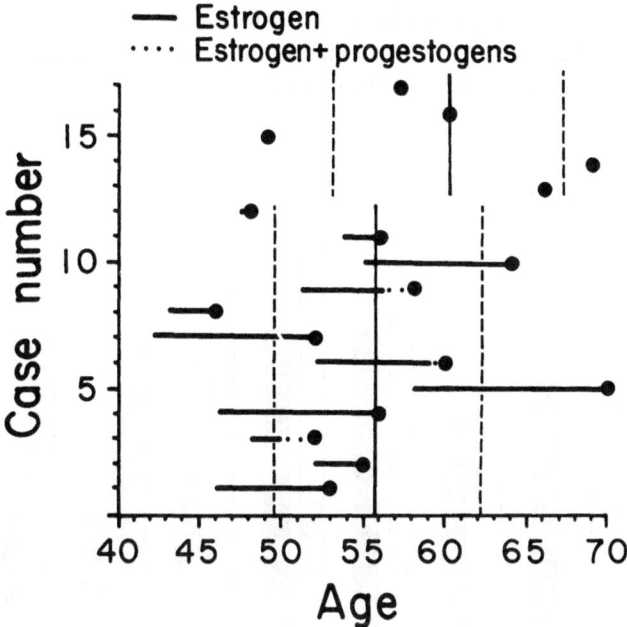

Figure 28.1 Age and duration of estrogen and estrogen–progestogen therapy in relation to diagnosis of endometrial cancer compared to age at diagnosis of cancer in untreated women

The number of endometrial cancers each year is compared to the number of estrogen-treated women in Figure 28.2. With ever-increasing estrogen usage, from approximately 1000 women in 1972 to 2300 women in 1975, the number of endometrial cancers each year stayed the same: six in 1972; five in 1973; and seven each during 1974 and 1975. However, with ever-increasing pro-gestogen usage among estrogen-treated women, from 10% in 1972 to 91.6% during 1978, the number of endometrial cancers decreased each year: seven in 1975; four in 1976; and three each during 1977 and 1978. In 1978, two of the adenocarcinomas of the endometrium occurred in untreated women and only one cancer was detected in an estrogen user.

It must now be accepted that estrogen therapy for postmenopausal women slightly increases the risk of endometrial cancer[3-11]. However, these retrospective case–control studies greatly magnified the risk because of the analytical methods used in these epidemiologic studies. To be told that estrogen therapy increased the risk of cancer 3.1- to 8.0-fold was alarming to both physicians and patients. To place this risk in a proper perspective, there is a three-fold to nine-fold increased risk of endometrial cancer in postmenopausal women who are from 25 to 50 pounds overweight[35]. The risk of dying from lung cancer is increased 17 times in those who smoke 20 cigarettes or more per day[36]. The lowest mortality for all gynecologic malignancies is from adenocarcinoma of the endometrium. At Wilford Hall USAF Medical Center, 116 of 121 patients are known to be living and well for 5 or more years after therapy for endometrial malignancy. Only one patient is known to have succumbed to her disease while the other four have been lost to follow-up.

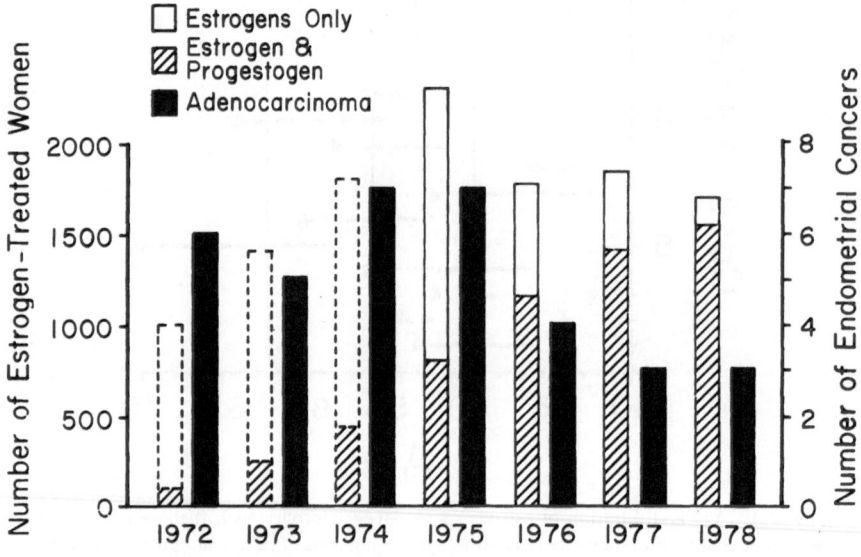

Figure 28.2 Number of estrogen and estrogen–progestogen users compared to number of endometrial cancers each year from 1972 to 1978

The greatest discrepancy in all these retrospective studies is the failure to give the natural incidence of endometrial cancer, thus greatly magnifying the extent of the problem. The probability for untreated postmenopausal women developing adenocarcinoma of the endometrium is 1 : 1000 per year[37]. Even if the risk from estrogen therapy is increased eight-fold[6], this would indicate that 992 of each 1000 estrogen-treated women do not develop endometrial cancer each year. In our study, although the risk of endometrial cancer was increased

1.4-fold, there was no statistically significant difference between the estrogen users (3.6:1000) and the untreated women (2.5:1000). Not only was the incidence of endometrial malignancy significantly lower in the estrogen-progestogen users (0.6:1000) than in the untreated women (2.5:1000) but it was also lower than that expected in the general population (1:1000)[37]. Other authors have confirmed that progestogens are protective against the carcinogenic effects of estrogen in postmenopausal women[38-40].

In one of the case–control studies of estrogens and adenocarcinoma of the endometrium, the authors used alternative analytic methods to eliminate the detection bias that arises from increased diagnostic attention received by women with uterine bleeding after estrogen use[9]. Utilizing conventional methods to choose cases and controls, the risk ratio was 12.0. However, when cases and controls consisted of patients who had undergone either dilatation and curettage or hysterectomy because of uterine bleeding, the risk ratio was only 1.7. Their study clearly demonstrated how detection bias was neglected in the other retrospective studies and concluded that the magnitude of the association between estrogens and endometrial cancer has been greatly overestimated. It is interesting to note that their risk ratio of 1.7 was very similar to what we observed (RR = 1.4) and thus is the only retrospective study that is in agreement with our prospective study.

ROLE OF ENDOGENOUS ESTROGENS IN ENDOMETRIAL CANCER

During the reproductive years, estradiol secretion by the ovary constitutes the major source of estrogen production. In addition, there is extraglandular production of estrone from circulating androstenedione, derived from both the adrenal glands and the ovaries in approximately equal quantities. When ovarian estradiol production diminishes at menopause, the principal source of estrogens is the peripheral conversion of adrenal androstenedione to estrone[41]. Two factors can increase endogenous estrogen production in postmenopausal women: (1) increased production rates of androstenedione, and (2) increased peripheral conversion of this hormone to estrone. Although the amount of androstenedione produced by normal postmenopausal women is one-half that of premenopausal women, the percentage conversion of androstenedione to estrone in postmenopausal women is almost one and one-half times that in premenopausal subjects[42]. The percentage conversion of androstenedione to estrone is increased by aging, obesity, liver disease and several other conditions[43]. Any excess production of androstenedione, such as from polycystic ovaries, hyperthecosis, or virilizing ovarian tumors, can lead to overproduction of estrone. These data provide some insight as to how the predisposing factors recognized for many years, such as obesity, liver disease and nulliparity, are related to endometrial cancer.

It has been demonstrated that excessive estrogen production more than 10 years after menopause may lead to endometrial neoplasia[41]. In eight obese women with a mean weight of 205 pounds and a mean age of 66.8 years, the production rate of androstenedione was similar to that of younger women, 1700 µg per 24 hours. However, the percentage conversion of androstenedione to estrone was much higher (4.4%) than in subjects with a normal weight, resulting in a total of 86 µg per 24 hours of estrone derived from androstenedione, compared to 40 µg of estrone produced daily by normal non-obese postmenopausal patients. Either adenomatous endometrial hyperplasia, with or without atypia, or cancer was found in seven of these eight women. There are certain changes in hormone production after menopause that may lead to increased endogenous estrogens, which may eventually result in either endometrial hyperplasia or neoplasia.

There are many numerators, such as infertility, nulliparity, obesity, liver disease and estrogen-secreting ovarian tumors; however, *the common denominator is the lack of progesterone*. It is recommended that these women at high risk for adenocarcinoma of the endometrium be identified and treated with either cyclic progestogens or by hysterectomy. Various tests can be performed, such as vaginal smears, endometrial biopsies, and either serum or urinary estrogen levels. The most important test is the *progestogen challenge test*. All postmenopausal women with an intact uterus should be given a trial of progestogen to see if withdrawal bleeding follows. The progestogen should be continued cyclically for 10 days each month for as long as withdrawal bleeding results. With this method, the majority of endometrial cancers can be prevented.

ROLE OF ORAL CONTRACEPTIVES IN ENDOMETRIAL CANCER

If progestogens are protective in postmenopausal women, both estrogen-treated and those with increased endogenous estrogens, why have so many cases of endometrial cancer been reported in oral contraceptive users? Including three cases from Wilford Hall USAF Medical Center, 42 adenocarcinomas of the endometrium have been associated with oral contraceptives, principally the sequential type[12–16,33]. In the largest study of patients collected by a tumor registry from all over the United States, the authors rightfully assigned eight patients to a separate group because of predisposing conditions such as polycystic ovaries, oral contraceptive therapy for abnormal bleeding, or a poor history[13]. In seven of these patients, the birth control pill use had discontinued for 8 months to 6 years before the diagnosis of malignancy. Contrary to the opinion of the authors, these patients should also receive separate consideration, since progestogens can only be effective in preventing malignancy while they are being used. In a prospective study of sequential birth control pill users, adenomatous hyperplasia was found in 15 of 111 (13.5%) consecutive endometrial biopsies during 8382 cycles of therapy[44]. No atypical hyperplasias or neoplasias were discovered and 96 (86.5%) of these patients had a perfectly normal endometrium.

Other factors are important in evaluating the sequential oral contraceptive–endometrial cancer controversy. The 100 μg of ethinyl estradiol in Oracon[R] (Mead-Johnson) is a considerably higher dosage than the 20 μg of this estrogen or the 0.625 mg of conjugated estrogens usually given to post-menopausal women. Dimethisterone is one of the weakest of all progestogens and is also the only progestogen that was not a 19-nor steroid like all the other progestogens in birth control pills available in the United States during the mid-1970s. Furthermore, the 5 days of dimethisterone therapy in this sequential pill was insufficient to produce complete endometrial shedding for some women, especially in view of the high dosage of estrogen present in that sequential oral contraceptive.

There are 10–13 million women in the United States taking oral contraceptives and most are under age 40[27, 28]. The annual incidence of endometrial malignancy in the United States is 21:100000 women of all ages[4, 5]. The incidence of endometrial cancer under age 40 is not greater than 1:100000 women per year[13]. If there are 10000000 women under age 40 in the United States using birth control pills and the incidence of endometrial malignancy is 1:100000 per year, the expected 100 cases per year is more than three times the number of cases reported during the past 3 years (Table 28.2). It has been suggested that the combined agents may be protective against and the sequential pills predispose toward endometrial cancer. A more logical conclusion is that the combination birth control pills are protective against developing adenocarcinoma of the endometrium while the sequential oral contraceptives afford less protection.

Table 28.2 Incidence of endometrial cancer in oral contraceptive users

	Under age 40	All ages
Oral contraceptive users in US	≤ 10000000	13000000
Incidence of endometrial cancer	≤ 1:100000	21:100000
Expected cancers in OC users (per year)	100	273*
Reported cancers in OC users (3 years)	28	42

* Based upon 10%, of endometrial cancers occurring before age 50 and few women taking oral contraceptives beyond age 50

ROLE OF EXOGENOUS ESTROGENS IN BREAST CANCER

A far more serious disorder than endometrial cancer is breast cancer, since it is the most frequent malignancy in females (26% of all cancers) and also the leading cause of death from cancer in women (20% of all female cancer deaths in the United States)[46]. There were approximately 90000 new cases of breast carcinoma in the United States during 1978 and 33800 women were expected to die that year from this tumor, which is ten times the number of deaths each year from uterine corpus cancer. The mortality rate from breast cancer of 23 : 100000 female population has not changed during the past 45 years, while death from uterine cancer has declined from 27 : 100000 in 1930 to 7 : 100000 in 1975. It has been speculated for many years that exogenous estrogens are causally related to breast cancer; however, two recent epidemiologic studies have failed to incriminate estrogen replacement therapy for postmenopausal women as a cause of breast cancer.[17, 18].

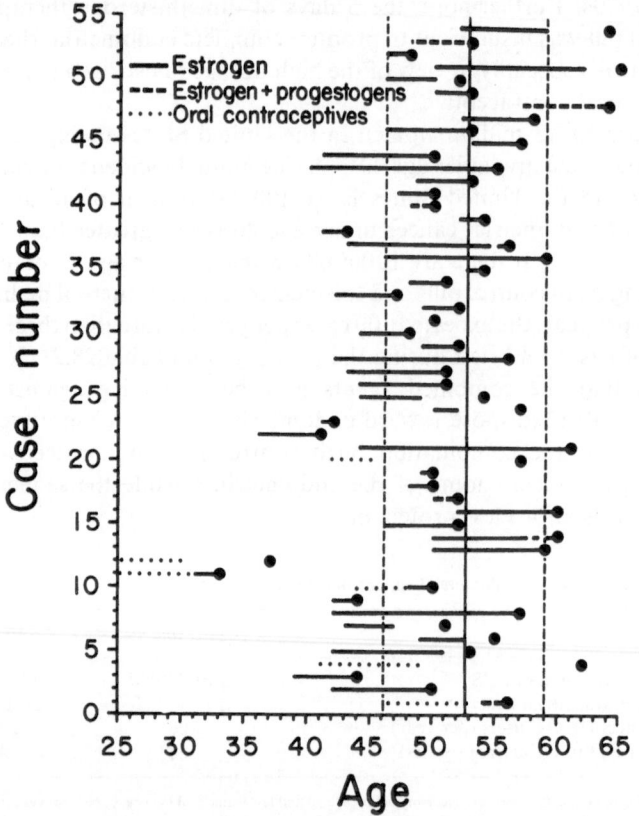

Figure 28.3   Age and duration of estrogen, estrogen–progestogen and oral contraceptive therapy in relation to age at diagnosis of breast cancer

As a part of the prospective study of estrogen usage among postmenopausal women at Wilford Hall USAF Medical Center, hormone use in patients with breast cancer from 1972 to 1978 was investigated. During these 7 years there were 295 cases of breast cancer identified from the tumor registry, including two males, 133 premenopausal females and 160 postmenopausal females. Figure 28.3 illustrates the time relationship of hormone therapy in 54 of the 56 postmenopausal women either using or giving a past history of hormone use when breast cancer was diagnosed. Excluded from the figure are two patients: one who received injectable medroxyprogesterone acetate for 2 years prior to detection of breast cancer and another patient who had used estrogen vaginal cream for 7 months prior to discovery of the malignancy. There were 35 women (21.9%) who were using estrogens when the breast cancer was diagnosed. Duration of treatment in this group varied from 5 months (Case No. 3) to 17 years (Case No. 21), with a mean of 5.7 years. Cases number 10 and 11

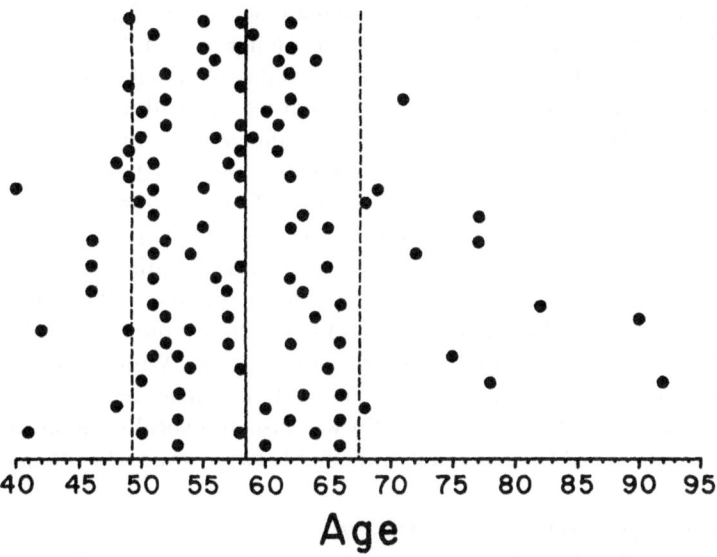

Figure 28.4 Age that breast cancer was diagnosed in 104 postmenopausal women never using hormones

had also used oral contraceptives for 4 and 6 years before estrogens were started. Another seven patients (4.4%) gave a past history of estrogen usage for 2 to 12 years (mean 6.1 years) before discontinuing therapy from 2 to 5 years (mean 3.7 years) before detection of cancer. Estrogens and progestogens were being used by nine women (5.6%) at diagnosis of breast malignancy. Cases number 17, 40, 48 and 53 had used both estrogens and progestogens for the 2–7 years before detection of cancer, while cases number 6, 14, 37 and 39 had used estrogens only for 3 to 11 years with the progestogen added the last 2 to 3 years before malignancy was diagnosed. Case number 1 used oral contraceptives for 8 years and then was treated with estrogens and progestogens for the last 2 years before discovery of breast cancer. There were three patients (Cases No. 4, 12, 20) who had used oral contraceptives for 3 to 8 years before breast cancer was discovered from 7 to 13 years later. The mean age at diagnosis of breast malignancy was 52.7 ± 6.52 years for these hormone users, including those patients with a past history of hormone use. Figure 28.4 illustrates the age at which the 104 untreated postmenopausal women (65%) developed breast cancer. The age in this group varied from 40 to 90 years, with a mean age of 58.4 ± 9.12 years.

During 1975–1978, data collected during the prospective postmenopausal estrogen survey made it possible to determine the incidence of breast cancer with various hormone therapies and compare these with the incidence in untreated women. There were 5263 registered patients followed for a total of 19 444 patient-years of observation (Table 28.3). During these 4 years there were 38 patients found to have breast malignancy, for an overall incidence of $1.9:1000$ women per year. This incidence is similar to the $1.9:1000$ females for ages 55–59 reported in the Third United States National Cancer Survey[45], since the mean age for our postmenopausal women with breast cancer was 56.5 years. There were 13 breast cancers in the group taking estrogens only during 9114 patient-years of observation for an annual incidence rate of $1.4:1000$ women. During 5424 patient-years of observation, there were nine breast cancers in the estrogen–progestogen users for an annual incidence of $1.7:1000$ women. With 14 breast cancers during 3168 patient-years of observation, the incidence in the untreated women was $4.4:1000$ women. The difference between the estrogen users ($1.4:1000$) and the untreated women ($4.4:1000$) was statistically significant with $p < 0.01$. With an incidence of $1.7:1000$ in the estrogen–progestogen users, the difference between this group and the untreated patients ($4.4:1000$) was also statistically significant with $p < 0.05$. There was no significant difference between any of the other groups.

Table 28.3   Incidence of breast cancer: 1975–1978

Therapy group	Patient-years of observation	Patients with cancer	Incidence
Estrogen users	9114	13	1.4:1000
Estrogen–progestogen users	5424	9	1.7:1000
Estrogen vaginal cream users	1287	1	0.8:1000
Other hormones*	451	1	2.2:1000
Untreated women	3168	14	4.4:1000
TOTAL	19 444	38	1.9:1000

* Progestogens – 388, androgens – 63

The short-term prognosis of breast cancer was better in the hormone users when compared to the non-users. To date, 32 of 157 patients from the total group (three were lost to follow-up) have already died, for a mortality rate of 20.4%. Among the hormone-treated women, including those with a past history of use, five out of 56 have died, for a mortality rate of 8.9%. In those women who had never used hormones, 27 of 101 have died, for a mortality rate of 26.7%. The difference between the hormone users and the untreated women was statistically significant with $p < 0.01$. Another study also found a lower mortality rate (decreased by 25%) in estrogen-treated women developing breast cancer[17]. Our study can only evaluate the short-term prognosis, since none of our patients have been followed for more than 7 years, most for considerably less. The better prognosis in hormone-treated women most likely reflects an earlier diagnosis, since these women are examined at least annually and are quickly subjected to breast biopsy when a mass is found.

ROLE OF ENDOGENOUS HORMONES IN BREAST CANCER

Breast cancer is a multifactorial disorder with genetic considerations, endocrine relationships, oncogenic factors, such as viruses, and environmental conditions, such as chemical carcinogens[47]. Lower values of androgen metabolites have been reported in patients with breast cancer who responded poorly to endocrine ablative procedures[48]. In women who eventually developed breast cancer, but at a time before the malignancy was evident, decreased urinary etiocholanolone was also found[49]. It has also been proposed that unopposed endogenous estrogens due to progesterone deficiency may provide a favorable setting for breast cancer[50]. However, no abnormalities in progesterone production have been reported, so this hypothesis needs confirmation. Most of the evidence linking prolactin to breast cancer is indirect by showing improvement from prolactin-suppressing drugs, such as L-dopa or bromocryptine in some patients with metastasis[51]. It has been suggested that there may be an association of thyroid hormone and breast cancer, especially since thyrotropin releasing hormone (TRH) can also increase prolactin levels[52]. An estriol hypothesis has been proposed from findings that women with breast cancer excreted less estriol than estradiol and estrone[53]. This hypothesis proposed that estriol impeded the action of estradiol and estrone at the cellular level. It is a paradox that some patients with metastatic carcinoma of the breast respond to endocrine ablative surgery while others may have remission with estrogen therapy. Two recent reviews conclude that despite many years of extensive investigation of endocrine factors, hormones, including androgens, estrogens, progesterone, prolactin and thyroid, have not been established as a cause of breast cancer[47, 52].

ROLE OF ORAL CONTRACEPTIVES IN BREAST CANCER

Over 10 000 000 women in the United States use oral contraceptives each year. Because of the uncertain role of sex steroids in breast cancer, speculation has arisen that any carcinogenic potential of birth control pills might not be detectable for 10 years or more. Of the 295 patients with breast cancer treated at Wilford Hall USAF Medical Center from 1972 through 1978, 133 occurred before menopause. There were 17 women (12.8%) who were using oral contraceptives at the time breast cancer was diagnosed and 23 additional patients (17.3%) gave a past history of birth control pill use. One other patient was taking medroxyprogesterone acetate for 7 days each month to regulate menstrual periods. However, 92 of these 133 women (69.2%) had never used hormones of any type. There were 31 patients with breast cancer during the 4 years from 1975 to 1978 in which oral contraceptive use could be estimated. A negative history of hormone usage was obtained in 18 of these 31 women (58.1%). There were 13 women in this group who either were using oral contraceptives when the breast cancer was detected or gave a past history of birth control pill use. In the 11 women who knew which oral contraceptive they had taken, there were eight different birth control pills that had been used. Duration of use varied from 3 months to 14 years and eight patients had discontinued use of birth control pills from 5 months to 15 years prior to detection of the breast cancer.

Table 28.4 Incidence of breast cancer in oral contraceptive users: 1975–1978

Oral contraceptive use	Patient-years of observation	Mean age (range)	Patients with cancer	Incidence
Current use	29 871	36.6 (35–39)	5	16.7
Use within 1 year	> 29 871	35.7 (31–39)	6	< 20.1
Any past history	> 29 871	38.8 (31–53)	13	< 43.5
Third National Cancer Survey		(35–39)		53.3

Estimation of oral contraceptive use from 1975 to 1978 was calculated from computerized pharmacy records and is based upon the number of birth control pills dispensed to patients. There were five women using oral contraceptives at the time the breast cancer was diagnosed during 29 871 patient-years of observation, for an annual incidence rate of 16.7 : 100 000 women (Table 28.4). One other patient had used a birth control pill until 5 months before detection of breast cancer. Including this patient, the incidence of breast cancer among oral contraceptive users was less than 20.1 : 100 000 women per year. Including all 13 women with a history of birth control pill use, the incidence of breast cancer was less than 43.5 : 100 000. All three of these incidence rates are lower than the 53.3 : 100 000 women, age range 35–39, of the Third National Cancer Survey of the United States[45]. This lower incidence of breast cancer in oral contraceptive users was statistically significant by the two-tail 'Student' t-test with $p < 0.05$. The short-term prognosis of breast cancer was better in the oral contraceptive users when compared to non-users. To date, 31 of the 133 premenopausal patients have died, for a mortality rate of 23.3%. Death has occurred in 30 of the 93 non-users (32.3%), compared to one of the 40 women (2.5%) either using oral contraceptives or giving a past history of use.

Epidemiologic studies indicate that oral contraceptives afford some protection from benign breast disease and there has been no evidence to associate birth control pills with an increased risk for carcinoma of the breast[20–25]. Some studies have not found an increased risk of breast cancer in oral contraceptive users while others observed lower rates of breast malignancy in those taking birth control pills[21–23, 54, 55]. None of these differences were statistically significant except one that observed a relative risk of 1.9 between 2 and 4 years of oral contraceptive use[22]. However, there was no risk $(RR = 1.0)$ between 4 and 6 years of use and the risk was not significantly increased $(RR = 1.3)$ with using birth control pills for more than 6 years. This study also found a significantly reduced risk of benign breast disease among oral contraceptive users $(RR = 0.8)$ which decreased further with longer duration of use $(RR = 0.2$ for more than 8 years taking birth control pills). In another study, none of the patients with breast cancer had used birth control pills for more than 3 years, yet 10% of the controls had used oral contraceptives longer than 5 years[21].

Benign breast diseases, such as fibrocystic disease and fibroadenomas, have been associated with an increased risk of breast cancer. All the epidemiologic studies have found a significantly decreased risk of fibrocystic and other benign breast diseases in oral contraceptive users[20–24]. It is logical then that birth control pills would afford some protection from breast cancer, since they reduce potentially precancerous conditions. The longer the duration of oral contraceptive use, the greater was the reduction in the incidence of fibrocystic disease of the breast[22, 24]. It is significant that only two of our patients with breast cancer had used birth control pills for longer than 5 years. Most studies list pregnancy, lactation and increased parity as potentially protective conditions for breast cancer[56]. Probably even more important than increasing parity is the age at which the woman had her first term child. Protection from breast cancer by early pregnancy is manifested at all ages, even among the older women[47]. Oral contraceptives, by simulating pregnancy, especially with long-term usage to simulate increasing parity, may exert a protective mechanism from subsequent carcinoma of the breast.

References

1. Speert, H. (1949). Cancer of the endometrium in young women. *Surg. Gynecol. Obstet.*, **88**, 332
2. Larson, J. A. (1954). Estrogen and endometrial carcinoma. *Obstet. Gynecol.*, **3**, 551
3. Quint, B. C. (1975). Changing patterns in endometrial adenocarcinoma. *Am. J. Obstet. Gynecol.*, **122**, 498
4. Smith, D. C., Prentice, R., Thompson, D. J. *et al.* (1975). Association of exogenous estrogen and endometrial carcinoma. *N. Engl. J. Med.*, **293**, 1164

5. Ziel, H. K. and Finkle, W. D. (1975). Increased risk of endometrial carcinoma among users of conjugated estrogens. *N. Engl. J. Med.*, **293**, 1167

6. Mack, T. M., Pike, M. C., Henderson, B. E. *et al.* (1976). Estrogens and endometrial cancer in a retirement community. *N. Engl. J. Med.*, **294**, 1262

7. Gray, L. A. Sr., Christopherson, W. M. and Hoover, R. N. (1977). Estrogens and endometrial carcinoma. *Obstet. Gynecol.*, **49**, 385

8. McDonald, T. W., Annegers, J. F., O'Fallow, W. M. *et al.* (1977). Exogenous estrogen and endometrial carcinoma: case-control and incidence study. *Am. J. Obstet. Gynecol.*, **127**, 572

9. Horwitz, R. I. and Feinstein, A. R. (1978). Alternative analytic methods for case-control studies of estrogens and endometrial cancer. *N. Engl. J. Med.*, **299**, 1089

10. Antunes, C. M. F., Stolley, P. D., Rosenshein, N. B. *et al.* (1979). Endometrial cancer and estrogen use. Report of a large case-control study. *N. Engl. J. Med.*, **300**, 9

11. Jick, H., Watkins, R. N., Hunter, J. R. *et al.* (1979). Replacement estrogens and endometrial cancer. *N. Engl. J. Med.*, **300**, 218

12. Lyon, F. A. (1975). The development of adenocarcinoma of the endometrium in young women receiving long-term sequential oral contraception. Report of four cases. *Am. J. Obstet. Gynecol.*, **123**, 299

13. Silverberg, S. G. and Makowski, E. L. (1975). Endometrial carcinoma in young women taking oral contraceptive agents. *Obstet. Gynecol.*, **46**, 503

14. Kelly, H. W., Miles, P. A., Buster, J. E. *et al.* (1976). Adenocarcinoma of the endometrium in women taking sequential oral contraceptives. *Obstet. Gynecol.*, **47**, 200

15. Cohen, C. J. and Deppe, G. (1977). Endometrial carcinoma and oral contraceptive agents. *Obstet. Gynecol.*, **49**, 390

16. Reeves, K. O. and Kaufman, R. H. (1977). Exogenous estrogens and endometrial carcinoma. *J. Reprod. Med.*, **18**, 297

17. Burch, J. C., Byrd, B. F. and Vaughn, W. K. (1976). Results of estrogen treatment in one thousand hysterectomized women for 14318 years. In P. A. van Keep, R. B. Greenblatt, M. Albeaux-Fernet (eds.). *Consensus on Menopause Research*, pp. 164-169. (Lancaster: MTP Press)

18. Hoover, R., Gray, L. A. Sr., Cole, P. *et al.* (1976). Menopausal estrogens and breast cancer. *N. Engl. J. Med.*, **295**, 401

19. Hertz, R. (1969). The problem of possible effects of oral contraceptives on cancer of the breast. *Cancer*, **24**, 1140

20. Arthes, F. G., Sartwell, P. E. and Lewison, E. P. (1971). The pill, estrogen, and the breast. Epidemiologic aspects. *Cancer*, **28**, 1391

21. Boston Collaborative Drug Surveillance Program (1973). Oral contraceptives and venous thromboembolic disease surgically confirmed, gall-bladder disease and breast tumours. *Lancet*, **1**, 1399

22. Fasal, E. and Pattenbarger, R. S. (1975). Oral contraceptives as related to cancer and benign lesions of the breast. *J. Natl. Cancer Inst.*, **55**, 757

23. Vessey, M. P., Doll, R. and Jones, K. (1975). Oral contraceptives and breast cancer. *Lancet*, **1**, 941

24. Ory, H., Cole, P., MacMahon, B. and Hoover, R. (1976). Oral contraceptives and reduced risk of benign breast disease. *N. Engl. J. Med.*, **294**, 419

25. Kretzschmar, R. M. (1978). Oral contraceptives and cancer. *Cancer*, **28**, 118

26. Gambrell, R. D. Jr. (1976). Estrogens, progestogens, and endometrial cancer. In P. A. van Keep, R. B. Greenblatt and M. Albeaux-Fernet (eds.). *Consensus on Menopause Research*, pp. 152-163. (Lancaster: MTP Press)

27. Gambrell, R. D. Jr. (1977). Postmenopausal bleeding. *Clin. Obstet. Gynaecol.*, **4**, 129

28. Gambrell, R. D. Jr. (1977). Estrogens, progestogens and endometrial cancer. *J. Reprod. Med.*, **18**, 301

29. Gambrell, R. D. Jr. (1978). The prevention of endometrial cancer in postmenopausal women with progestogens. *Maturitas*, 1, 107

30. Gambrell, R. D. Jr. (1978). The role of hormones in endometrial cancer. *South. Med. J.*, 71, 1280

31. Gambrell, R. D. Jr., Castaneda, T. A. and Ricci, C. A. (1978). Management of postmenopausal bleeding to prevent endometrial cancer. *Maturitas*, 1, 99

32. Gambrell, R. D. Jr., Massey, F. M., Castaneda, T. A. *et al.* (1979). Breast cancer and oral contraceptive therapy in premenopausal women. *J. Reprod. Med.* (In press)

33. Gambrell, R. D. Jr., Massey, F. M., Castaneda, T. A. *et al.* (1979). The reduction of endometrial cancer in postmenopausal women with progestogens. *J. Am. Geriatr. Soc.* (In press)

34. Gambrell, R. D. Jr., Massey, F. M., Castaneda, T. A. *et al.* (1979). Estrogen therapy and breast cancer in postmenopausal women. *Obstet. Gynecol.* (In press)

35. Gusberg, S. B. (1976). The individual at high-risk for endometrial carcinoma. *Am. J. Obstet. Gynecol.*, 126, 535

36. Ryan, K. J. (1975). Cancer risk and estrogen use in the menopause. *N. Engl. J. Med.*, 293, 1199

37. Weiss, N. S. (1975). Risks and benefit of estrogen use. *N. Engl. J. Med.*, 293, 1200

38. Nachtigall, L. E., Nachtigall, R. H., Nachtigall, R. B. *et al.* (1976). Letter: Estrogens and endometrial carcinoma. *N. Engl. J. Med.*, 294, 848

39. Whitehead, M. I. (1978). The effects of oestrogens and progestogens on the postmenopausal endometrium. *Maturitas*, 1, 87

40. Hammond, C. B., Jelovsek, F. R., Lee, K. L. *et al.* (1979). Effects of long-term estrogen replacement therapy. II. Neoplasia. *Am. J. Obstet. Gynecol.*, 133, 537

41. Siiteri, P. K. and McDonald, P. C. (1973). Role of extraglandular estrogen in human endocrinology. In R. O. Greep and E. B. Astwood (eds.). *Handbook of Physiology*, Vol. II, part I, pp. 615–629. (American Physiology Society)

42. Hemsell, D. L., Grodin, J. M., Brenner, P. F. *et al.* (1974). Plasma precursors of estrogen. II. Correlation of the extent of conversion of plasma androstenedione to estrone with age. *J. Clin. Endocrinol. Metab.*, 38, 467

43. Shoemaker, E. S., Forney, J. P. and MacDonald, P. C. (1977). Estrogen treatment of postmenopausal women. Benefits and risks. *J. Am. Med. Assoc.*, 238, 1524

44. Kreuter, A. Jr., Johnson, D. and Williamson, H. O. (1976). Histology of the endometrium in long-term use of a sequential oral contraceptive. *Fertil. Steril.*, 27, 905

45. Cutler, S. J. and Young, J. L. Jr. (1975). Third National Cancer Survey: Incidence data. *Natl. Cancer Inst. Monogr.*, 41

46. Silverberg, E. (1978). Cancer statistics. *Cancer*, 28, 17

47. Vorherr, H. and Messer, R. H. (1978). Breast cancer: potentially predisposing and protecting factors. *Am. J. Obstet. Gynecol.*, 130, 335

48. Bulbrook, R. D., Greenwood, F. C. and Hayward, J. L. (1960). Selection of breast cancer patients for adrenalectomy or hypophysectomy by determinations of 17-hydroxy-corticosteroids and aetiocholanolone. *Lancet*, 2, 1154

49. Bulbrook, R. D. and Hayward, J. L. (1967). Abnormal steroid excretion and subsequent breast cancer. A prospective study in the Island of Guernsey. *Lancet*, 2, 519

50. Sherman, B. M. and Korenman, S. C. (1974). Inadequate corpus luteum function: a pathophysiological interpretation of human breast cancer epidemiology. *Cancer*, 33, 1306

51. Dickey, R. P. and Minton, J. P. (1972). L-dopa effect on prolactin, follicle-stimulating hormone, and luteinizing hormone in women with advanced breast cancer: a preliminary report. *Am. J. Obstet. Gynecol.*, 114, 267

52. Kirschner, M. A. (1977). The role of hormones in the etiology of human breast cancer. *Cancer*, 39, 2716

53. Lemon, H. M., Wotiz, H. H., Parsons, I. *et al.* (1966). Reduced estriol secretion in patients with breast cancer prior to endocrine therapy. *J. Am. Med. Assoc.*, 196, 112

54. Keifer, W. S. and Scott, J. C. (1975). A clinical appraisal of patients following long-term contraception. *Am. J. Obstet. Gynecol.*, **122**, 446
55. Wynder, E. L., MacCormack, F. A. and Stellman, S. D. (1978). The epidemiology of breast cancer in 785 United States Caucasian women. *Cancer*, **41**, 2341
56. MacMahon, B., Cole, P. and Brown, J. (1973). Etiology of human breast cancer: a review. *J. Natl. Cancer Inst.*, **50**, 21

Discussion

The following is an abbreviated transcript of some of the most relevant parts of the discussions which took place throughout the symposium.

SECTION I: DISCUSSION TO CHAPTERS 1-5

P. G. Crosignani (Moderator), R. Deghenghi, J. Fishman, C. Orlandi, P. Paoletti, A. E. Schindler and M. I. Whitehead

Question: Dr Whitehead has mentioned two progestogens which were added sequentially to the oestrogen therapy: norethisterone and medroxyprogesterone acetate. Have the two been compared statistically? Was one of them used predominantly or were they prescribed equally?

Whitehead: About 80% of the patients were receiving norethisterone. The number receiving medroxyprogesterone acetate is too small for any valid statistical conclusions to be drawn as to comparative effects. There is further data on this in Chapter 28.

Question: Were the same changes observed with other progestogens, such as norgestrel, as with norethisterone?

Whitehead: We have not looked at other progestins. However, in a dose-dependency study we have a series of 15 patients, all of them taking Premarin 1.25 mg daily continuously and differing doses of norethisterone for 7 days each calendar month. We have obtained biopsies on Day 6. We have found that we can reduce the dose of norethisterone to 1 mg daily and still see nuclear channel systems – a marker of progestogen activity.

Question: What is the biological basis for the suggestion that certain estrone:estradiol ratios are favorable but others are not.

Schindler: Having read Dr Fishman's chapter (5), we have learned that it may be necessary to revise my simple statement which concerned only the three main estrogens.

Without it being possible to measure the other metabolites, from a biological standpoint it is of interest that there is a certain amount of estradiol working in the cell. If a compound such as estrone is administered and it does not change into estradiol, then one would expect to see less biological effect. That is why I said that to get a favorable ratio with Premarin, for instance, is to get an increase of estradiol. The estrone sulfate

305

in the preparation converts to estradiol and produces the favorable biological situation – something that is not the case when free estrone is used. When free estrone is given, the ratio can be as high as 4.0, and from my point of view that would not be as favorable.

Deghenghi: Dr Schindler has shown conclusively that the conjugated estrogens, present in Premarin or Presomen, are not superimposable on a similar preparation including estrone sulfate, and this in spite of the fact that conjugated estrogens contain 50% estrone sulfate.

In my view this can be explained in one of two ways. Either the pharmaceutical preparation given is responsible for the difference in the metabolism, or the additional estrogens present in conjugated estrogens of equine origin are responsible for the modulation of the metabolism of estrone sulfate present in Premarin.

Question: Are the conclusions of chapter 5 valid? Dr Fishman has compared eight cancers of the male breast, a rare disease, with five healthy men. Is good health a rarity in his country?

Fishman: Healthy men who are old are a rarity in any country. 'Healthy' does not necessarily mean in complete and perfect health. For these studies we have to identify individuals who are generally healthy and who have no defects of liver metabolism or of their kidneys, or many other diseases. Individuals of this type are not too easy to find, and they are even more difficult to find when we bear in mind that we want them to sit still for the study, which takes about 3 days. The number 'five' is then quite justifiable.

I was rather impressed that we were able to get eight cancers of the male breast, which is, I would agree, a rare disease. The same considerations were found in women with breast cancer, although not quite to the same extent. The women with breast cancer did metabolize estradiol more towards estriol than the women without the disease. It is not so much that the findings are positive, but they are important because they negate the previous studies that have been published over and over again, suggesting that high estriol is protective against breast cancer, and that women with breast cancer have low estriol levels. These studies are important because they show that the opposite is true.

The issue is one that has come up again and again, and is still very prevalent throughout the world – that estriol is a safe estrogen. Estriol behaves almost exactly as estradiol. It is a potent estrogen, and it too will induce cancer under the same test conditions as estradiol.

I think it is important to remind everyone that estriol is not a safe estrogen.

Question: Could Dr Whitehead give more information on the definition of hyperplasia? How often, and how long, after stopping estrogen therapy was the hyperplasia reversible? In cervical cancer, some dysplasias are reversible. Could Dr Whitehead comment on similarities in endometrium?

Whitehead: Our pathologists' definition of cystic hyperplasia is predominantly cystic change without really marked atypical changes in the glands. Atypical hyperplasia has cellular atypia, glandular reduplication and back-to-back formation.

I have presented our data on the ability of sequential therapy to reverse endometrial hyperplasia. We observed a return to normal endometrium in 19 of 20 patients so treated and the one patient in whom the desired effect was not achieved had atypical hyperplasia. In addition, we investigated whether estrogen-induced hyperplasia persisted after exogenous estrogen therapy was withdrawn in half a dozen patients. Biopsies were obtained at 2-monthly intervals after stopping therapy and we found that atypical hyperplasia first reverted to cystic hyperplasia and eventually to normal endometrium. This transition usually occurred over a period of 6 months.

On the question of the importance of hyperplasia *vis-a-vis* the risk of subsequently developing endometrial carcinoma, I personally am not desperately worried about cystic hyperplasia. Statements to the effect that any woman given unopposed estrogens for a period of time will develop cystic hyperplasia are often made but our data do not support this concept. Some of our patients have had very high doses of estrogens for very long periods of time and have a completely atrophic endometrium. There is enormous interpatient variation in end-organ response.

I suspect that patients with cystic hyperplasia have endometrium which is slightly more sensitive to estrogens than those who have atrophic endometrium. We have previously presented evidence (King, R. J. B., Whitehead, M. I., Campbell, S. and Minardi, Jane (1979), *Cancer Res.*, **39**, 1094) that biochemically atypical hyperplasia demonstrates increased end-organ sensitivity to estrogen. For this reason I believe that atypical hyperplasia is a much more worrying condition and clinically cannot be detected from the pattern of vaginal bleeding.

Question: Do the catechol estrogens compete for the catecholamine receptors in a similar fashion to their capacity to be metabolized by transferase (COMT) or to inhibit tyrosine hydroxylase?

Fishman: The answer is rather a confusing one. They do not compete normally for the catecholamine receptors. However, 2-hydroxy-estradiol does compete for the pituitary dopamine receptor and will induce prolactin release. It is the only one that does. Whether that is the mechanism of action we do not know at this stage.

Question: Can progestogens eliminate hot flushes through hypophyseal gonadotropin inhibition?

Fishman: Possibly. Nevertheless, the mechanisms by which the progestogens and the catechol estrogens work are probably quite different in that one will work at the hypothalamic levels while the other presumably works at the pituitary.

Whitehead: I would like to comment on the 'safety' of estriol with regard to endometrium. We have given patients estriol succinate and found using 2 mg or 4 mg daily that although endometrial proliferation was minimal these doses did not control vasomotor symptoms. To relieve very bad hot flushes, perhaps 20 a day and three each night, we had to give 10 mg daily of estriol succinate and at these doses we observed marked endometrial proliferation after only 3 months' therapy.

SECTION II: DISCUSSION TO CHAPTERS 6–11

F. Gasparri (Moderator), P. Boemi, L. de Cecco, M. Maneschi, P. Smith, J. M. Wenderlein, K. Wood, L. Zichella

Wood: I would comment that the short trial that I described in Chapter 6 incorporated measurements of plasma-free tryptophan. We found that when the patients were on the estrogen cycle rather than the placebo cycle, their plasma-free tryptophans increased. More tryptophan entering the brain means more 5HT is formed, and this may increase the wellbeing of the patients.

Estrogens would therefore seem to have an effect on both noradrenergic and serotonergic mechanisms in depressed patients.

Question: Is prophylactic treatment for urinary dystrophy repeatable as needed?

Smith: Yes, it can be repeated. Again it is on a somewhat empirical basis. We wait for a period of approximately 3 months following completion of treatment, i.e. 6 months from starting the original therapy, and if the symptoms recur, we give another 3 months. Whether we should give it for longer is difficult to say. In certain cases we have continued treatment in individual patients for as much as 2 years, with very satisfactory results.

As regards prophylaxis, it is a very difficult question. I am not in a position to answer it today because I have insufficient information.

In summary, a 3-month course appears to be effective for the majority of patients, but where symptoms persist a urethral dilatation is indicated, and where symptoms recur at regular intervals, prolonged hormone therapy may be required.

Campbell: Let me reply to the question of how long do we continue treatment and are we certain that we shall not cause more serious long-term consequences by giving estrogen treatment – which is a very serious question and one to which we must devote all our attention.

I believe that I have demonstrated that there is a dramatic and clearcut improvement in symptomatology and we shall therefore need to show definite and serious side-effects before we can say that the treatment should not be given and that it should not continue to be given. That is why I raised the point. We need to investigate whether there is any difference between the effect of natural estrogens and synthetic estrogens on the metabolism of the woman. There is little doubt that synthetic estrogens will cause serious side-effects, especially in high-risk patients, obese patients, women who smoke, etc. The same risks of myocardial infarction, venous thrombosis and thromboembolism have not been demonstrated with natural estrogens. Of course, not as many women have taken natural estrogens as synthetic estrogens as contained in the pill, yet I still believe that most of the evidence we have so far has shown that the effects on plasma lipids and the effects on the clotting factors, e.g. antithrombin-3, are not as severe as the effects of synthetic estrogens.

There is the further question of whether we are looking at equivalent dosages of the two types of estrogen, synthetic and natural, but I think that the evidence is still quite strong and that the natural estrogens have a less profound effect on these metabolic features. I am quite hopeful that in the long term there will not be these serious effects.

I accept these risks. I accept the evidence and I think that there is an increased risk, which is why we have to use progestogens. But I believe that progestogens can protect, given for the right length of time each month, and in the right dosage.

Question: What is the real effect of placebo treatment in comparison to estrogen therapy?

Campbell: Because a patient has a placebo response, that does not mean that she will not get a greater response from Premarin or any natural estrogen. Just because there is a placebo response, it does not mean that she should not get estrogen. But, there are some women in whom it is not possible to distinguish any difference between their response on placebo and their response to estrogen. In such patients I would regard it as not worthwhile pursuing estrogen treatment. There are other patients who benefit from estrogen therapy.

Question: How should progestogen be prescribed?

Campbell: We administer it in a sequential fashion to cause a shedding of the endometrium. That is one of the principal modes of its protective action. But there is little doubt that it will reduce the amount of cytosol estrogen receptor, thus preventing estrogen getting into the cell. It also affects the estradiol dehydrogenase levels and this subject is covered in Chapter 21.

Question: What are the indications for treating patients suffering from severe depression with estrogen?

Wenderlein: It is important to find out whether estrogen therapy removes the depression. If that is not successful, the patient should be referred to a specialist, a psychiatrist. Most such patients had depressions before their menopauses – psychoses – and such are not the province of the gynecologist.

Question: How long can long-term therapy last?

Campbell: Where my own patients are concerned, we have been treating patients for 7 or 8 years. Some have discontinued treatment and are very happy to discontinue treatment, and some have continued for as long as 7 or 8 years. All that I can do is to review the situation every year in relation to possible complications and evidence, and I would obviously alter my treatment accordingly. We cannot make didactic statements on that, but we must continue to monitor these patients very closely in all aspects.

Question: Is it advisable to carry out curettage on a yearly basis, to monitor long-term estrogen treatment?

Campbell: We do perform curettage on all our patients on a 6-monthly or yearly basis depending on the particular regimen that the patient is on. We do it by Vabra curettage as an outpatient, and in over 80% of patients on estrogen therapy this can be performed as an outpatient procedure, so that there is no need to admit the patient into hospital.

Until we can prove that we have a regime that is absolutely safe, and Mr Studd seems to be confident that 13 days of progestogen each month is absolutely safe, I believe that even patients on a sequential regime should have the procedure. When we have a regime that is proven to be safe we can perhaps discontinue it. However, 13 days of progestogen to a large extent will nullify the beneficial effects of the estrogen. There is no doubt that women do not like that amount of progestogen.

I think we shall have to play around with different doses of progestogen to find a shorter course that will protect the endometrium.

Question: Is atypical hyperplasia due to estrogen therapy reversible with progestogen treatment?

Campbell: The question probably relates to estrogen-induced hyperplasia. We always give these patients progestogens if they have been on cyclical unopposed estrogens, and we have been able to reverse almost all of these hyperplasias. There have been a few patients on 1 week of progestogen each month which have not reversed, but the vast majority have been reversed.

Of course, if the hyperplasia is not reversed with a prolonged course of progestogens, then the patients does require hysterectomy.

One point on the rise of endometrial cancer, particularly in the USA : I agree that the rate of endometrial cancer has risen, even if we allow for the fact that pathologists may be over-diagnosing for protection. But the number of deaths from such cancers has fallen. If there is an increase in endometrial cancer from estrogen, it seems to be a very benign form, usually stage one lesions which are usually treatable, and because these patients are being monitored very carefully they are dealt with quickly and the death rate is falling.

SECTION III: DISCUSSION TO CHAPTERS 12–18

A. Onnis (Moderator), C. Andreoli, G. B. Candiani, G. Gordan, P. Klotz, R. Lindsay, G. Montanari, N. Pasetto and J. Studd

Question: How well do women tolerate 13 days of progestogen?

Studd: In Chapter 13 I have discussed the protective effect of progestogen. It is true that some women have difficulty in tolerating 13 days of 5 mg norethisterone because this does produce breast discomfort, depression, irritability, and the same sort of symptoms which cause younger women to complain in the premenstrual syndrome. The symptoms are very similar to the symptoms of premenstrual tension.

Our combined therapy is a compromise between 5 days of progestogen, to which very few patients will object, and 13 days, when about half the women will have fairly unpleasant symptoms of breast discomfort. But it will protect the endometrium.

We must find some progestogen or progesterone which will not give rise to these worrying and symptomatic side-effects so that we can, with the combination therapy, maximize the benefits of estrogen therapy and minimize the risks of endometrial carcinoma, and yet at the same time not do away with that feeling of wellbeing that women get with estrogen alone.

Question: What about using 10 mg progestin for 5 days instead of 5 mg for 13 days?

Studd: I believe that the usefulness of progestogen is duration-dependent rather than dose-dependent. Although I did not mention it in my chapter, the protective effect of 13 days of norethisterone was in doses of 1.25–2.5 mg. It was a smaller total dose causing fewer side-effects, but used over a longer period of time and therefore protective.

My experience is that 10 mg norethisterone does produce more side-effects and if used for 5 days will not protect the endometrium.

Question: What is the incidence of physical inactivity of women in the pathogenesis of osteoporosis?

Gordan: The question of inactivity is an important one. The osteoporosis of disuse is a very serious disease in women who have been immobilized for a long time because they have been put in a cast or because they have a paralysis, or perhaps because they have had a paraplegia. There is no relationship between the osteoporosis of inactivity and the osteoporosis of estrogen deficiency. They have very different kinetics. They look different on X-rays and they have very different chemistry. For example, in inactivity one finds an immediate rise in the alkaline phosphatase which gradually subsides, but one does not find this in postmenopausal osteoporosis. Actually, Dr Picchi and I took activity histories in our osteoporotic women and found that they had been remarkably vigorous until painful fractures slowed them down.

Question: What limits are there for estrogen therapy in obese menopausal women, and what is the alternative for such women?

Pasetto: An obese woman is a patient at risk because of the several complications of estrogen treatment. One possibility of doing away with this risk is to administer the estrogen in low doses. Such patients maintain greater quantities of estrone in their bodies as compared to other women.

We should be precise as to what we mean by low-dose treatment. Until quite recently certain dose levels, now thought to be high, were thought to be low.

As to the other alternative, it could be a progestogen/estrogen combination treatment with low doses.

Question: What is the influence of menopausal estrogen therapy on the incidence of myocardial infarction?

Pasetto: On the basis of the statistical surveys available, it seems as though this incidence remains the same, although according to some of the surveys incidence might even be reduced with low doses. There is no consensus here. But there is consensus on the fact that low dosage does not produce any variations in the age-dependent physiological pattern.

Question: It is suggested that the change of estrogen schedule to weekdays on and weekends off therapy, rather than the traditional 3 weeks on and 1 week off, is more beneficial, preventing the estrogen letdown that occurs during the week off the treatment and the first days of resuming treatment until the estrogen is recompensated.

Studd: Where unopposed estrogens are given cyclically, patients do usually have their symptoms return in the 7 tablet-free days. I know that the weekdays on weekends off is recommended by some people. I have used it occasionally, but I have not enough patients to give any information on the rate of hyperplasia. It is certainly convenient, but what we want to know is the percentage risk of hyperplasia in patients having unopposed estrogen even with this regimen.

Gordan: Five days on and 2 days off is not cyclic therapy. In 2 days the endometrium will not reverse at all. Five days on and 2 days off is continuous estrogen therapy.

Lindsay: I should like to return to the question of side-effects in those patients who were taking 12 mg estriol per day. In Chapter 17 I commented on the fact that there were significant menopausal symptoms in the group of patients taking these fairly large doses of estriol. In those patients who maintained that they were happy to take 8–12 mg/day, after 1 year we began to see evidence of some endometrial hypertrophy. However, we did not really see anything in the way of symptomatic side-effects.

It is true that 12 mg of estriol as the hemi-succinate is not effective in halting osteoporosis in postmenopausal women (*Maturitas* (1979), **1**, 279). Additionally, in our study approximately 25% of women came off the end of the trial complaining that 12 mg of estriol hemi-succinate was not sufficient to control their symptoms. Most of them complained of symptoms nocturnally, I suspect due to the short biological halflife of the compound. In that study the median dose required for control of symptoms was 8 mg/day, and all those patients who required more than 12 mg were adequately controlled on either 1.25 mg of Premarin or 2 mg of estradiol valerate.

Gordan: There are a few women who develop endometrial hyperplasia and breakthrough bleeding even with small doses of estrogen. Not all of these women in our study could be controlled with the intramuscular progestins then available. In view of the anxiety produced by breakthrough bleeding and the fact that estrogen-induced hyperplasia can closely resemble an early carcinoma, we now strongly recommend adding a progestational agent for 10–13 days of each treatment cycle of estrogen. We did not include a progestational agent in our long-term treatment study of osteoporosis because, in 1948 when I began this study, there were no good oral progestins available. Now we have a number of excellent agents so if I were to start a similar study today I would add a progestational agent for the last 10–13 days of each 21–25-day estrogen cycle.

I am very pleased to have Dr Lindsay's data and other data which show that a progestational agent alone, or a progestational agent in combination with estrogen, is beneficial to bone.

Question: What dosage of estrogen did Professor Gordan use for the prevention of osteoporosis, and what did he use following its onset, and for what length of time?

Did these high doses of estrogen bring about untoward side-effects since some of them are transformed into testosterone?

Gordan: The published doses of estrogen found effective in preventing postmenopausal or post-oophorectomy bone loss are mestranol 20 μg daily (Lindsay *et al.*); ethynyl estradiol 20 μg daily, *or* Premarin 0.6 mg with methyltestosterone 5 mg daily (Recker *et al.*).

There are unpublished data, from Judd in Los Angeles, that 10 μg ethynyl estradiol or 0.3 mg Premarin will prevent the rise in the urinary calcium to creatinine ratio in castrated women. These are very low doses that do not affect the maturation index in the vagina, do not cause endometrial hyperplasia, do not produce bleeding, and have not been incriminated in causing cancer.

We are now conducting a prospective study measuring bone mass by four methods to determine the lowest prophylactic dose of estrogens. Our women are receiving Premarin in doses of 0.15, 0.3, 0.45 and 0.6 mg daily; a fifth group receives an inert placebo. From the preliminary data, without breaking the double-blind, it seems to be clear that women who are taking any dose of estrogen are protected and actually show an increase in bone mass after oophorectomy.

As I indicated previously, estrogen prophylaxis must be continued for life to avoid further bone loss and fractures. The treatment dose of estrogen for established osteoporosis is two to four times as great as that needed for prevention.

I know of no evidence that estrogens increase androgenic activity, have never seen any such effects clinically and, in fact, have noted considerable published and personal evidence that all estrogens are anti-androgenic in women after the menopause or oophorectomy.

Question: Has Dr Studd always performed preventive biopsy of the endometrium in those subjects that he has treated? Secondly, has cyclic estrogen with progestogen treatment brought about pseudo-menstruation?

Studd: Do we always do a curettage on our patients? We like to have a routine of doing a curettage every year. I do not normally do a pretreatment curettage unless there has been some menstrual irregularity, although I will always do a curettage if the patient comes to me having had any postmenopausal estrogen therapy from elsewhere, so that I know my starting point.

That is my practice at the moment, but I am sure it will change once we have established the risk of hyperplasia in the different treatment regimens. At the moment I am collecting material, so every patient has her curettage every year, but my prediction will be that those patients who have unopposed cyclic estrogens will need a curettage every year. Patients who have irregular bleeding will have a curettage there and then, and patients who are taking 10 or 13 days of progestogen will not need a curettage, although perhaps every 5 years would be a worthwhile compromise.

I feel that if this treatment that we are giving is so dangerous that we have to expose a woman to a curettage every year, we should not be doing it. There must be a compromise where we can give a combination of estrogen and progestogen, abolish any risk of hyperplasia and cancer, and the patient will then not need a curettage.

The second question was whether the patients have a bleed with the cyclical therapy. Patients having unopposed cyclical therapy for 3 weeks out of 4 will usually have a withdrawal bleed, although not always. If they have a very low dose of Premarin, such as 0.625 mg or 0.3 mg, then about 30% will have a bleed. Patients having progestogen will all, 98%, have withdrawal bleeding.

Question: During therapy, on the days when progestogen is added, does the climacteric symptomatology re-appear or not? If it does re-appear, is it superimposed on the symptoms of 7-day suspension?

Secondly, when is it advisable to implant estrogens?

Pasetto: I would agree that during the short period when progestogen is added to estrogen therapy there are no changes in menopausal symptoms. On the contrary, in the period between the two cycles, although it is difficult to quantify the percentage, there is frequently a reappearance of some menopausal symptoms.

As to implants, I have no experience and I do not know of any experience with implants in Italy.

SECTION IV: DISCUSSION TO CHAPTERS 19–28 AND ROUND TABLE DISCUSSION

A. Bompiani (Moderator), J. Ambrus, K. Bland, J. B. Buchanan, J. Fishman, R. I. Horwitz, R. D. Gambrell, A. Onnis, N. Pasetto, S. Robboy, J. Studd, R. Vokaer, W. Völker and M. Whitehead

Question: Speaking of breast symptomatology, pain is the reaction to a replacement estrogen therapy in oophorectomized women. Would this have any pathological meaning after a few months, and what kind of therapy should be instituted?

Bland: The question is: should patients who develop symptoms on estrogens, particularly those who become symptomatic in the classification we designated as those with mastalgia – meaning they have pain because of swelling, engorgement of the breast, lobular increase – should those patients be removed from estrogens to evaluate them?

In fact, those patients whom we considered symptomatic we evaluated and submitted to biopsies – 90 patients out of 129 had biopsies and they represent 70% of the entire group in whom we biopsied. The group that were biopsied came up with a total incidence of cancer which was approximately 10% of the entire group that was diagnosed. In other words, in 10% of patients whom we thought had a lesion worthy of biopsy, it proved to be carcinoma.

Our current measures and what we suggest are that patients who develop lesions, that is engorgement, pain, mass or thickening, should probably be withdrawn from estrogen replacement and have biopsies done immediately. Dr Völker may hold a different opinion.

Völker: We take it as symptoms of an overdose and reduce the dose. This is also the recommendation of the Drug Commission of the German Medical Society.

Question: Rudali has reported the induction of mammary cancers in mice following administration of estriol. How are these data to be explained?

Fishman: The Rudali experiment was carried out by the implantation of pellets containing estriol and this precisely duplicated a physiological situation in that continuous estriol was used to induce the cancers. If the estriol is given as individual injections it does not do so.

Question: Dr Bland found fewer cancers after 8 years of estrogen therapy, but how many patients developed carcinoma during that time, and particularly in the first 2 years? Is there a bimodal distribution of onset?

Bland: Actually it was 7.6 years, and the incidence of total cancers in the group was seven. From our study design, I cannot say if there is a bimodal distribution – in other words, more cancers developing in the first part of the therapy treatment. All I can say is that in the group who were symptomatic users of estrogens, their total duration of therapy was 12 months longer.

Question: Can androgen play any role in the control of the negative action performed by estrogens?

Gambrell: We have had a limited experience with androgens and have had no cancers, but we did not have enough patients to show any significant differences as to whether or not they should develop cancers.

One of the reasons we started to use androgens was to see if when the androgen was given with the estrogen the patient would not have withdrawal bleeding when given the progestogen. This did not work. If we used 0.625 mg Premarin or more then the patient would develop withdrawal bleeding even though she was given androgen every time we gave the challenge with the progestogen.

Whitehead: I would like to comment on the anti-estrogenic effects of androgens at cellular levels. Thijssen from Utrecht has shown that patients with endometrial carcinoma have decreased urinary excretion of etiocholanolone and androsterone. He has suggested (*Endometrial Cancer* (1978), ed. Brush, M. G., p. 375. Baillière Tindall, London) that decreased production of 11-deoxo-17-oxosteroids results in enhanced estrogenic activity within the cell – these androgens being potent inhibitors of the binding of estradiol to its specific receptor.

Question: Has Dr Gambrell any experience at comparing the efficacy of different types of progestin in either preventing or reversing hyperplasia, e.g. comparing norethisterone against medroxyprogesterone acetate, for example?

Gambrell: We have some studies comparing medroxyprogesterone acetate and northindrone acetate. The northindrone acetate, when the acetate is added, is a little more potent than the group without the acetate. Between these two compounds, our data would indicate that approximately 5 mg northindrone acetate is equal to 10 mg medroxyprogesterone acetate.

We did have a difference in treating hyperplasias with 7 days of therapy and 10 days. Equal days of therapy with the two compounds indicated that norlutate or northindrone acetate was superior in reversing hyperplasia. However, the greatest difference was in the duration of dosage and we feel that should be a minimum of 10 days each month.

Question: Many of us are perhaps now using the estrogen and progesterone receptors when we diagnose breast cancer as an index or guide to possible responsiveness to hormonal ablation. Has anybody had the opportunity to do a biopsy on a patient who has been on or off Premarin or sequential progestational agents and then to repeat the analysis in subsequent possibilities? Had there been any changes in the reactivity of the ER binding? If it was positive and the patient had ablation, were they more responsive? I might add that it is only that several studies have been carried out and there is no relationship between circulating estrogens and the receptor level in breast tissue.

Onnis: Do the panellists know anything of the hypothesis that suggests a blocking action of progesterone on the estrogen-dependent sites in both endometrium and breast? This might explain the usefulness of the association of progesterone with estrogens in replacement therapy in the menopause.

Whitehead: I can answer the question for endometrium. Progestogens reduced the binding capacity of both nuclear estrogen receptor and cytosol progesterone receptor and the latter is an index of estrogenic stimulation. The mechanism whereby these effects are mediated is in part via the induction of dehydrogenase activity. In addition, progestogens induce – as Dr King showed in Chapter 21 – various lysosomal enzymes which are involved in cell autolysis and thus increase the efficiency of endometrial shedding at menstruation. Acid phosphatase and isocitric dehydrogenase will probably be very important in this role.

CLOSING COMMENTS

Professor Bompiani

I could only attend part of these proceedings, but I found those sections that I was able to be present at particularly interesting. This discussion which closes the symposium has had something to say on the meaning of estrogen and progestogen therapy in the menopause.

My conclusions are as follows:

(1) treatment must be personalized;

(2) control must be periodical, and the methods of control must be better developed so as to avoid risks.

Both the doctor and the patient must exercise caution in the use of longterm therapies. In the last section of our symposium this has been clearly shown at the epidemiological level. It has been shown that therapy administered with those estrogens known to be highly active on the receptors at an age which might be critical in regard to balance of receptor actions is not so dangerous a treatment as has sometimes been made out. I believe, however, that the problem of achieving perfect health is a basic problem, and the more so when the therapy is optional rather than essential.

Having said that, I think I can speak on behalf of all those present by thanking the organizers of the symposium for giving us all the opportunity to have this update and to verify our own results. For us Italians it has been very interesting to see the Anglo-Saxon capacity and depth at first hand.

We hope that there will soon be another such meeting so that we can be given further information and exchange information and data as interesting as the data that has been presented here today, and so that we might improve our knowledge of this extremely important period in the life of women. Today, taking into account the social implications of the lives of women at any stage, at any age, their working lives, their independence, we can appreciate that women need the support of medicine and of pharmacology to be able to live in perfect balance and to function better within society.

Index